Imaging of Bone Tumors in Wrist, Hand, Ankle and Foot

Xiaoguang Cheng • Yongbin Su
Mingqian Huang

Imaging of Bone Tumors in Wrist, Hand, Ankle and Foot

中国协和医科大学出版社
Peking Union Medical College Press

Springer

Xiaoguang Cheng
Department of Radiology,
Beijing Jishuitan Hospital, Capital
Medical University
Beijing, China

Yongbin Su
Department of Radiology
Beijing Jishuitan Hospital,
Capital Medical University
Beijing, China

Mingqian Huang
Department of Diagnostic,
Molecular and Intervention Radiology
Icahn School of Medicine
at Mount Sinai
NY, NY, USA

ISBN 978-981-99-6409-3 ISBN 978-981-99-6407-9 (eBook)
https://doi.org/10.1007/978-981-99-6407-9

Jointly published with Peking Union Medical College Press
The print edition is not for sale in China (Mainland). Customers from China (Mainland) please order the print book from: Peking Union Medical College Press.

This Springer imprint is published by the registered company Springer Nature Singapore Pte Ltd.
The registered company address is: 152 Beach Road, #21-01/04 Gateway East, Singapore 189721, Singapore

Paper in this product is recyclable.

Contents

Authors and Contributors

Authors

Xiaoguang Cheng, MD Department of Radiology, Beijing Jishuitan Hospital, Beijing, People's Republic of China

Capital Medical University, Beijing, People's Republic of China

Yongbin Su, MD Department of Radiology, Beijing Jishuitan Hospital, Beijing, People's Republic of China

Mingqian Huang, MD Department of Diagnostic, Molecular, and Interventional Radiology, Mount Sinai Health System, New York, NY, USA

Contributors

Wei Cai Department of Radiology, Beijing Jishuitan Hospital, Beijing, People's Republic of China

Guangming Cao Department of Radiology, Yan'an University Affiliated Hospital, Taiyuan, Shanxi, People's Republic of China

Xiangshu Chen Department of Radiology, Beijing Jishuitan Hospital, Beijing, People's Republic of China

Yi Ding Department of Pathology, Beijing Jishuitan Hospital, Beijing, People's Republic of China

Qiangqiang Feng Department of Radiology, Beijing Jishuitan Hospital, Beijing, People's Republic of China

Lihua Gong Department of Pathology, Beijing Jishuitan Hospital, Beijing, People's Republic of China

Zhe Guo Department of Radiology, Beijing Jishuitan Hospital, Beijing, People's Republic of China

Xue Hou Department of Radiology, Beijing Jishuitan Hospital, Beijing, People's Republic of China

Pengju Huang Department of Radiology, Beijing Anding Hospital, Beijing, People's Republic of China

Shanqing Huang Department of Radiology, Taizhou Hospital of Zhejiang, Taizhou, Zhejiang, People's Republic of China

Meiyu Hu Department of Radiology, The Sixth Affiliated Hospital of Sun Yat-Sen University, Guangzhou, Guangdong, People's Republic of China

Yanping Hu Department of Medical Imaging, Kaifeng People's Hospital, Kaifeng, Henan, People's Republic of China

Kai Li Department of Radiology, Beijing Jishuitan Hospital, Beijing, People's Republic of China

Qing Li Department of Medical Imaging, Beijing Anzhen Hospital, Beijing, People's Republic of China

Baoyue Liu Department of Pathology, Beijing Jishuitan Hospital, Beijing, People's Republic of China

Weifeng Liu Department of Orthopaedic Oncology, Beijing Jishuitan Hospital, Beijing, People's Republic of China

Yandong Liu Department of Radiology, Beijing Jishuitan Hospital, Beijing, People's Republic of China

Xinmin Li Department of Radiology, Beijing Jishuitan Hospital, Beijing, People's Republic of China

Ying Li Department of MRI, The First Affiliated Hospital of Zhengzhou University, Zhengzhou, Henan, People's Republic of China

Luxin Lou Department of Radiology, Beijing Jishuitan Hospital, Beijing, People's Republic of China

Ning Ma Department of Radiology, Beijing Hepingli Hospital, Beijing, People's Republic of China

Yimin Ma Department of Radiology, Beijing Jishuitan Hospital, Beijing, People's Republic of China

Zhanhua Qian Department of Radiology, Beijing Jishuitan Hospital, Beijing, People's Republic of China

Yanbo Rong Department of Hand Surgery, Beijing Jishuitan Hospital, Beijing, People's Republic of China

Songming Wang Department of Radiology, Beijing Hepingli Hospital, Beijing, People's Republic of China

Tao Wang Department of Orthopaedic Oncology, Beijing Jishuitan Hospital, Beijing, People's Republic of China

Yongquan Wang Department of Radiology, Chinese Medicine Hospital of Chongqing, Chongqing, People's Republic of China

Hairong Xu Department of Orthopaedic Oncology, Beijing Jishuitan Hospital, Beijing, People's Republic of China

Li Xu Department of Radiology, Beijing Jishuitan Hospital, Beijing, People's Republic of China

Xiaoming Xu Department of Radiology, Beijing Jishuitan Hospital, Beijing, People's Republic of China

Dong Yan Department of Radiology, Beijing Jishuitan Hospital, Beijing, People's Republic of China

Li Yang Department of Radiology, The No.4 People's Hospital of Hengshui, Hengshui, Hebei, People's Republic of China

Honghong Zhang Department of Radiology, The First Hospital of Fangshan District, Beijing, People's Republic of China

Huili Zhan Department of Radiology, Beijing Jishuitan Hospital, Beijing, People's Republic of China

Zikun Zong Department of Radiology, Integrated Traditional Chinese and Western Medicine, Hospital of Tongzhou District, Beijing, People's Republic of China

Yuhong Zuo Department of Radiology, Guizhou Provincial Orthopedics Hospital, Guiyang, Guizhou, People's Republic of China

Part I

Wrist

1 Bizarre Parosteal Osteochondromatous Proliferation: Case 1

1.1 Medical History

Patient is a 30-year-old female. She presented with a mass at the ulnar aspect of the left hand at the outpatient clinic.

1.2 Physical Examination

Not done.

1.3 Imaging Findings

1.3.1 Radiograph(Figs. 1.1 and 1.2)

Radiographs of the left hand demonstrated a bony protuberance along the ulnar cortex of the distal fifth metacarpal with clear margin.

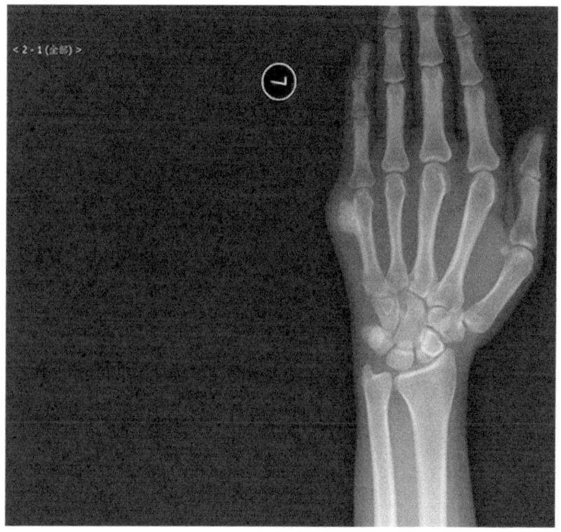

Fig. 1.1 Frontal view of the left hand

1.3.2 CT Imaging (Figs. 1.3, 1.4, 1.5 and 1.6)

CT images of the left hand demonstrated a focal broad-based bony protuberance along the ulnar cortex of the fifth metacarpal. There is no medullary continuity. There are internal heterogeneous densities with predominant sclerosis and peripheral thin rim of lower densities. No enhancement is noted.

X. Cheng et al., *Imaging of Bone Tumors in Wrist, Hand, Ankle and Foot*,
https://doi.org/10.1007/978-981-99-6407-9_1

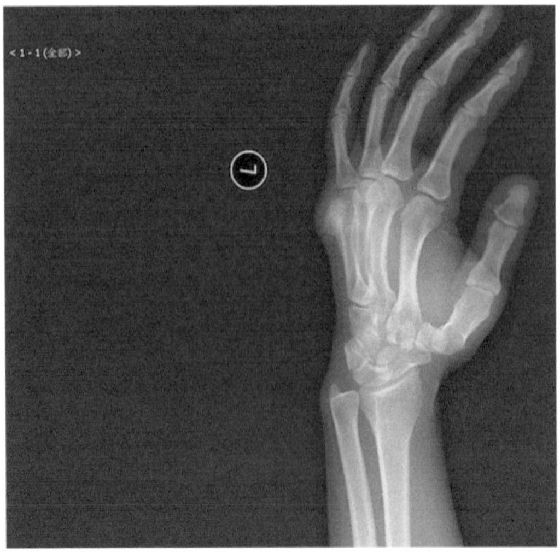

Fig. 1.2 Oblique view of the left hand

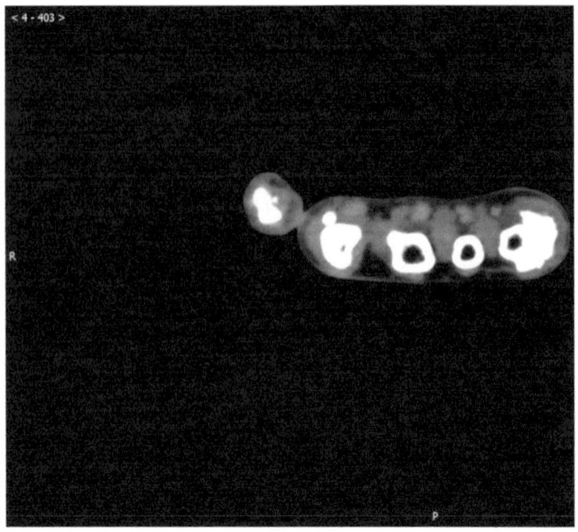

Fig. 1.4 Axial CT image of the left hand in soft tissue window

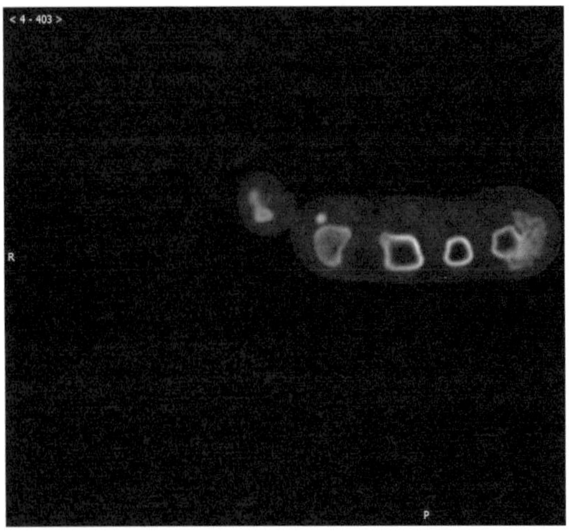

Fig. 1.3 Axial CT image of the left hand in bone window

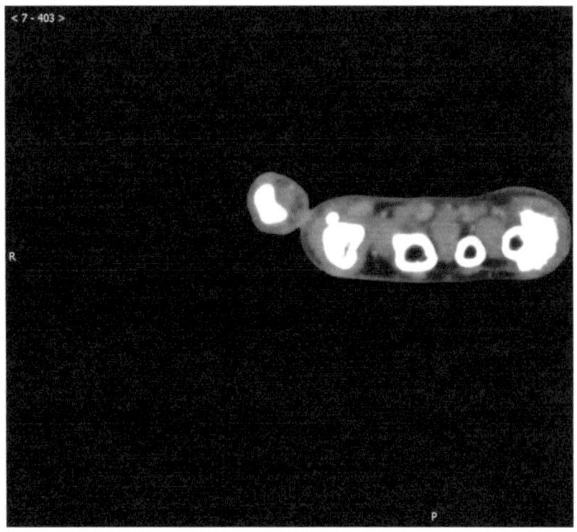

Fig. 1.5 Axial post-contrast CT image of the left hand in soft tissue window

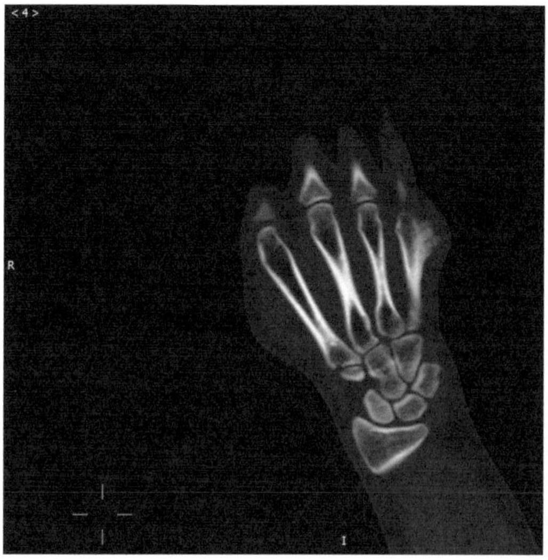

Fig. 1.6 Coronal CT image of the left hand in bone window

1.4 Description and Discussion from Residents

Radiographs demonstrated a bony protuberance along the ulnar cortex of the fifth metacarpal distally, appeared to originating from the cortex with mild thickening of the adjacent periosteum. CT images demonstrated relatively homogenous bony densities of the lesion and lack of associated soft tissue mass and no enhancement. Differential diagnosis of a bony protuberance along the cortex includes (1) myositis ossificans; (2) periosteal chondroma (3) bizarre parosteal osteochondromatous proliferation (BPOP), also known as Nora's disease; (4) subperiosteal osteoid osteoma or osteoblastoma. Usually, there is a space between myositis ossificans and the adjacent cortex, and the lesion commonly shows zonal calcification, not consistent with the current case. Periosteal chondroma usually shows calcifications with "saucerization" of the adjacent cortex, not present of the current case. Nora's disease is similar to periosteal chondroma without the typical "saucerization" and calcifications. Subperiosteal osteoid osteoma and osteoblastoma usually are morphologically round or lumpy, not seen here. Overall, periosteal chondroma and Nora's disease are at the top of our differential diagnosis.

1.5 Analysis and Comments from Professor Cheng Xiao-Guang

Focal osseous protuberance at distal fifth metacarpal originating from the cortex without any bony destruction noted on radiographs. CT images better delineated the relationship between the lesion and the cortex and the medullary cavity, aiding differential diagnosis. Nora's disease is at the top of the differential diagnosis. Differential diagnosis is well discussed by the residents, however, osteochondroma should be included in the differential diagnosis. There is medullary continuity in osteochondroma with typical cartilaginous cap. There is no medullary continuity of the current case, thus can exclude osteochondroma.

1.6 Diagnosis

Bizarre Parosteal Osteochondromatous Proliferation, BPOP, (Nora's Disease).

Suggested Reading

Berber O, Dawson-Bowling S, Jalgaonkar A, et al. Bizarre parosteal osteochondromatous proliferation of bone: clinical management of a series of 22 cases. J Bone Joint Surg Br. 2011; 93(8):1118-21.

Cocks M, Helmke E, Meyers CA, et al. Bizarre parosteal osteochondromatous proliferation: 16 Cases with a focus on histologic variability. J Orthop. 2018; 15(1):138-142.

2 Fibro-Osseous Pseudotumor of Digits: Case 2

2.1 Medical History

Patient is a 19-year-old female. She presented with a mass at the ulnar aspect of the left hand for half a year with pain and swelling and restricted motion for 1 month.

2.2 Physical Examination

Swelling along the hypothenar of the left palm.

2.3 Imaging Findings

2.3.1 Radiograph(Figs. 2.1 and 2.2)

Radiographs of the left hand demonstrated irregular densities of the proximal left fifth metacarpal with adjacent soft tissue densities.

2.3.2 CT Imaging(Figs. 2.3, 2.4, 2.5, and 2.6)

CT images of the left hand demonstrated extensive periosteal reaction along the fifth metacarpal in the volar aspect. The periosteal reaction is thick with irregular margin. Soft tissue mass is noted proximally. Multiple calcifications are noted at the base with surrounding soft tissue swelling.

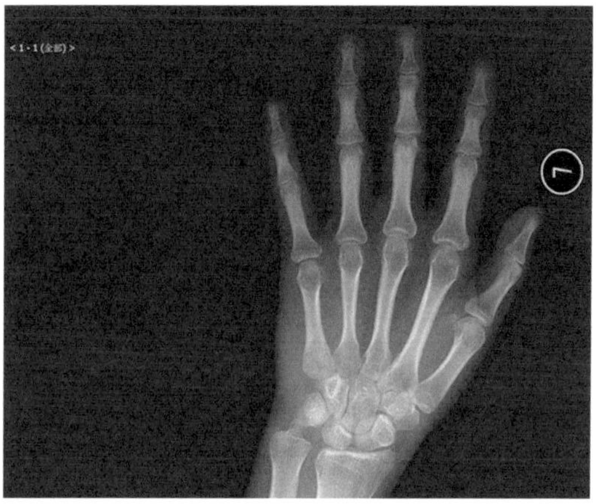

Fig. 2.1 Frontal view of the left hand

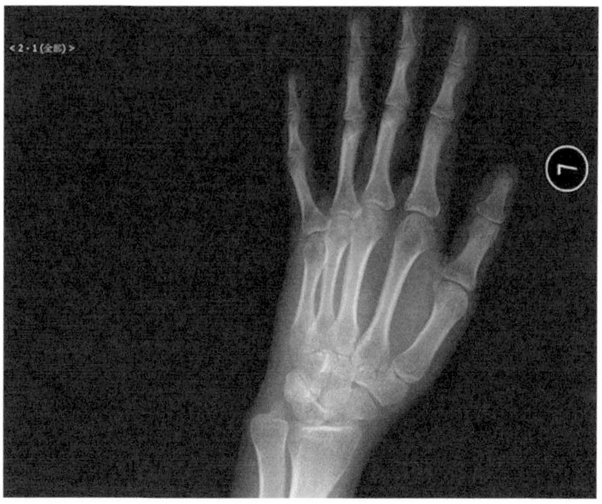

Fig. 2.2 Oblique view of the left hand

X. Cheng et al., *Imaging of Bone Tumors in Wrist, Hand, Ankle and Foot*,
https://doi.org/10.1007/978-981-99-6407-9_2

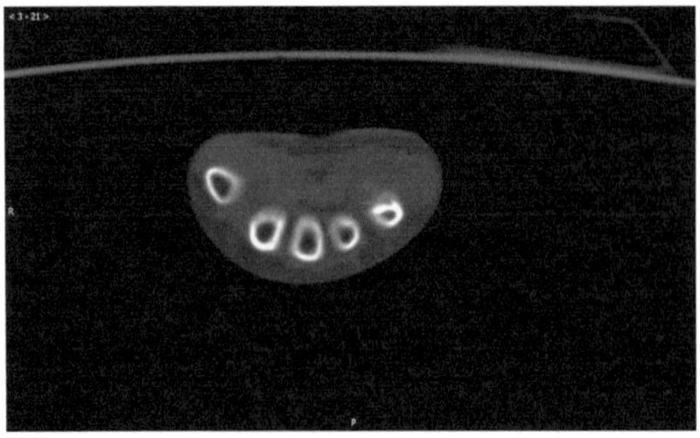

Fig. 2.3 Axial CT image of the left hand in bone window

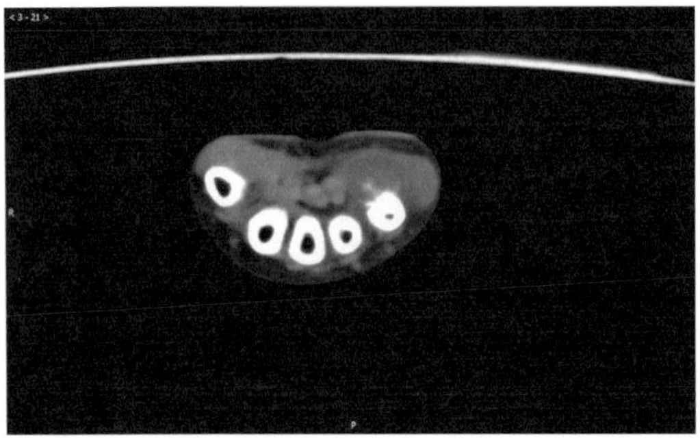

Fig. 2.4 Axial CT image of the left hand in soft tissue window

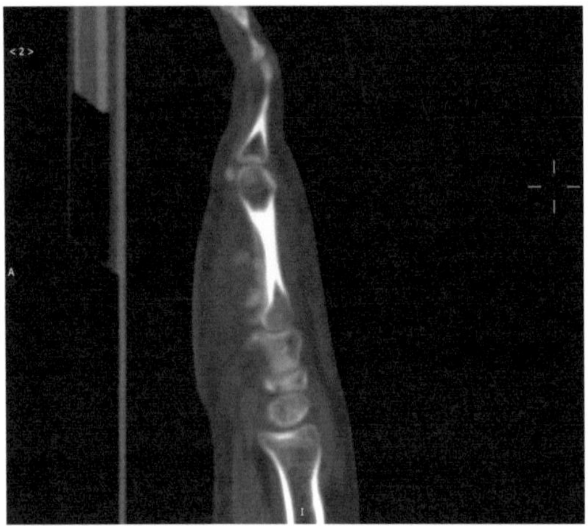

Fig. 2.5 Sagittal CT image of the left hand in bone window

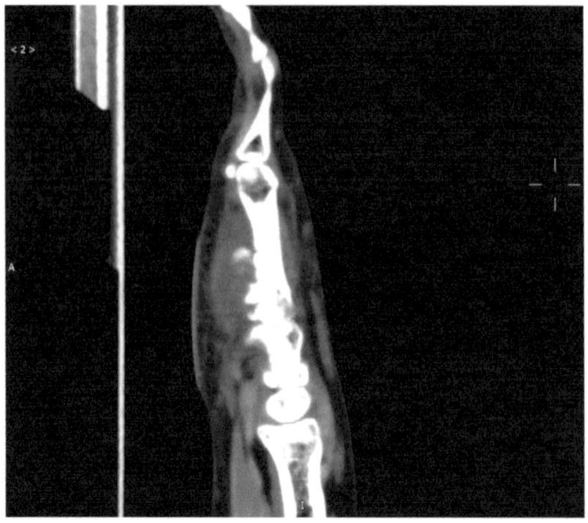

Fig. 2.6 Sagittal CT image of the left hand in soft tissue window

2.4 Description and Discussion from Residents

Radiographs demonstrated irregular densities at the proximal fifth metacarpal with adjacent soft tissue densities. CT images demonstrated soft tissue mass along the proximal fifth metacarpal, in proximity to the cortex with associated continuous, mature periosteal reaction. This type of cortical thickening is usually reactive to the soft tissue mass. Based on these findings, benign etiology is most likely. Given the location of hypothenar with calcification, vascular lesion is favored.

2.5 Analysis and Comments from Professor Cheng Xiao-Guang

The patient presented with relatively long history and the lesion located at the volar aspect of the fifth metacarpal. There is internal osteoid or calcification and surrounding periosteum thickened due to reaction from adjacent volar soft tissue mass. The periosteal reaction is extensive. Even without known history of trauma, myositis ossificans should be considered. However, we usually see zonal calcification with myositis ossificans and not present here. Periosteal or paro-osteal tumors should be included in the consideration. With soft tissue mass and adjacent periosteal reaction, malignant causes can't be entirely excluded. However, malignancy along the hand is rare. Contrast enhanced CT images and MRI images would be helpful for narrowing down the differential diagnosis.

2.6 Diagnosis

Fibro-osseous pseudotumor of digits.

Suggested Reading

Broski SM, Wenger DE. Multimodality imaging features of USP6-associated neoplasms. Skeletal Radiol. 2022, 52(3):297-313. doi: https://doi.org/10.1007/s00256-022-04146-x.

Švajdler M, Michal M, Martínek P, et al. Fibro-osseous pseudotumor of digits and myositis ossificans show consistent COL1A1-USP6 rearrangement: a clinicopathological and genetic study of 27 cases. Hum Pathol. 2019;88:39-47.

Periosteal Chondroma: Case 3

3

3.1 Medical History

Patient is a 16-year-old female. She presented with swelling of the left palm for about 1 month.

3.2 Physical Examination

There is a palpable mass at the left second metacarpal, size of a date, solid, non-mobile with clear margin.

3.3 Imaging Findings

3.3.1 Radiograph (Figs. 3.1 and 3.2)

Radiographs of the left hand demonstrated focal high-density lesion along the second metacarpal volarly with irregular margin and multiple patch calcifications.

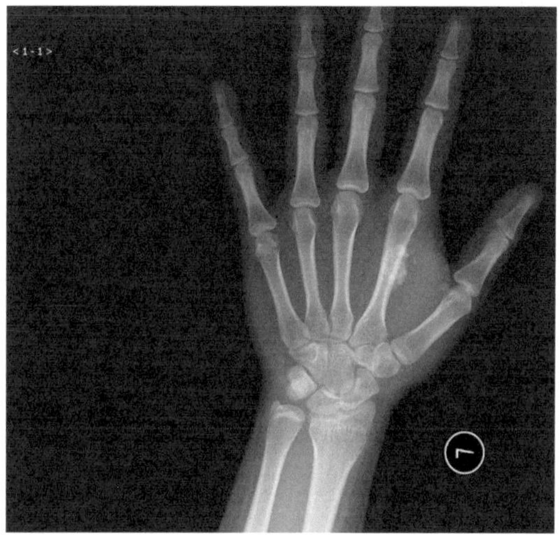

Fig. 3.1 Frontal view of the left hand

3.3.2 CT Imaging (Figs. 3.3, 3.4, 3.5, 3.6, 3.7, and 3.8)

CT images of the left hand demonstrated volar soft tissue mass along the periosteum of the left second metacarpal. There is high density at the base of the lesion. There is low density at the soft tissue portion of the lesion with multiple patch calcifications. No invasion into the cortex or medullary cavity. No enhancement.

X. Cheng et al., *Imaging of Bone Tumors in Wrist, Hand, Ankle and Foot*,
https://doi.org/10.1007/978-981-99-6407-9_3

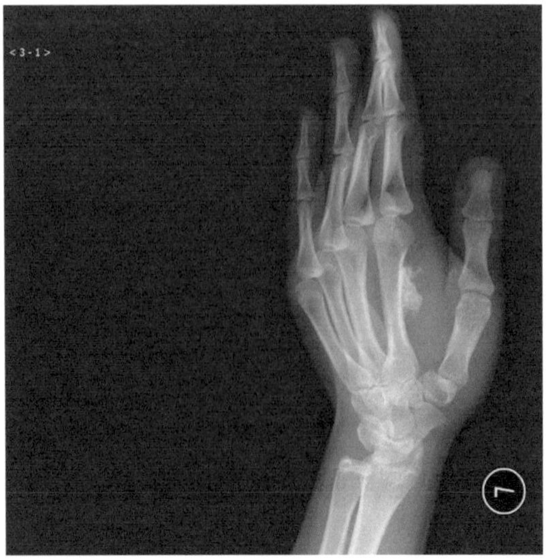

Fig. 3.2 Oblique view of the left hand

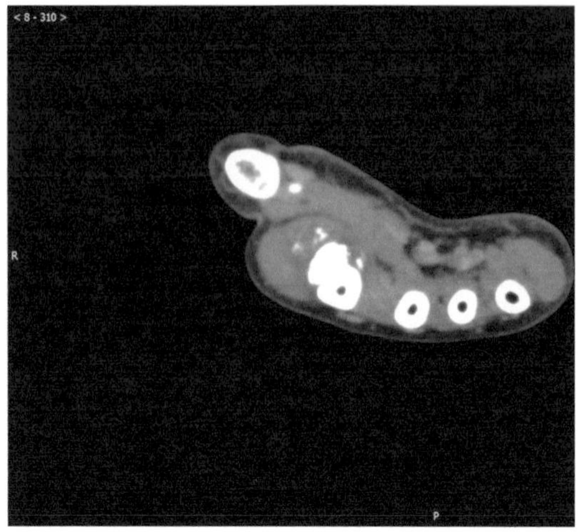

Fig. 3.4 Axial CT image of the left hand in soft tissue window

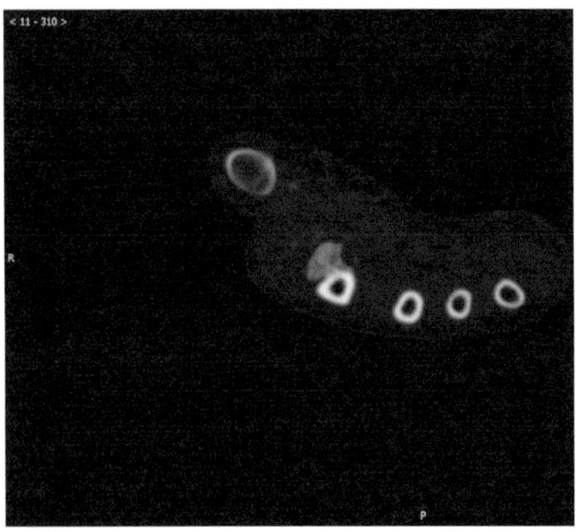

Fig. 3.3 Axial CT image of the left hand in bone window

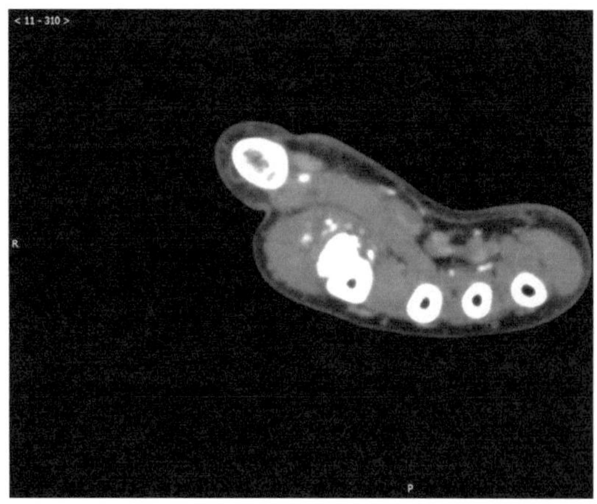

Fig. 3.5 Axial post-contrast CT image of the left hand in soft tissue window

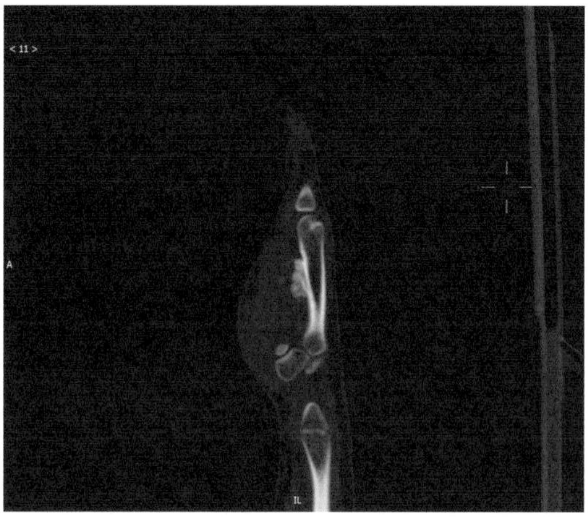

Fig. 3.6 Sagittal CT image of the left hand in bone window

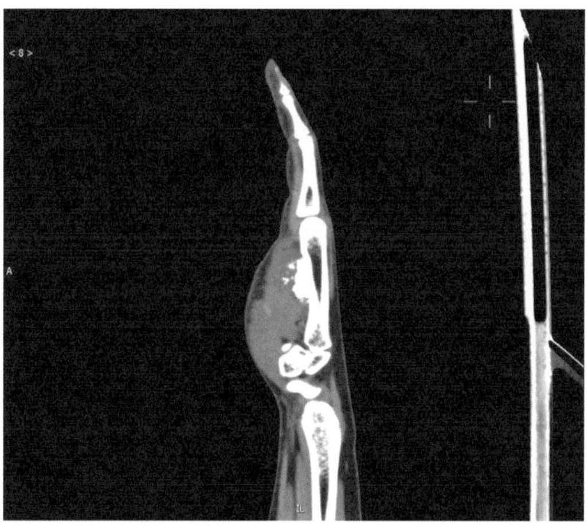

Fig. 3.7 Sagittal CT image of the left hand in soft tissue window

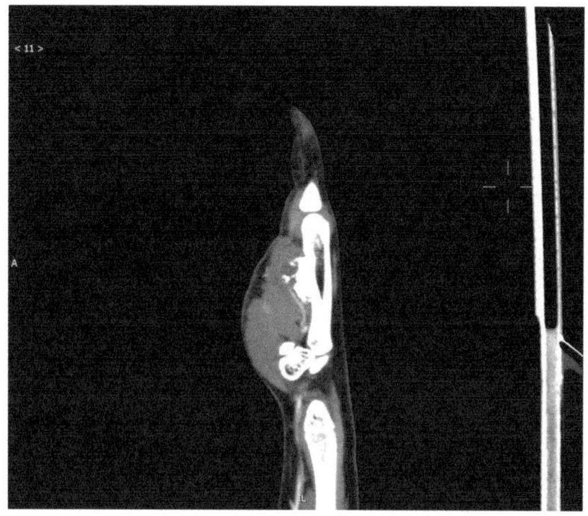

Fig. 3.8 Sagittal post-contrast CT image of the left hand in soft tissue window

3.4 Description and Discussion from Residents

High density lesion was noted along the volar aspect of the left second metacarpal with mild periosteal reaction, and adjacent soft tissue mass with calcification. In contrast to the zonal calcification from peripheral to center of myositis ossificans, this lesion demonstrated mineralization of the chondroid lesion. Differential diagnosis includes tumor and tumor-like lesion. In tumor category, we would consider the ones originate from periosteum, such as periosteal chondroma; for aggressive tumor, we would consider parosteal osteosarcoma or periosteal chondrosarcoma.

However, these aggressive lesions are rare in the hand. For tumor-like lesion, we should consider fibro-osseous pseudotumor (florid reactive periostitis) or Nora's disease. However, there is usually history of trauma with these entities.

3.5 Analysis and Comments from Professor Cheng Xiao-Guang

The lesion located at the volar aspect of the left second metacarpal, with close association with the cortex, and soft tissue mass and patchy calcification. On the post-contrast images, there is mild enhancement of surrounding muscle, without much enhancement of the lesion. This is most likely of chondrogenic tumor, first consideration is periosteal chondroma and Nora's disease in the differential diagnosis.

3.6 Diagnosis

Periosteal chondroma.

Suggested Reading

Flint JH, McKay PL, et al. Bizarre parosteal osteochondromatous proliferation and periosteal chondroma: a comparative report and review of the literature. J Hand Surg Am. 2007;32(6):893–8.

Rabarin F, Laulan J, Cast YS, et al. Focal periosteal chondroma of the hand: a review of 24 cases. Orthop Traumatol Surg Res. 2014;100(6):617–20.

Robinson P, White LM, Sundaram M, et al. Periosteal chondroid tumors: radiologic evaluation with pathologic correlation. AJR Am J Roentgenol. 2001;177(5):1183–8.

4 Enchondromatosis: Case 4

4.1 Medical History

Patient is a 25-year-old female. She presented with a mass around the proximal ring finger for 4 years without clear inciting event.

4.2 Physical Examination

There are bony protuberances around the proximal and middle phalanges of the ring finger, hard, non-mobile with point tenderness.

4.3 Imaging Findings

4.3.1 Radiograph (Figs. 4.1 and 4.2)

Radiographs of the left hand demonstrated bony destruction around middle phalanx of the ring finger with soft tissue mass, adjacent periosteal elevation with clear margin. There is multiple small nodular destruction of the cortex adjacent to the proximal phalanx.

4.3.2 CT Imaging (Figs. 4.3, 4.4, 4.5, 4.6, 4.7, and 4.8)

CT images of the left hand demonstrated multiple areas of bony destruction around the middle and proximal phalanges of the ring finger. The

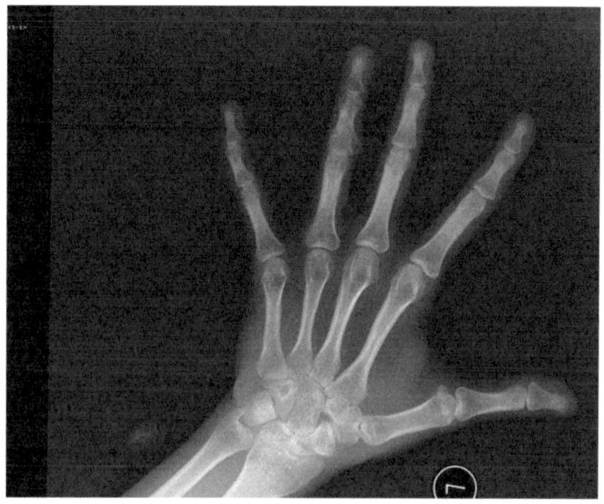

Fig. 4.1 Frontal view of the left hand

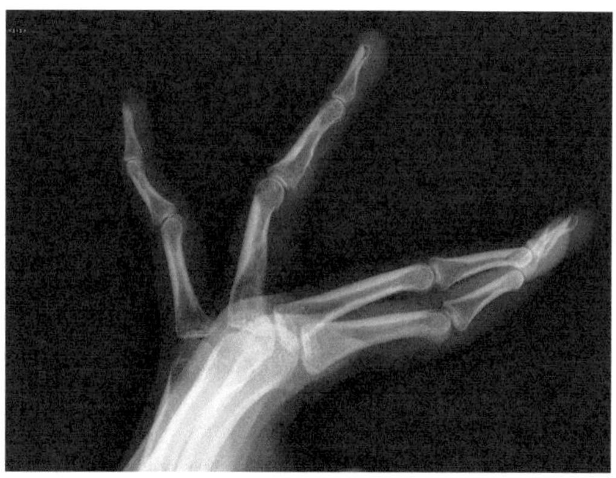

Fig. 4.2 Lateral view of the left ring finger

X. Cheng et al., *Imaging of Bone Tumors in Wrist, Hand, Ankle and Foot*,
https://doi.org/10.1007/978-981-99-6407-9_4

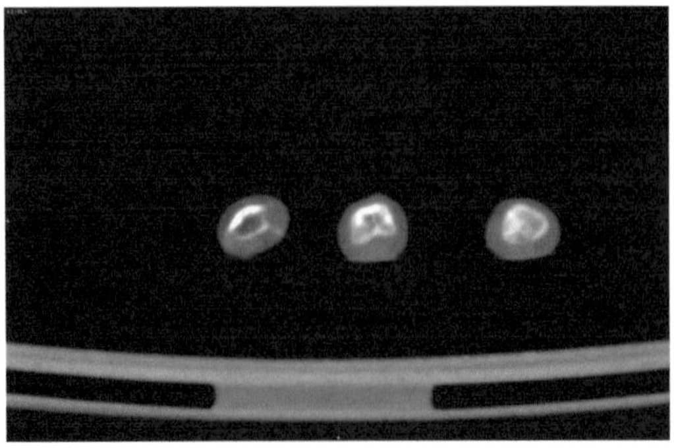

Fig. 4.3 Axial CT image of the left hand in bone window (middle phalanx level)

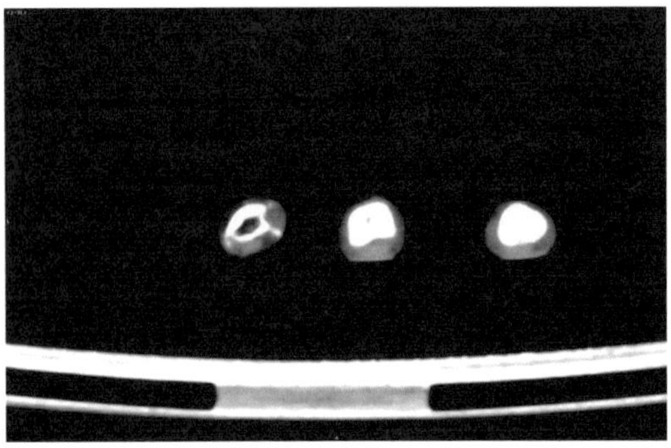

Fig. 4.4 Axial CT image of the left hand in soft tissue window (middle phalanx level)

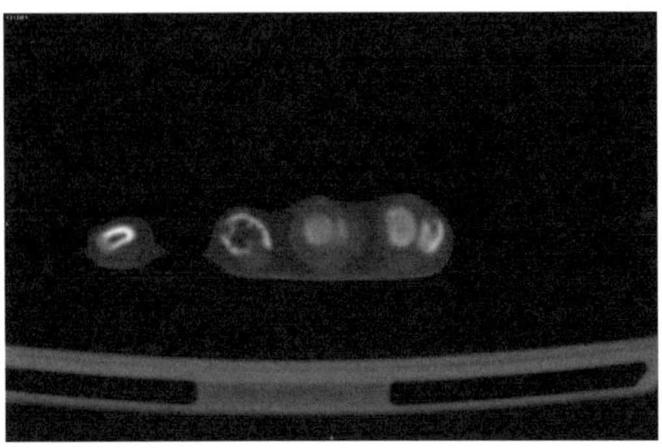

Fig. 4.5 Axial CT image of the left hand in bone window (proximal phalanx level)

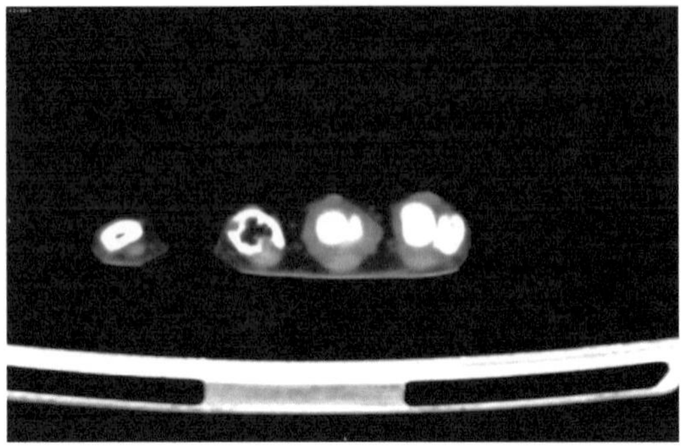

Fig. 4.6 Axial CT image of the left hand in soft tissue window (proximal phalanx level)

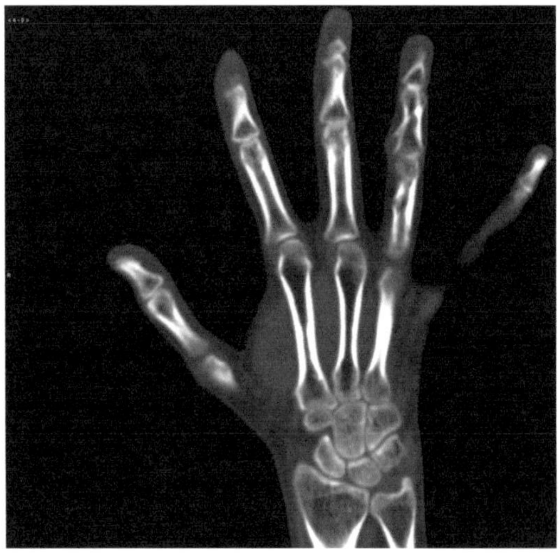

Fig. 4.7 Coronal CT image of the left hand in bone window

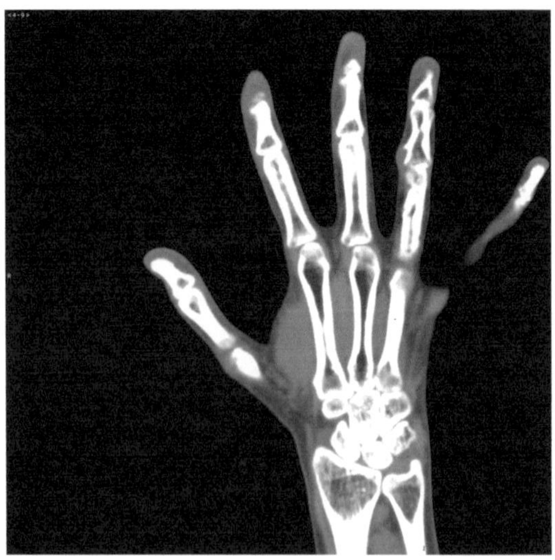

Fig. 4.8 Coronal CT image of the left hand in soft tissue window

lesions protruded beyond the cortex with periosteal elevation. There are clear margins around the lesion with focal peripheral sclerosis.

4.4 Description and Discussion from Residents

The radiographs demonstrated bony destruction around the base of middle phalanx of the ring finger with volar side soft tissue swelling and compression to the adjacent cortex without periosteal reaction or sclerosis. CT images demonstrated soft tissue mass around the proximal middle phalanx of the ring finger with invasion of the proximal middle phalanx and distal proximal phalanx, suggesting soft tissue or periosteal origin of the lesion. There is smooth articular surface of the proximal phalanx without narrowing of the interphalangeal joint space, thus exclude arthropathy. We favor non-aggressive process, given the long course of the disease and our top consideration is giant cell tumor of the tendon sheath with periosteal chondroma in the differential diagnose.

4.5 Analysis and Comments from Professor Cheng Xiao-Guang

When we evaluate the radiographs, first, we need to pay attention to the overall condition of the osseous structure, such as the presence of osteopenia. The bone mineralization of this case is normal. There is density change at the proximal middle phalanx of the ring finger without clear margin with elevation of the periosteum and surrounding soft tissue swelling. There is no destruction around the joint, indicating focal disease. The lesion appears to be well circumscribed with soft tissue mass and no associated calcification on CT images, indicating non-aggressive process. This could be a periosteal chondroma without obvious calcification. The lesion is along the lateral aspect of the phalanx, not adjacent to the tendon sheath, unlikely to be giant cell tumor of the tendon sheath. Additionally, the patient is a young adult, gout need to be excluded.

4.6 Diagnosis

Enchondromatosis.

Suggested Reading

Sharif B, Lindsay D, Asif Saifuddin A. Update on the imaging features of the enchondromatosis syndromes. Skeletal Radiol. 2022;51(4):747–762.

Sharif B, Rajakulasingam R, Sharifi S, et al. MRI features of low-grade and high-grade chondrosarcoma in enchondromatosis. Skeletal Radiol. 2021;50(8):1637–1646.

5 Enchondroma: Case 5

5.1 Medical History

Patient is a 35-year-old male. He presented with a mass at the right ring finger for over 2 years. Initially, he was asymptomatic and later pain developed.

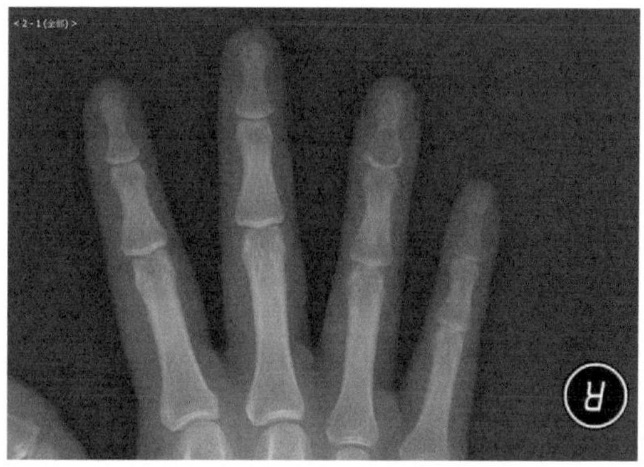

Fig. 5.1 Frontal view of the right ring finger

5.2 Physical Examination

Enlargement along the distal interphalangeal joint of the right ring finger without clear margin, with point tenderness and normal range of motion at the joint.

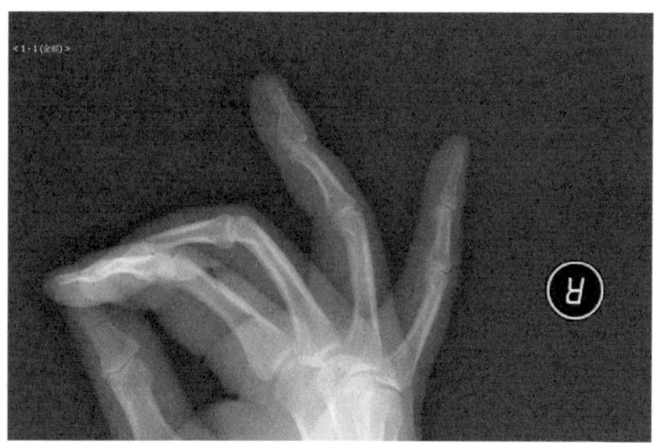

Fig. 5.2 Lateral view of the right ring finger

5.3 Imaging Findings

5.3.1 Radiograph (Figs. 5.1 and 5.2)

Radiographs of the right ring finger demonstrated expansion with lytic destruction of the proximal aspect of the distal phalanx with clear margin and thinning of the cortex with sclerosis.

5.3.2 CT Imaging (Figs. 5.3, 5.4, 5.5, 5.6 and 5.7)

CT images of the right hand demonstrated expansile and lytic lesion at the proximal aspect of the distal phalanx of the ring finger with thinning of the cortex, peripheral sclerosis and no associated soft tissue mass or periosteal reaction. The lesion is well circumscribed.

X. Cheng et al., *Imaging of Bone Tumors in Wrist, Hand, Ankle and Foot*,
https://doi.org/10.1007/978-981-99-6407-9_5

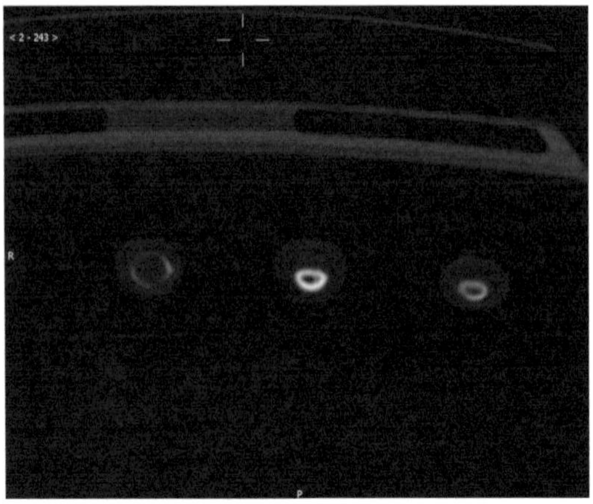

Fig. 5.3 Axial CT image of the right hand in bone window

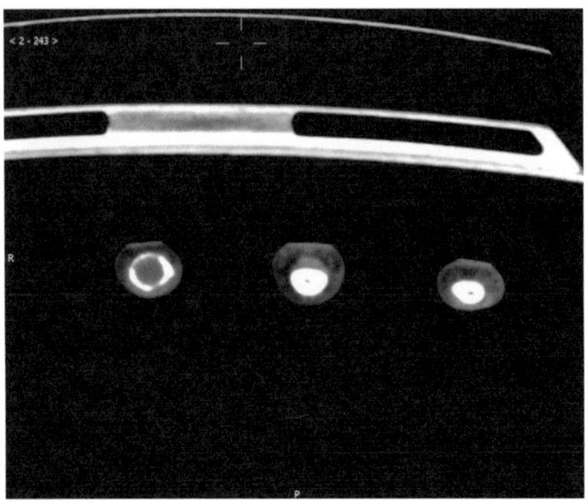

Fig. 5.4 Axial CT image of the right hand in soft tissue window

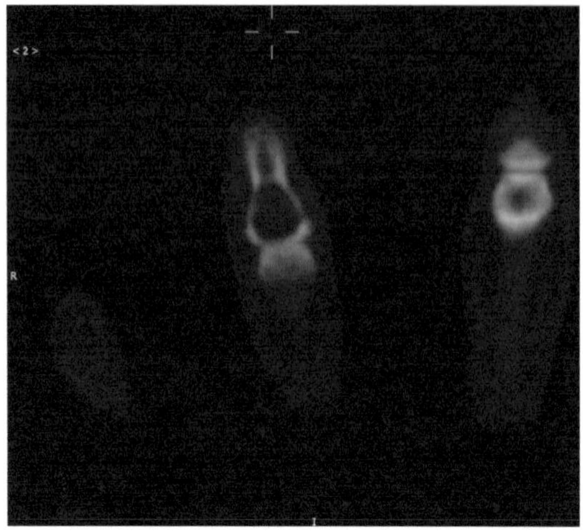

Fig. 5.5 Coronal CT image of the right hand in bone window

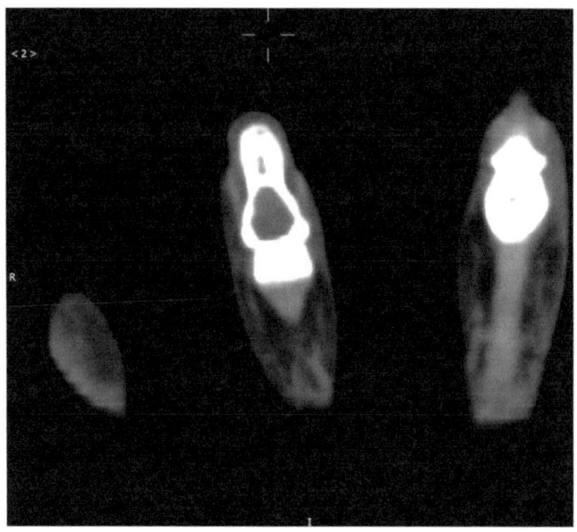

Fig. 5.6 Coronal CT image of the right hand in soft tissue window

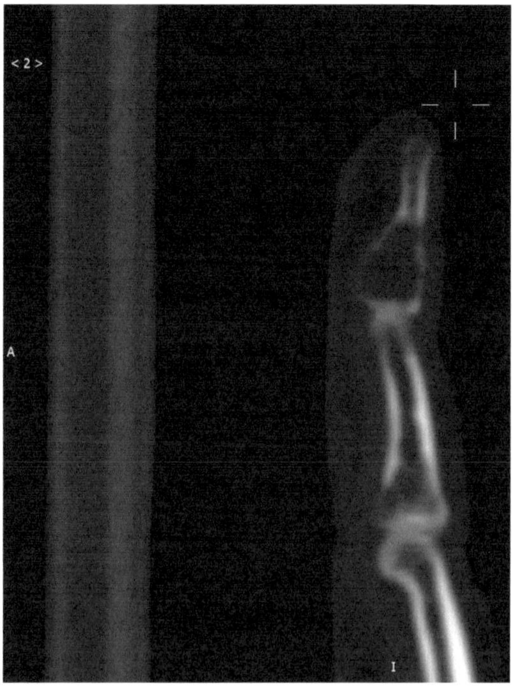

Fig. 5.7 Sagittal CT image of the right hand in bone window

5.4 Description and Discussion from Residents

The patient is a young male. There is an expansile, lytic lesion at the proximal aspect of the distal phalanx of the ring finger with clear margin, thinning of the cortex, peripheral sclerosis, and lack of calcification. The most common lesion in this location is enchondroma, which is our top consideration. Giant cell lesion of small bones is in the differential diagnoses and if patient has history of trauma in the region, intra-osseous epidermoid cyst is also in the differential diagnose.

5.5 Analysis and Comments from Professor Cheng Xiao-Guang

Patient presented with prolonged history. There is an expansile, lytic lesion with clear margin, and no soft tissue mass or swelling and no involvement of the joint, indicating slow growth and non-aggressive nature, most likely of enchondroma. There is no internal calcification and given the location, other etiologies need to be excluded, such as giant cell reparative granuloma of small bones (solid aneurysmal bone cyst), tuberculous dactylitis (spina ventosa), giant cell tumor of tendon sheath invading the bone. Contrast-enhanced CT scan and MRI would be helpful for differential diagnose.

5.6 Diagnosis

Enchondroma.

Suggested Reading

Jacobson ME, Ruff ME. Solitary enchondroma of the phalanx. J Hand Surg Am. 2011;36(11):1845–7.

Larbi A, Viala P, Omoumi P, et al. Cartilaginous tumours and calcified lesions of the hand: a pictorial review. Diagn Interv Imaging. 2013;94(4):395–409.

6 Epidermoid Cyst of Bone: Case 6

6.1 Medical History

Patient is a 43-year-old male. He presented at outpatient clinic with gradual enlargement of the right distal ring finger after trauma.

6.2 Physical Examination

Not done.

6.3 Imaging Findings

6.3.1 Radiograph (Figs. 6.1 and 6.2)

Radiographs of the right ring finger demonstrated expansile, lytic lesion of the distal phalanx with destruction of the majority of the cortex.

6.3.2 CT Imaging (Figs. 6.3, 6.4, 6.5, 6.6, 6.7, 6.8, 6.9, and 6.10)

CT images of the right ring finger demonstrated expansile, lytic lesion at the distal phalanx. The margin is clear with destruction of the distal cortex and internal low density with mild enhancement.

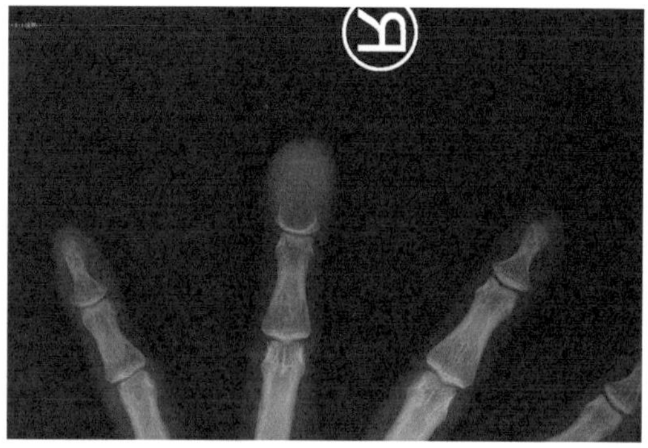

Fig. 6.1 Frontal view of the right ring finger

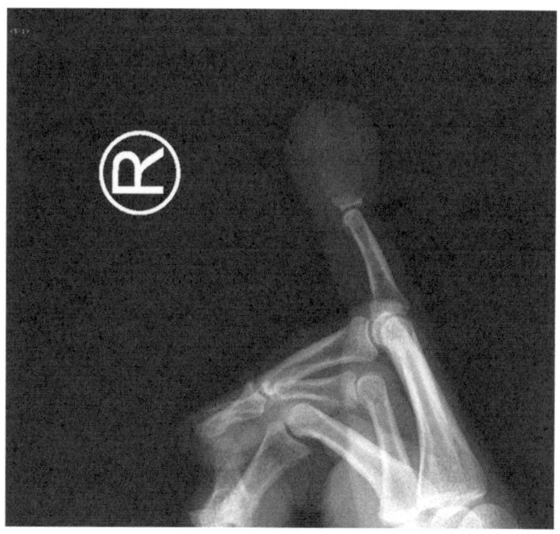

Fig. 6.2 Lateral view of the right ring finger

X. Cheng et al., *Imaging of Bone Tumors in Wrist, Hand, Ankle and Foot*,
https://doi.org/10.1007/978-981-99-6407-9_6

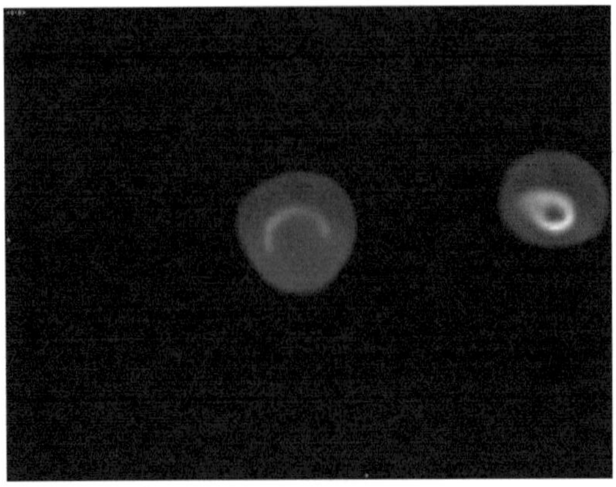

Fig. 6.3 Axial CT image of the right ringer finger distal phalanx in bone window (proximal)

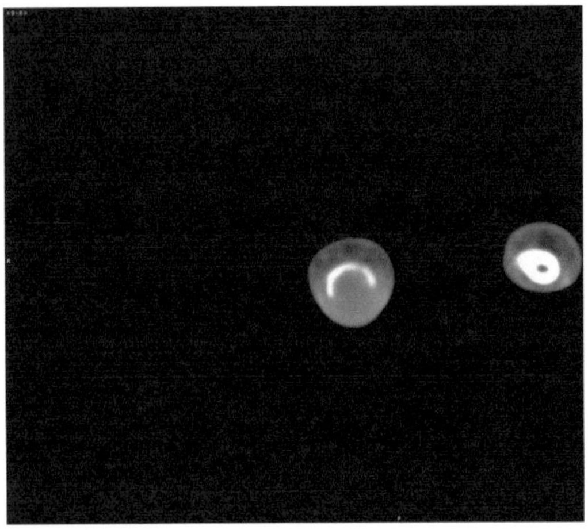

Fig. 6.4 Axial CT image of the right ringer finger distal phalanx in soft tissue window (proximal)

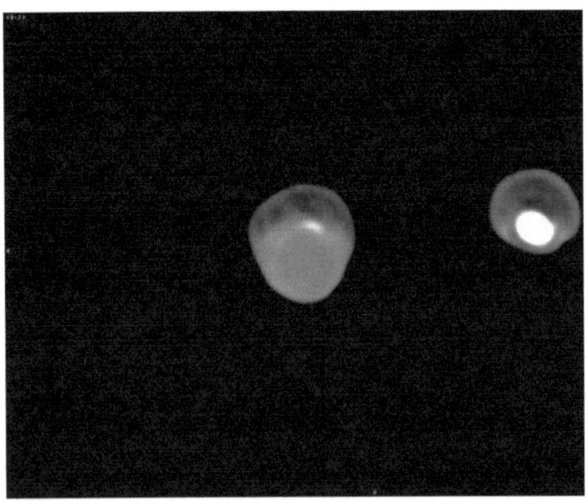

Fig. 6.5 Axial CT image of the right ringer finger distal phalanx in soft tissue window (distal)

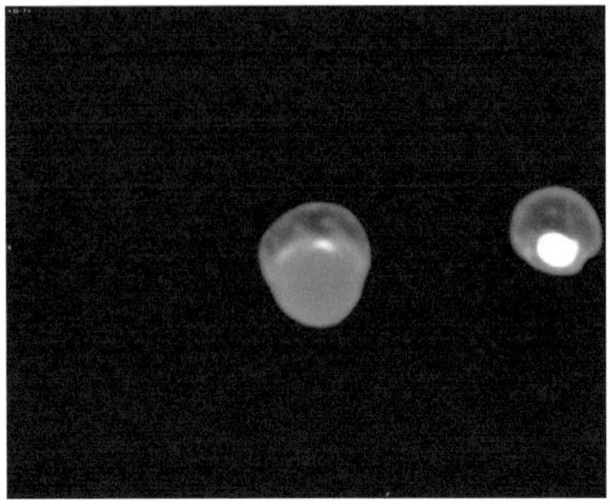

Fig. 6.6 Axial post-contrast CT image of the right ringer finger distal phalanx in soft tissue window (distal)

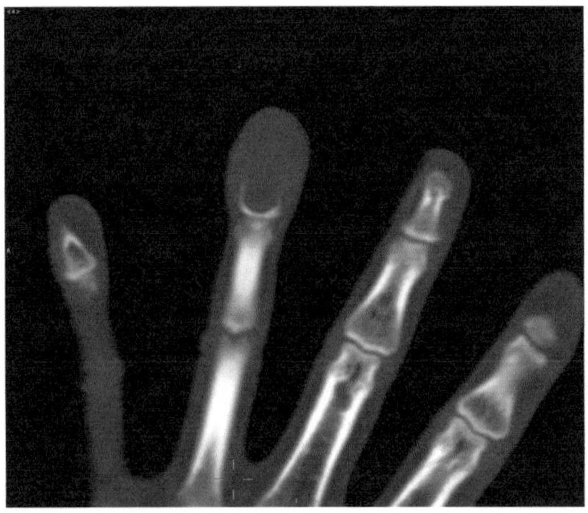

Fig. 6.7 Coronal CT image of the right ringer finger distal phalanx in bone window

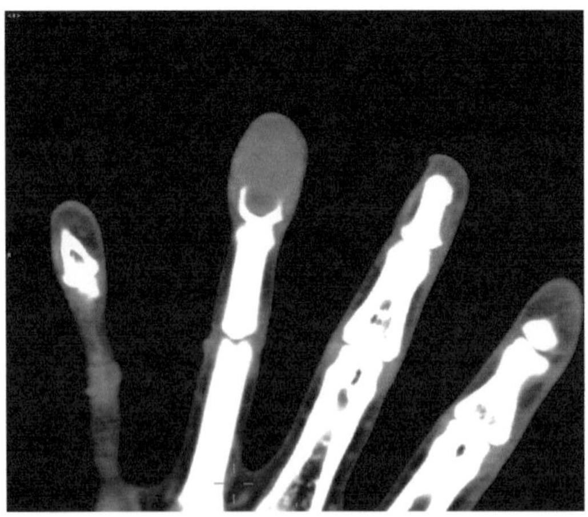

Fig. 6.8 Coronal CT image of the right ringer finger distal phalanx in soft tissue window

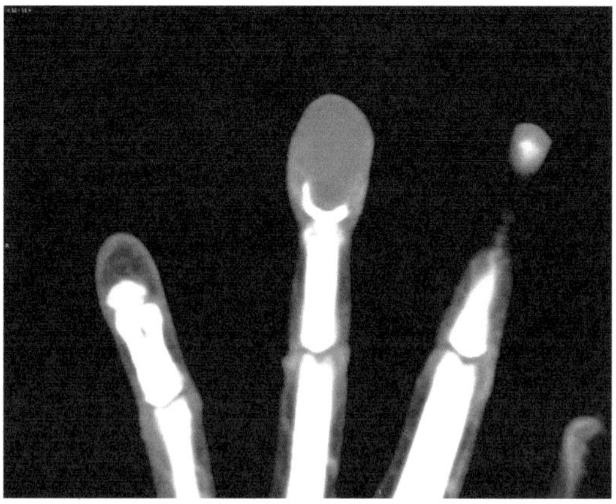

Fig. 6.9 Coronal post-contrast CT image of the right ringer finger distal phalanx in soft tissue window

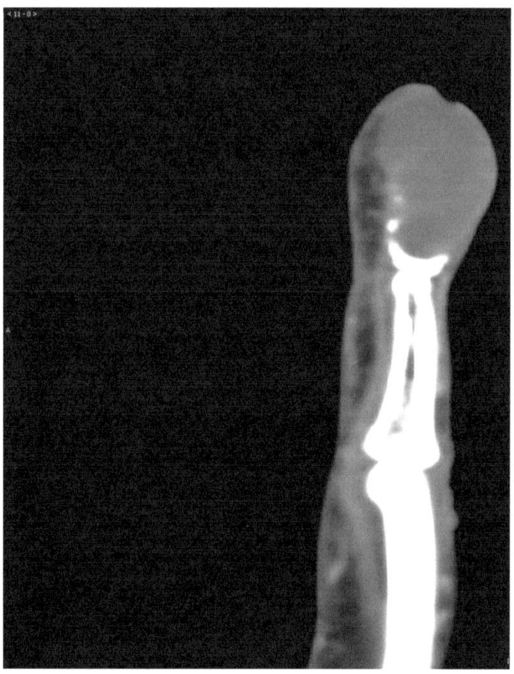

Fig. 6.10 Sagittal post-contrast CT image of the right ringer finger distal phalanx in soft tissue window

6.4 Description and Discussion from Residents

The lesion is expansile and lytic at distal phalanx of the right ring finger distally with clear margin and peripheral sclerosis. There was thinning and disruption of the distal cortex with internal mixed low densities and no periosteal reaction or internal calcification. Overall, this is consistent with a non-aggressive process. Given patient's history of trauma, infection is a possibility. Additionally, giant cell reparative granuloma (solid aneurysmal bone cyst) or epidermoid cyst is in the differential diagnose.

6.5 Analysis and Comments from Professor Cheng Xiao-Guang

The lesion is expansile and lytic at distal part of the distal phalanx of the right ring finger with clear margin and no involvement of the distal interphalangeal joint. Thus, infection excluded and benign neoplasm is top consideration. Glomus tumor is common at distal portion of the finger but not associated with trauma. No clear enhancement after contrast does not support giant cell reparative granuloma. Given patient's history of trauma, clear margin of the lesion, low density and focal sclerosis, and no clear enhancement, top considerations are epidermoid cyst and glomus tumor.

6.6 Diagnosis

Epidermoid cyst of bone.

Suggested Reading

Patel K, Bhuiya T, Chen S, et al. Epidermal inclusion cyst of phalanx: a case report and review of the literature. Skeletal Radiol. 2006;35(11):861–3.

Umana GE, Scalia G, Palmisciano P, et al. Acrometastases to the hand: a systematic review. Medicina (Kaunas). 2021;57(9):950.

7 Ollier's Disease: Case 7

7.1 Medical History

Patient is a 15-year-old boy who presented to outpatient clinic with multiple bone complaints.

7.2 Physical Examination

Not done.

7.3 Imaging Findings

7.3.1 Radiograph (Figs. 7.1, 7.2, 7.3, and 7.4)

Radiographs of both hands and left tibia and fibula demonstrated multiple areas of expansion of the intramedullary cavity with expansile bony destruction along the periosteum and some lesions with multiple calcifications and focal soft tissue swelling.

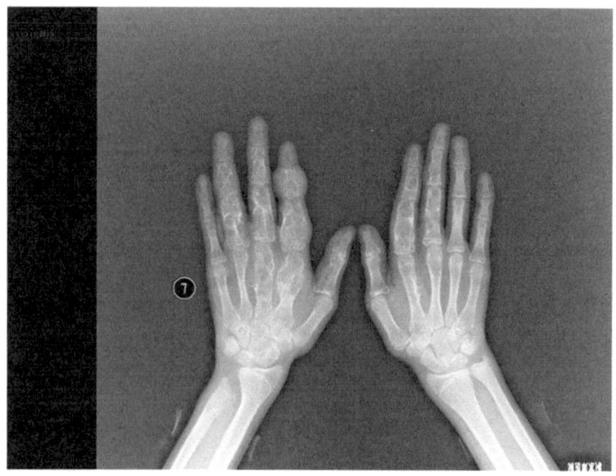

Fig. 7.1 Frontal view of both hands

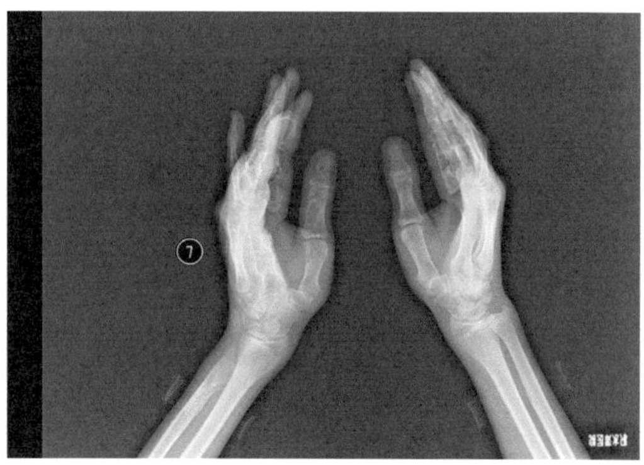

Fig. 7.2 Lateral view of both hands

7.3.2 CT Imaging (Figs. 7.5, 7.6, 7.7, 7.8, 7.9, and 7.10)

CT images of the hands demonstrated multiple expansile lesions involving the medullary cavity and cortex with destruction. There were multiple internal calcifications of some lesions. Focal soft tissue swelling was noted. Heterogeneous enhancements present.

X. Cheng et al., *Imaging of Bone Tumors in Wrist, Hand, Ankle and Foot*,
https://doi.org/10.1007/978-981-99-6407-9_7

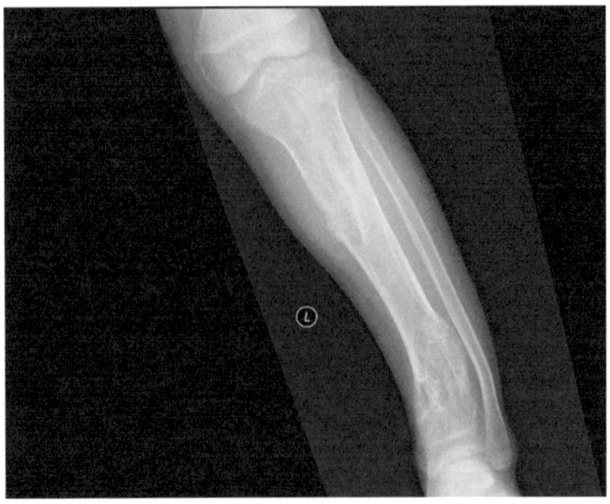

Fig. 7.3 Frontal view of the left tibia and fibula

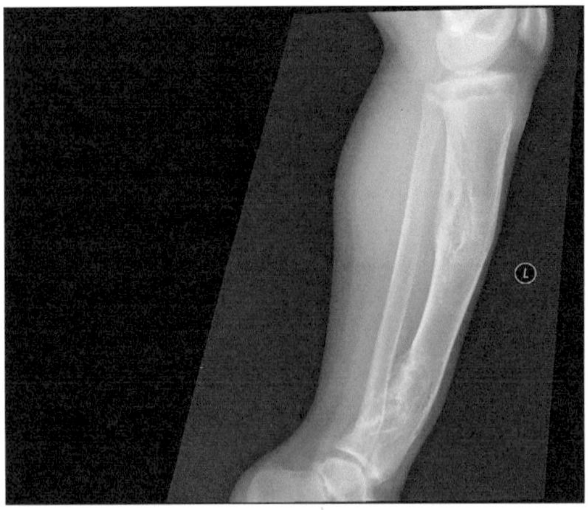

Fig. 7.4 Lateral view of the left tibia and fibula

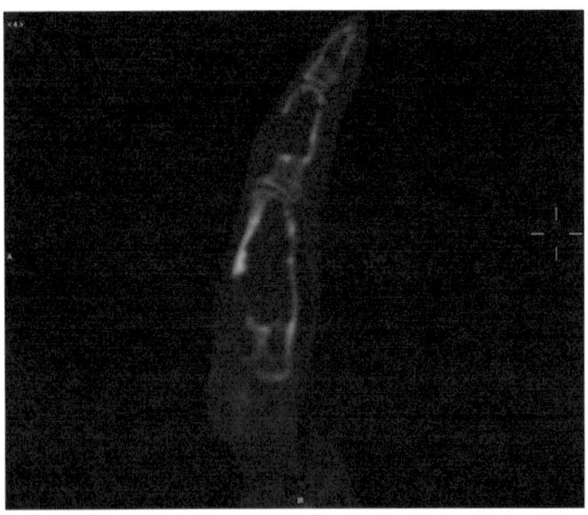

Fig. 7.5 Sagittal CT image of the right middle finger in bone window

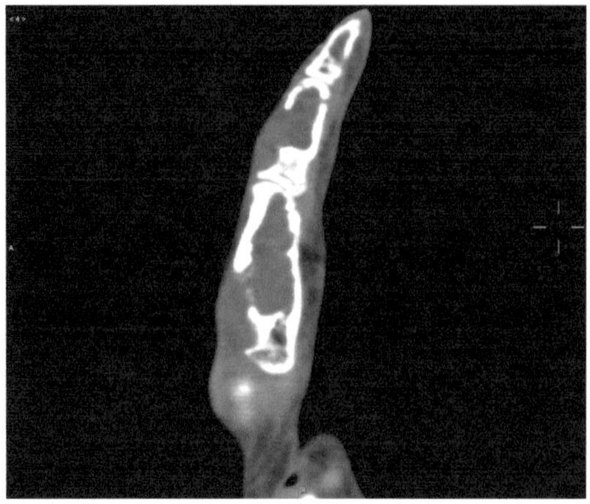

Fig. 7.6 Sagittal CT image of the right middle finger in soft tissue window

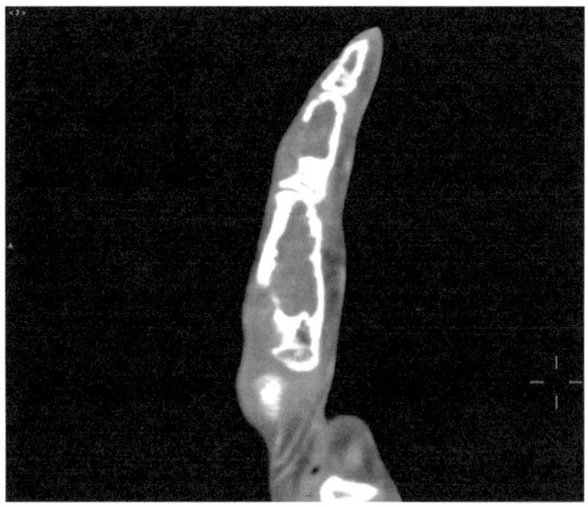

Fig. 7.7 Sagittal post-contrast CT image of the right middle finger in soft tissue window

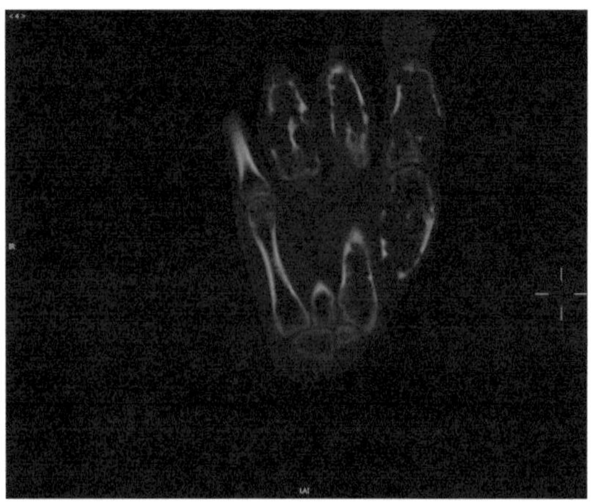

Fig. 7.8 Coronal CT image of the left hand in bone window

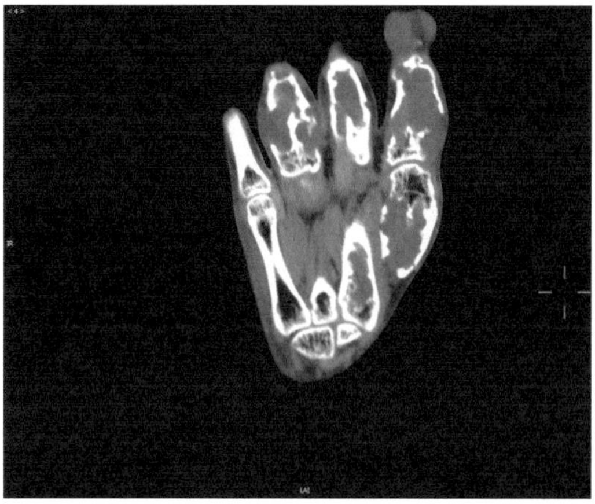

Fig. 7.9 Coronal CT image of the left hand in soft tissue window

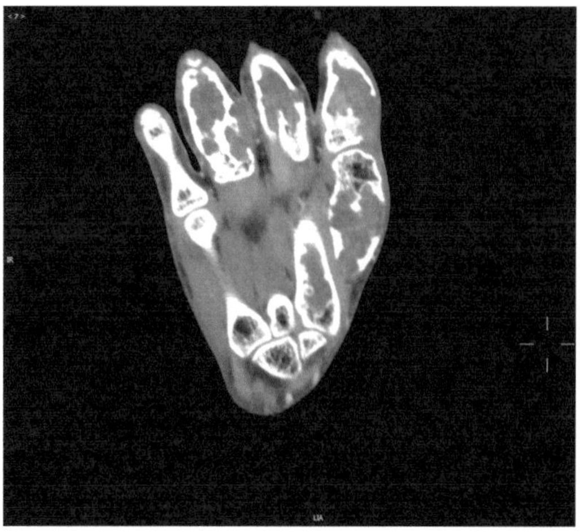

Fig. 7.10 Coronal post-contrast CT image of the left hand in soft tissue window

7.4 Description and Discussion from Residents

Radiographs show multiple lesions involving small and long tubular bones. Some lesions show expansile bony destructive changes with calcifications and focal soft tissue abnormalities. On the CT images, soft tissue was noted extending beyond the bony destruction with mild heterogeneous enhancement. The above findings are most suggestive of multiple enchondromas. Differential diagnoses include other processes that can affect multiple bones, such as fibrous dysplasia, and hyperparathyroidism. However, soft tissue mass is rarely seen with fibrous dysplasia and osteopenia is common with hyperparathyroidism.

7.5 Analysis and Comments from Professor Cheng Xiao-Guang

The patient is an adolescent. There are multiple bone lesions with bilateral involvement, slightly more on the left side. The affected bones show normal mineralization and development, thus hyperparathyroidism excluded. Soft tissue changes were noted along the metacarpal and phalanges on radiographs. This could be soft tissue changes or soft tissue mass extended beyond the destructed cortex. Based on the CT scan, these abnormalities were noted as mass adjacent to bone destruction and not soft tissue changes, indicating multiple enchondromas of Ollier's disease, classic form. When there is soft tissue hemangioma with multiple enchondromas, the diagnosis is Maffucci syndrome.

7.6 Diagnosis

Enchondromatosis (Ollier's disease).

Suggested Reading

Sharif B, Rajakulasingam R, Sharifi S, et al. MRI features of low-grade and high-grade chondrosarcoma in enchondromatosis. Skeletal Radiol. 2021;50(8):1637–1646.

Sharif B, Lindsay D, Asif Saifuddin A. Update on the imaging features of the enchondromatosis syndromes. Skeletal Radiol. 2022;51(4):747–762.

Gout: Case 8

8

8.1 Medical History

Patient is a 65-year-old male. He presented with a mass at the right middle finger without clear cause about 2 years ago, painless, and enlarging.

8.2 Physical Examination

Mass at the right middle finger with engorged veins noted in the skin, no skin break or drainage, point tenderness and rubbery.

8.3 Imaging Findings

8.3.1 Radiograph (Figs. 8.1 and 8.2)

Radiographs of the right middle finger demonstrated soft tissue swelling with increased densities about the proximal interphalangeal joint, multiple areas of bony destruction around the joint with clear margin, and overhanging edge. The joint spaces are relatively preserved.

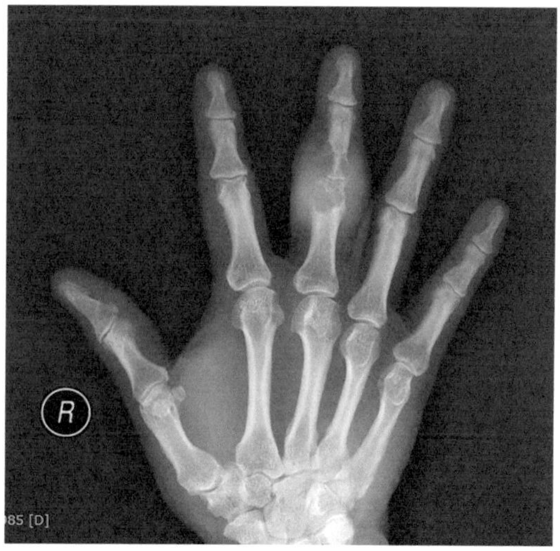

Fig. 8.1 Frontal view of the right middle finger

8.3.2 CT Imaging (Figs. 8.3 and 8.4)

CT images of the right middle finger demonstrated multiple erosions around the proximal interphalangeal joint with clear margin and associated high density soft tissue mass.

X. Cheng et al., *Imaging of Bone Tumors in Wrist, Hand, Ankle and Foot*,
https://doi.org/10.1007/978-981-99-6407-9_8

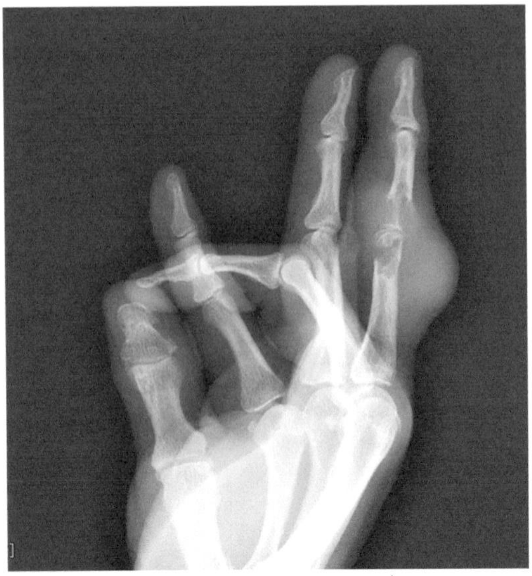

Fig. 8.2 Lateral view of the right middle finger

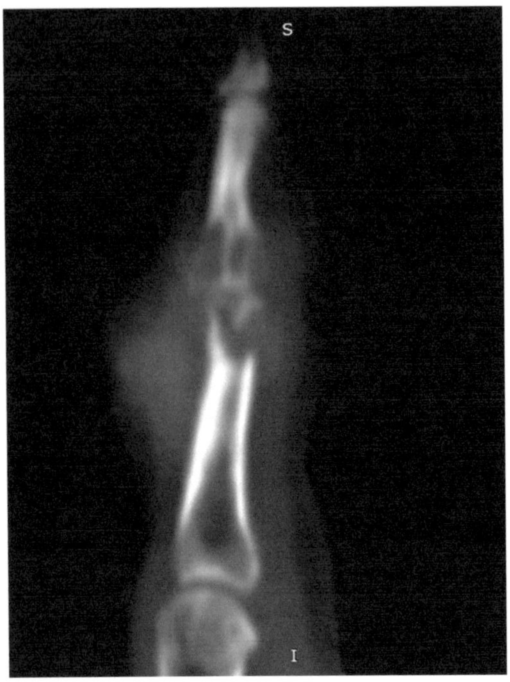

Fig. 8.3 Sagittal CT image of the right middle finger in bone window

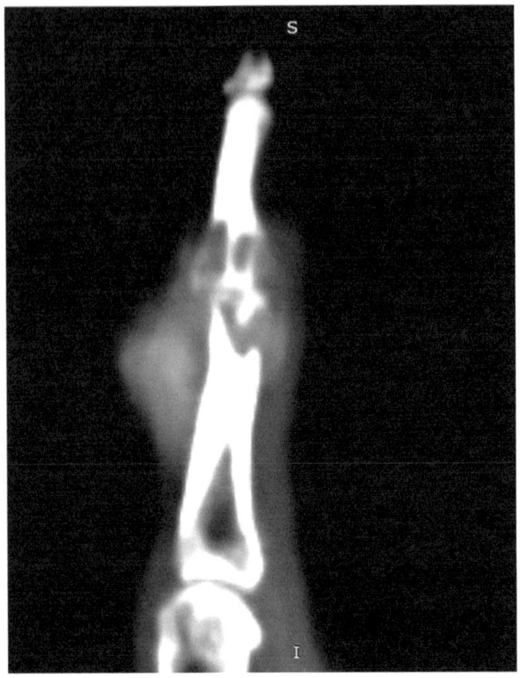

Fig. 8.4 Sagittal CT image of the right middle finger in soft tissue window

8.4 Description and Discussion from Residents

The bone mineral density of the right hand is normal. There was soft tissue swelling with increased densities around the proximal interphalangeal joint with preserved joint spaces. There were multiple erosions around the joint with clear margin and overhanging edge, indicating arthropathy. Given patient's sex and age, gout is the top consideration. However, no history of pain, not typical of gout.

8.5 Analysis and Comments from Professor Cheng Xiao-Guang

Normal bone mineralization on right hand radiographs can exclude rheumatoid arthritis. The lesions were centered around the proximal interphalangeal joint of the right middle finger with para-articular erosions and overhanging edge, relatively smooth articular surface in the unaffected region with preserved joint space. There were soft tissue swelling with increased density, consistent with tophi. Usually, patient with gout is symptomatic, however, this case is not. Increased soft tissue densities could also be seen in pigmented villonodular synovitis (PVNS) and asymptomatic. Many amorphous high densities within the soft tissues around the joint on CT images support tophi. In PVNS, usually just mildly increased densities in the soft tissues, not consistent with the current case.

8.6 Diagnosis

Gout.

Suggested Reading

Girish G, Glazebrook KN, Jacobson JA. Advanced imaging in gout. AJR Am J Roentgenol. 2013;201(3):515–25.

Teh J, McQueen F, Eshed I, et al. Advanced imaging in the diagnosis of gout and other crystal arthropathies. Semin Musculoskelet Radiol. 2018;22(2):225–236.

Benign Fibrous Tumor (Soft Tissue Tumor): Case 9

9

9.1 Medical History

Patient is a 47-year-old female. She presented with pain around the distal interphalangeal joint of the right fifth finger in the radial aspect for more than 2 months.

9.2 Physical Examination

Radial deviation of the right fifth finger around the distal interphalangeal joint with apparent point tenderness.

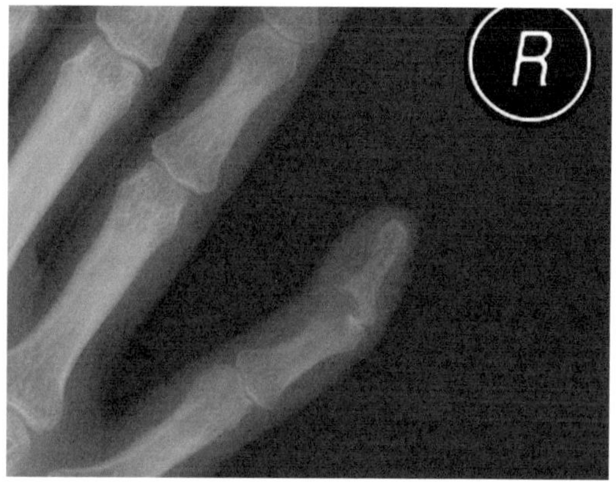

Fig. 9.1 Frontal view of the right fifth finger

9.3 Imaging Findings

9.3.1 Radiograph (Figs. 9.1 and 9.2)

Radiographs demonstrated bony destructive changes around the distal interphalangeal joint of the right fifth finger in the radial aspect with clear margin.

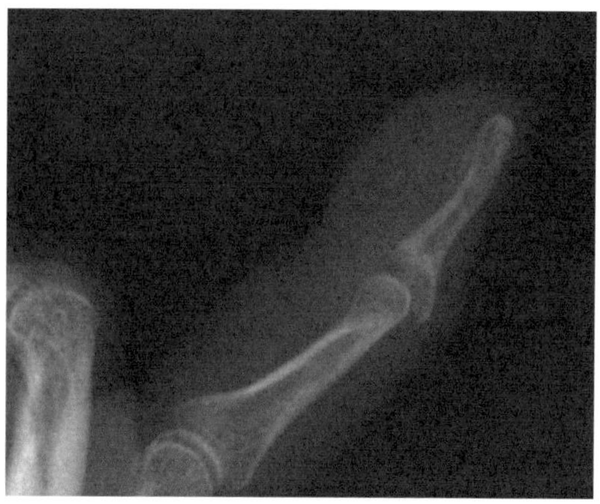

Fig. 9.2 Lateral view of the right fifth finger

9.3.2 CT Imaging (Figs. 9.3, 9.4, 9.5, 9.6, 9.7, and 9.8)

CT images of the right fifth finger demonstrated soft tissue mass at radial side of the distal interphalangeal joint, with bony destruction along distal middle phalanx and proximal distal phalanx with clear margin.

X. Cheng et al., *Imaging of Bone Tumors in Wrist, Hand, Ankle and Foot*,
https://doi.org/10.1007/978-981-99-6407-9_9

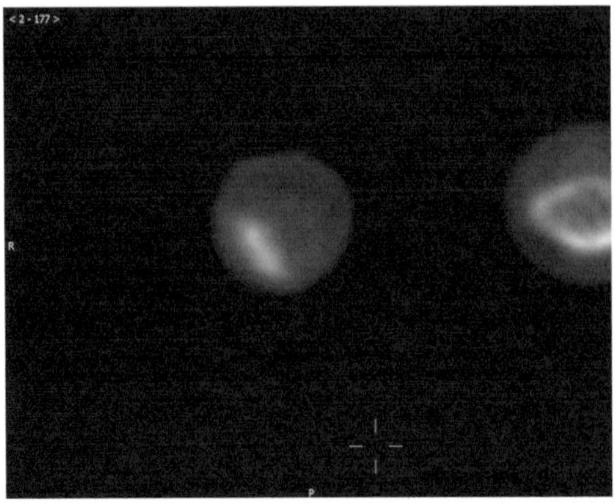

Fig. 9.3 Axial CT image of the right fifth finger in bone window

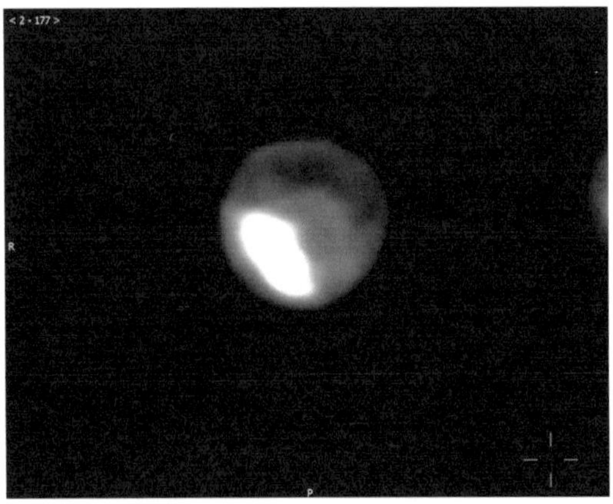

Fig. 9.4 Axial CT image of the right fifth finger in soft tissue window

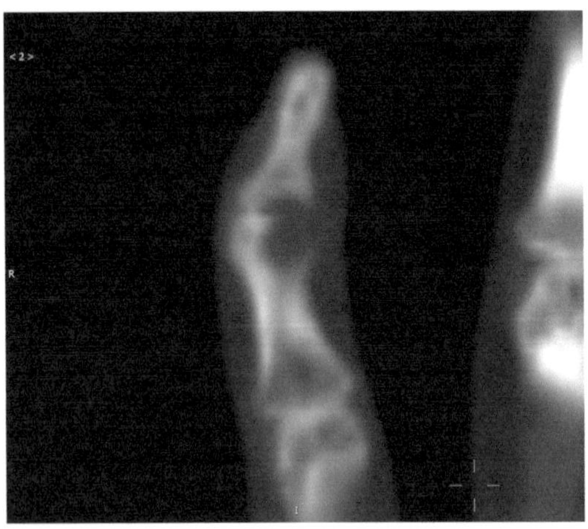

Fig. 9.5 Coronal CT image of the right fifth finger in bone window

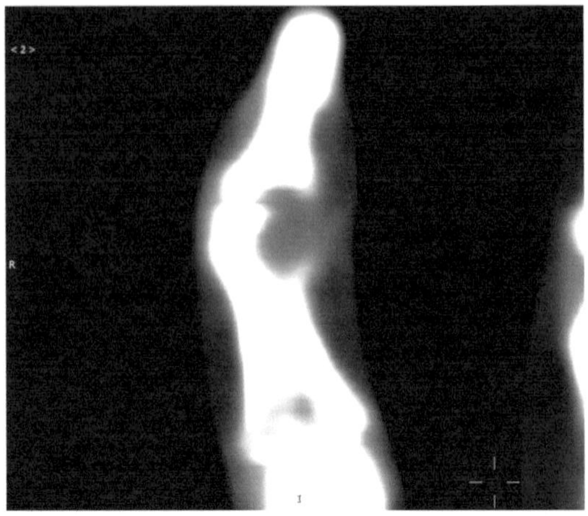

Fig. 9.6 Coronal CT image of the right fifth finger in soft tissue window

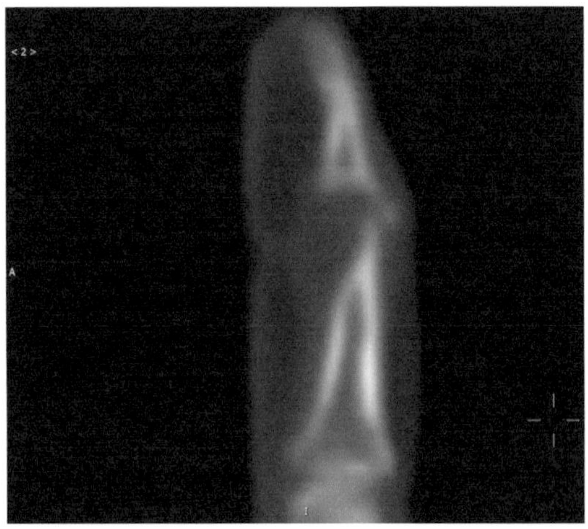

Fig. 9.7 Sagittal CT image of the right fifth finger in bone window

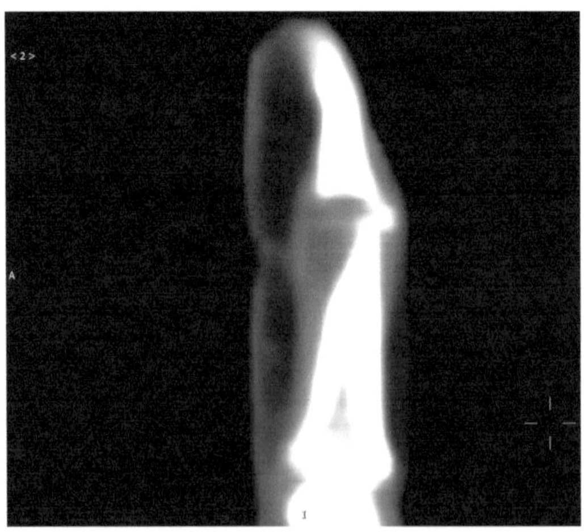

Fig. 9.8 Sagittal CT image of the right fifth finger in soft tissue window

9.4 Description and Discussion from Residents

The lesion is around the distal interphalangeal joint of the right fifth finger with bony compressive changes along the distal middle phalanx and proximal distal phalanx with clear margin and sclerotic border. Rheumatoid arthritis and gout commonly affect interphalangeal joints, however, this case demonstrated benign soft tissue compression, and resorption of the adjacent bone. Among soft tissue mass, giant cell tumor of the tendon sheath is most common and thus, our top consideration.

9.5 Analysis and Comments from Professor Cheng Xiao-Guang

Radiographs demonstrated bony compressive changes around radial aspect of the distal interphalangeal joint of the right fifth finger with clear margin. Soft tissue mass noted on the CT images with flexor tendon thickening, top consideration is related to tendon sheath, such as giant cell tumor of the tendon sheath. However, gout is common in this area and should be included in the differential diagnosis. Rheumatoid usually involves multiple joints, not consistent with the current case and can be excluded.

9.6 Diagnosis

Benign fibrous tumor (soft tissue tumor).

Suggested Reading

Kitagawa Y, Tamai K, Tsunoda R, et al. Bone changes associated with soft-tissue tumors of the hand. J Nippon Med Scheme 2012;79(4):267–73.

Simon MJK, Pogoda P, Hövelborn F, et al. Incidence, histopathologic analysis and distribution of tumours of the hand. BMC Musculoskelet Disord. 2014;15:182.

Brown Tumor from Hyperparathyroidism: Case 10

10

10.1 Medical History

Patient is a 23-year-old male. He had history of right clavicle fracture more than 3 months ago and right upper extremity and left lower extremity fractures more than 1 month ago with hypercalcemia for 2 weeks.

10.2 Physical Examination

Not done.

10.3 Imaging Findings

10.3.1 Radiograph (Figs. 10.1 and 10.2)

Radiographs of the right wrist demonstrated bony destructive changes at distal radius with clear margin and peripheral sclerosis.

10.3.2 CT Imaging (Figs. 10.3, 10.4, 10.5, 10.6, 10.7, 10.8, and 10.9)

CT images of the right wrist demonstrated bony lytic changes at the distal radius with clear margin, mild peripheral sclerosis, and no enhancement.

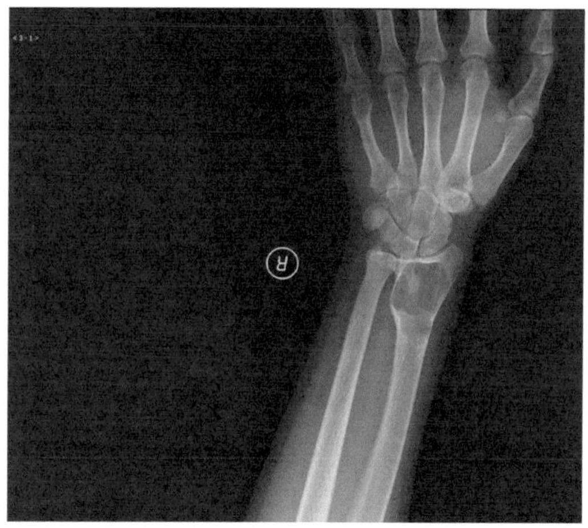

Fig. 10.1 Frontal view of the right wrist

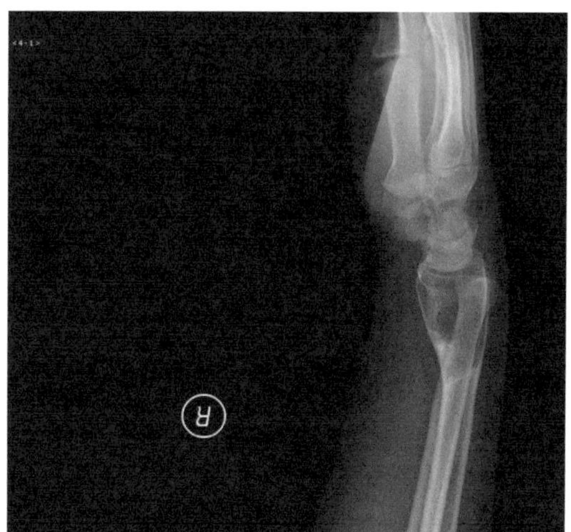

Fig. 10.2 Lateral view of the right wrist

X. Cheng et al., *Imaging of Bone Tumors in Wrist, Hand, Ankle and Foot*,
https://doi.org/10.1007/978-981-99-6407-9_10

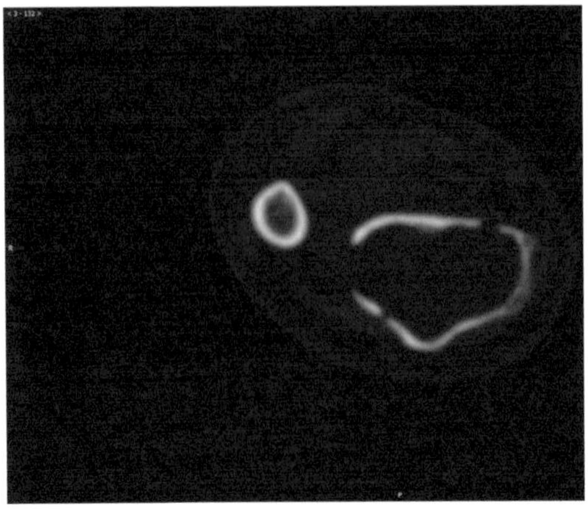

Fig. 10.3 Axial CT image of the right wrist in bone window

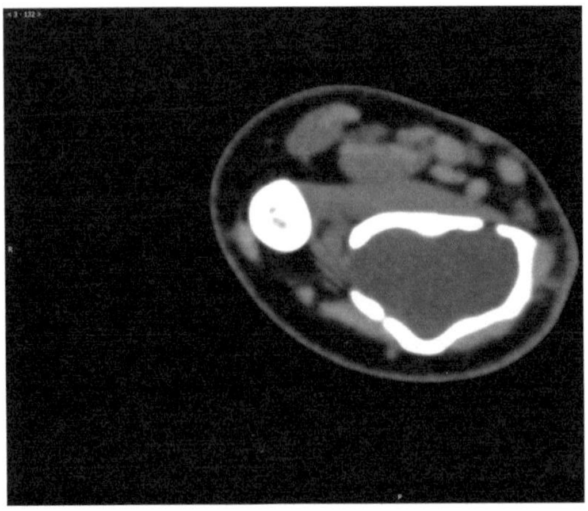

Fig. 10.4 Axial CT image of the right wrist in soft tissue window

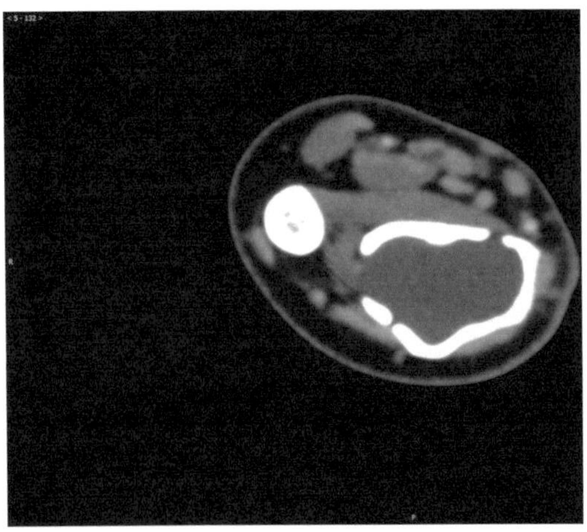

Fig. 10.5 Axial post-contrast CT image of the wrist in soft tissue window

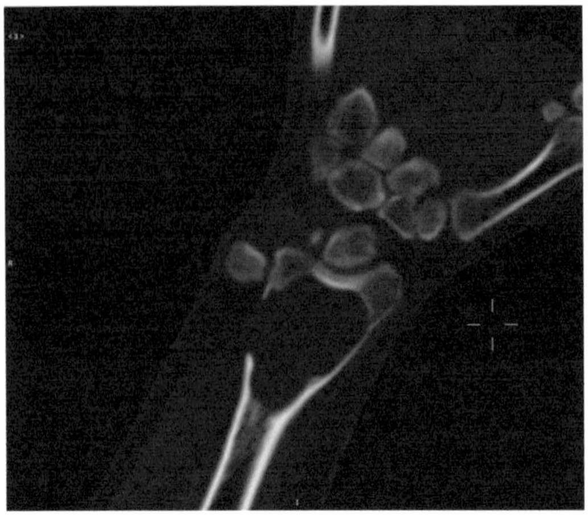

Fig. 10.6 Coronal CT image of the right wrist in bone window

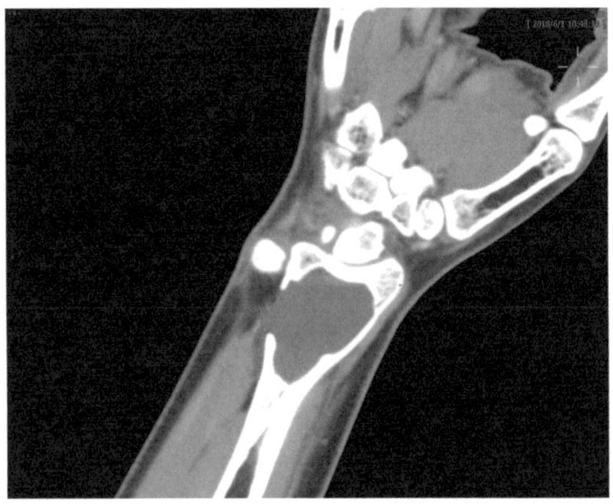

Fig. 10.7 Coronal CT image of the right wrist in soft tissue window

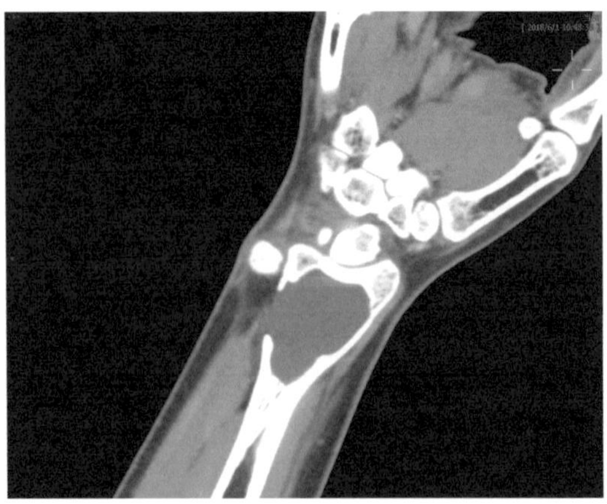

Fig. 10.8 Coronal post-contrast CT image of the right wrist in soft tissue window

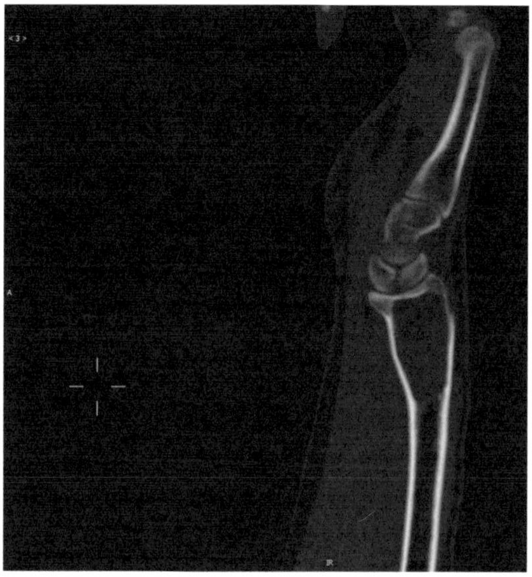

Fig. 10.9 Sagittal CT image of the right wrist in bone window

10.4 Description and Discussion from Residents

Radiographs demonstrated expansile lytic bony changes at distal radius with clear margin and internal residual bony trabeculae. Bony cortical disruption was demonstrated on CT images without associated soft tissue mass and no enhancement with CT value of 12HU. Patient is a young male with history of multiple fractures and hypercalcemia, brown tumor from hyperparathyroidism is our top consideration. It would be helpful to evaluate the images of other affected area. If this is the only lesion, we would consider aneurysmal bone cyst or giant cell tumor of bone, however, the enhancement pattern is not consistent with these two entities.

10.5 Analysis and Comments from Professor Cheng Xiao-Guang

Patient is a young male with history of multiple fractures and hypercalcemia. Lytic bone lesion at distal right radius with clear margin and osteopenia around the carpal bone and distal radius and ulna are noted. When there are cystic changes on the background of osteopenia, brown tumor from hyperparathyroidism is the top consideration. Given patient's age and affected area, differential diagnosis will include giant cell tumor of bone, but the lesion is not expansile and the enhancement pattern is not consistent with giant cell tumor, thus can be excluded.

10.6 Diagnosis

Brown tumor from hyperparathyroidism.

Suggested Reading

Bennett J, Suliburk JW, Morón FE. Osseous manifestations of primary hyperparathyroidism: imaging findings. Int J Endocrinol. 2020:3146535.

Hong WS, Sung MS, Chun KA, et al. Emphasis on the MR imaging findings of brown tumor: a report of five cases. Skeletal Radiol. 2011;40(2):205–13.

11 Giant Cell Tumor of Bone: Case 11

11.1 Medical History

Patient is a 33-year-old male. He presented with mild discomfort around the second metacarpal after exercise, without redness about 5 months ago. He had radiographs done at local hospital at the time and showed no abnormalities. About 3 months ago, he felt increasing pain after excessive use of the right hand with local mass and focal tenderness and restricted motion. He had radiographs at local hospital and demonstrated lesion around the second metacarpal.

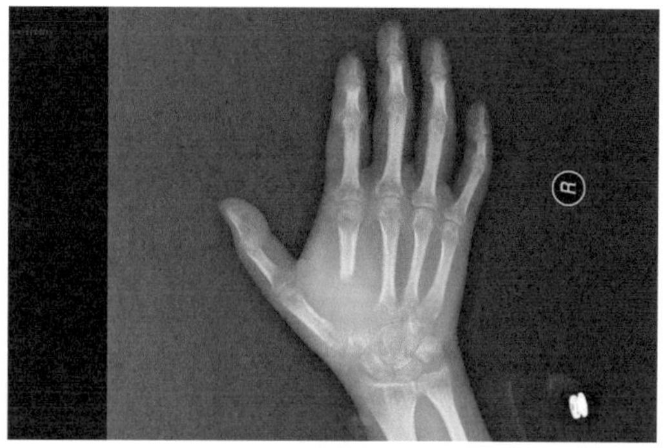

Fig. 11.1 Frontal view of the right hand

11.2 Physical Examination

4.5 cm × 3 cm × 3 cm mass by the right second metacarpal.

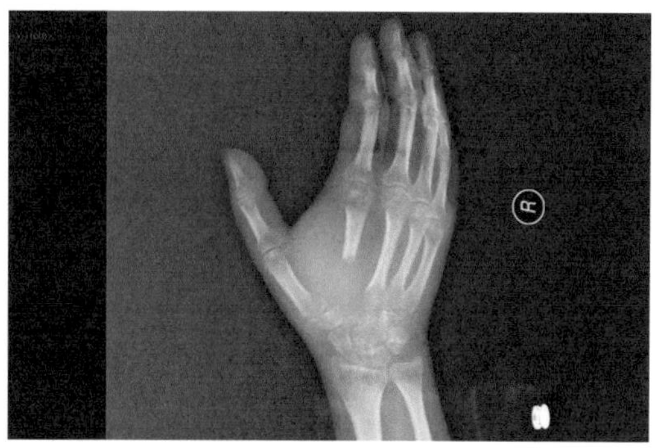

Fig. 11.2 Oblique view of the right hand

11.3 Imaging Findings

11.3.1 Radiograph (Figs. 11.1 and 11.2)

Radiographs of the right hand demonstrated bony destructive changes at the proximal second metacarpal with indistinct margin and adjacent soft tissue swelling. There was general osteopenia.

11.3.2 CT Imaging (Figs. 11.3, 11.4, 11.5, 11.6 and 11.7)

CT images of the right hand demonstrated lytic bony destructive changes of the second metacarpal with associated soft tissue mass of internal heterogenous

X. Cheng et al., *Imaging of Bone Tumors in Wrist, Hand, Ankle and Foot*,
https://doi.org/10.1007/978-981-99-6407-9_11

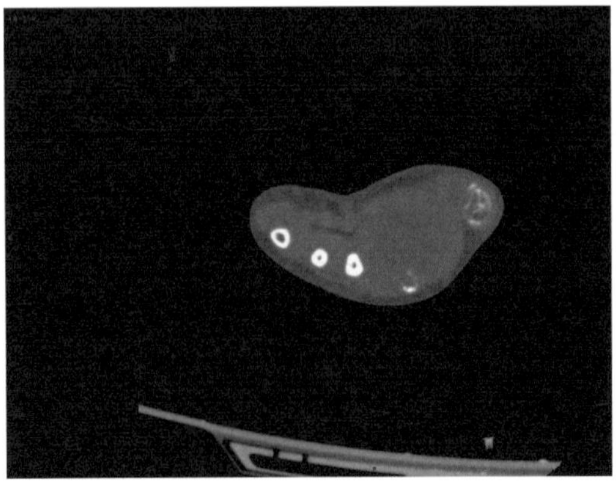

Fig. 11.3 Axial CT image of the right hand in bone window

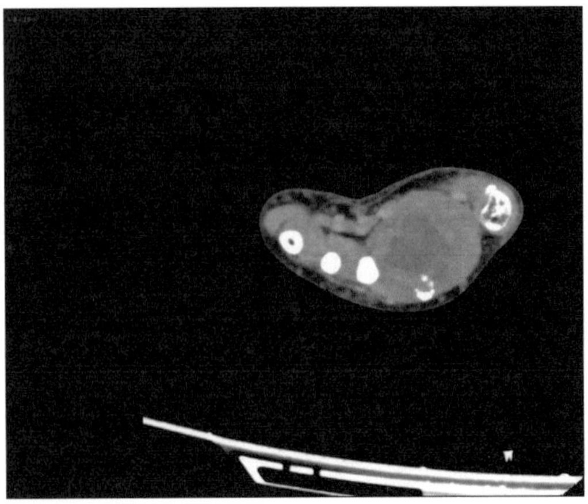

Fig. 11.4 Axial CT image of the right hand in soft tissue window

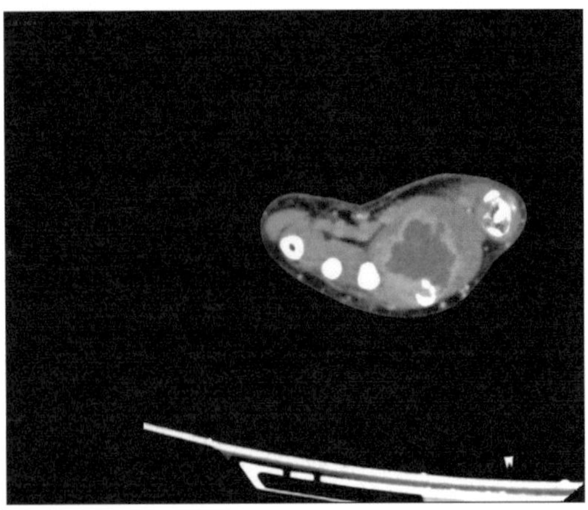

Fig. 11.5 Axial post-contrast CT image of the right hand in soft tissue window

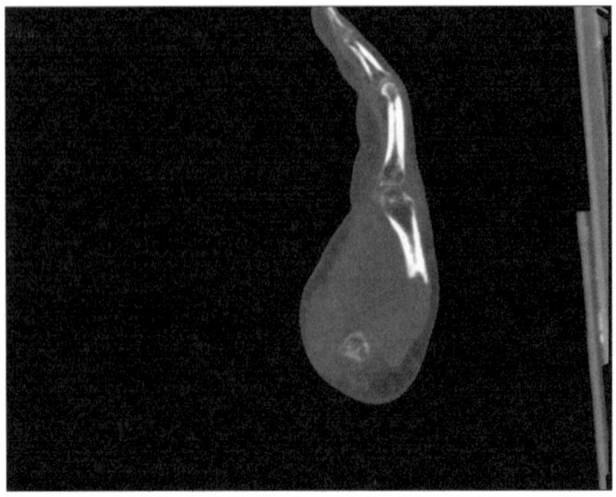

Fig. 11.6 Sagittal CT image of the right hand in bone window

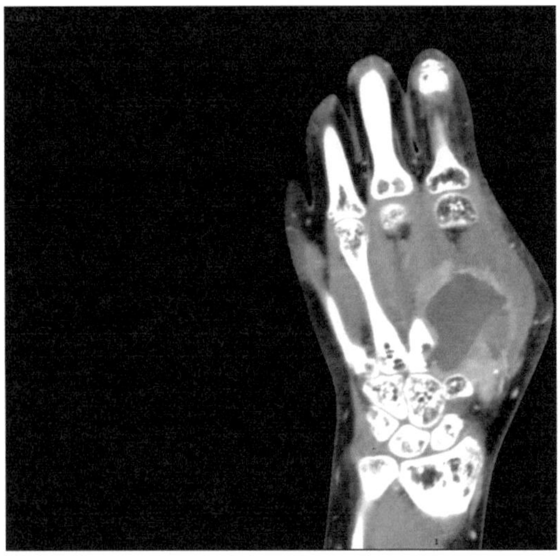

Fig. 11.7 Coronal post-contrast CT image of the right hand in soft tissue window

density with area of fluid density. There was peripheral discontinuous cortex with eggshell-like appearance and patchy high densities and clear margin along the residual cortex. Avid enhancement was noted. Additionally, there was involvement at the base of the third metacarpal with bony destruction.

11.3.3 MR Imaging (1 Month After Treatment) (Figs. 11.8, 11.9, 11.10, and 11.11)

MR images of the right hand demonstrated heterogenous signal of the soft tissue mass around the second metacarpal with multiple areas of hemor-

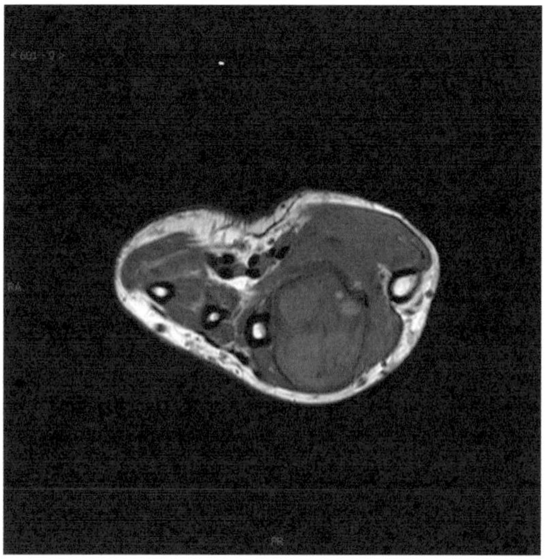

Fig. 11.8 Axial T1-weighted MR image of the right hand

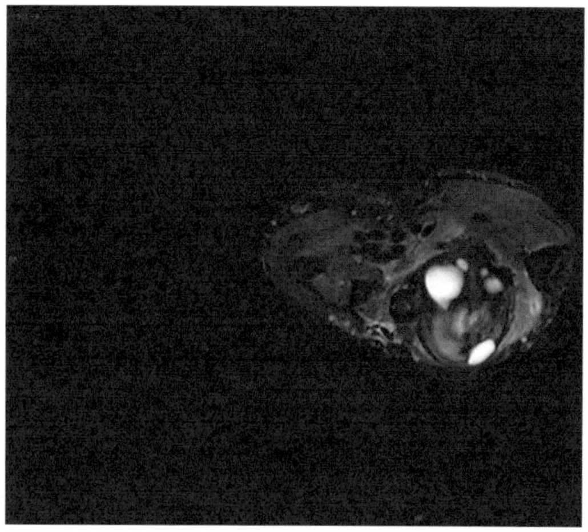

Fig. 11.10 Axial fat-suppressed T2-weighted MR image of the right hand

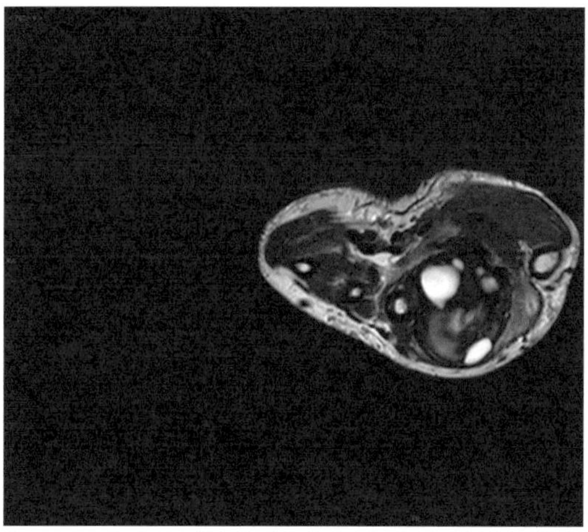

Fig. 11.9 Axial T2-weighted MR image of the right hand

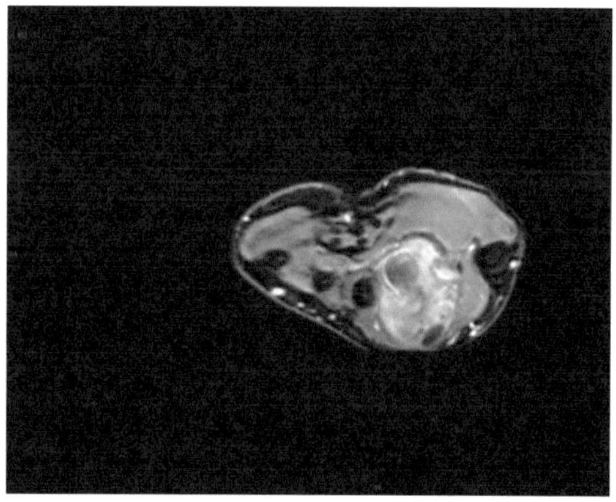

Fig. 11.11 Axial post-contrast fat-suppressed T1-weighted MR image of the right hand

rhage and cystic changes. The solid component area demonstrated majority low T1 signal with surrounding soft tissue edema. Enhancement was noted in the solid portion of the mass.

11.4 Description and Discussion from Residents

Right hand radiographs demonstrated overall background of osteopenia and lytic bony destruction at proximal second metacarpal with sharp margin and no sclerosis or calcification. No periosteal reaction was noted. Surrounding soft tissue swelling was noted. CT images demonstrated soft tissue mass with heterogenous densities, fluid density area of necrosis, and heterogenous enhancement with area of avid enhancement. There were heterogenous signals of the soft tissue mass on MR images with areas of necrosis and cystic changes; patchy area of low T2 and high T1 signal noted in the solid area, suggesting hemorrhage. Avid enhancement was noted in the solid portion of the mass. Our first consideration is giant cell tumor of bone. However, with osteopenia noted, brown tumor from hyperparathyroidism is included in the differential diagnosis.

11.5 Analysis and Comments from Professor Cheng Xiao-Guang

The patient is a young male with 5 months of history. There was complete lytic destruction of the bone at proximal second metacarpal. Osteopenia was noted of the remaining visualized osseous structures with relatively preserved cortex thickness, not typical of osteopenia from hyperparathyroidism, indicating disuse osteopenia. Common process that can lead to destruction of proximal metacarpals include giant cell tumor of bone and giant cell reparative granuloma (solid aneurysmal bone cyst); usually with avid enhancement of the solid portion of the mass, as demonstrated by current case. However, there was complete destruction of the bone of the current case, without a bony shell and soft tissue mass invades the base of the third metacarpal, raising concern for more aggressive etiology and correlation with pathology is recommended.

11.6 Diagnosis

Giant cell tumor of bone.

Suggested Reading

James SLJ, Davies AM. Giant-cell tumours of bone of the hand and wrist: a review of imaging findings and differential diagnoses. Eur Radiol. 2005;15(9):1855–1866.

Mavrogenis AF, Panagopoulos GN, Angelini A, et al. Tumors of the hand. Eur J Orthop Surg Traumatol. 2017;27(6):747–762.

12 Giant Cell Tumor of Bone: Case 12

12.1 Medical History

Patient is an 11-year-old girl. She presented with mass around the left second metacarpal.

12.2 Physical Examination

Not done.

12.3 Imaging Findings

12.3.1 Radiograph (Figs. 12.1 and 12.2)

Radiographs of the left hand demonstrated expansile and lytic bony changes at the second metacarpal with thinning of the cortex without sclerosis and adjacent soft tissue swelling.

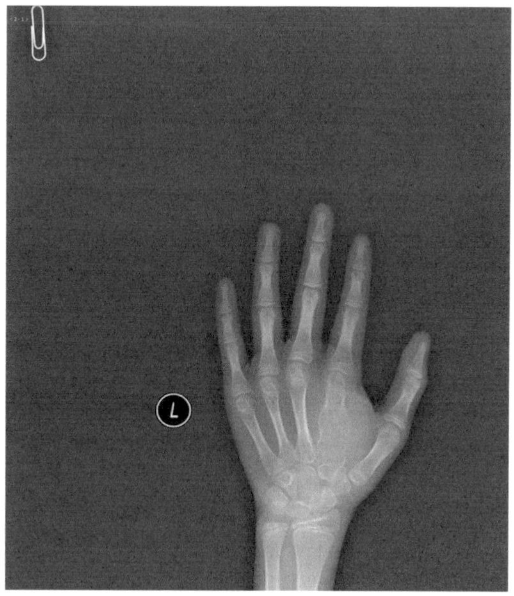

Fig. 12.1 Frontal view of the left hand

12.3.2 CT Imaging (Figs. 12.3, 12.4, 12.5, 12.6, 12.7, 12.8, and 12.9)

CT images of the left hand demonstrated vertically expansile and lytic lesion of the second metacarpal with bone destruction and homogenous internal density without calcification and peripheral bony shell with focal continuous disruption and associated soft tissue mass. Diffuse avid enhancement was noted. Base of the third metacarpal was involved.

X. Cheng et al., *Imaging of Bone Tumors in Wrist, Hand, Ankle and Foot*,
https://doi.org/10.1007/978-981-99-6407-9_12

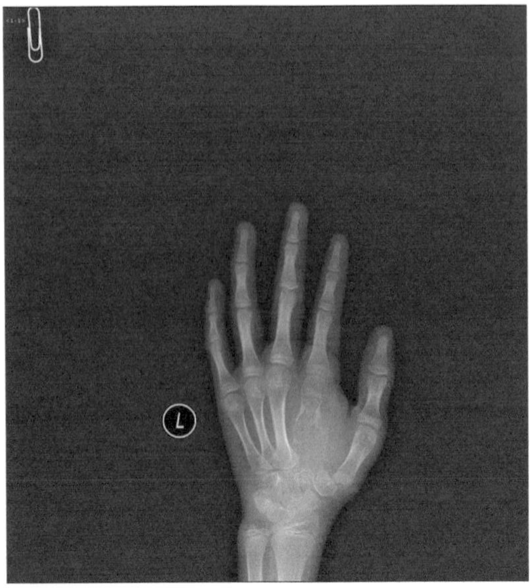

Fig. 12.2 Oblique view of the left hand

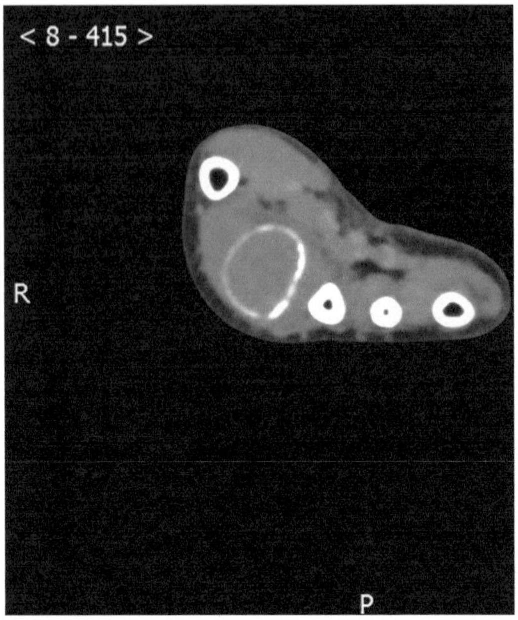

Fig. 12.4 Axial CT image of the left hand in soft tissue window

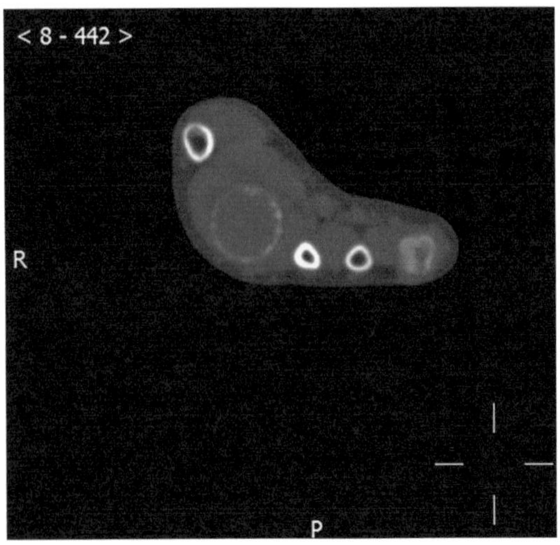

Fig. 12.3 Axial CT image of the left hand in bone window

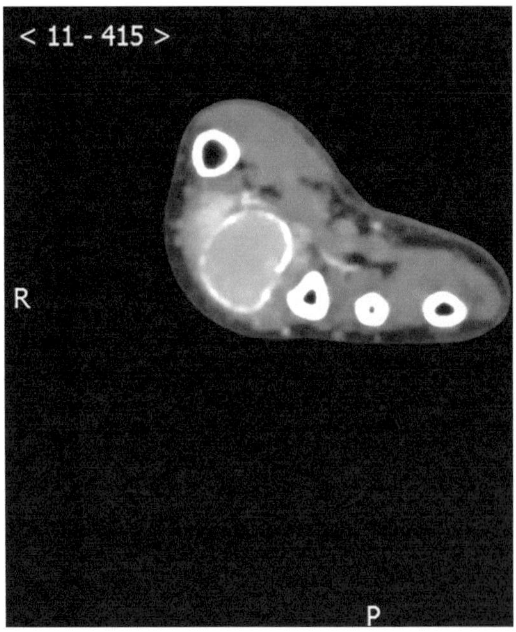

Fig. 12.5 Axial post-contrast CT image of the left hand in soft tissue window

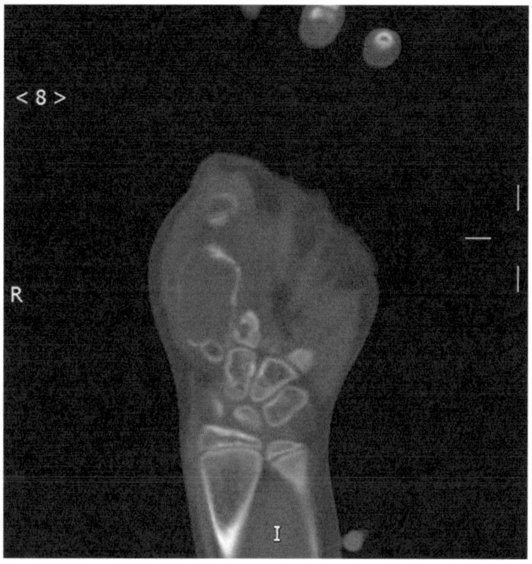

Fig. 12.6 Coronal CT image of the left hand in bone window

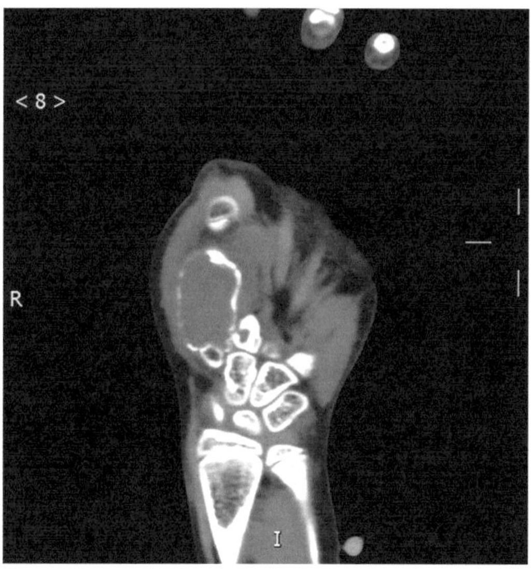

Fig. 12.7 Coronal CT image of the left hand in soft tissue window

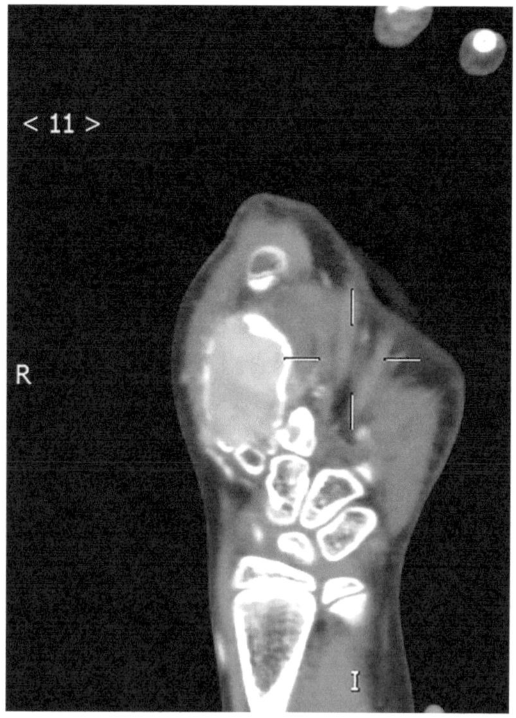

Fig. 12.8 Coronal post-contrast CT image of the left hand in soft tissue window

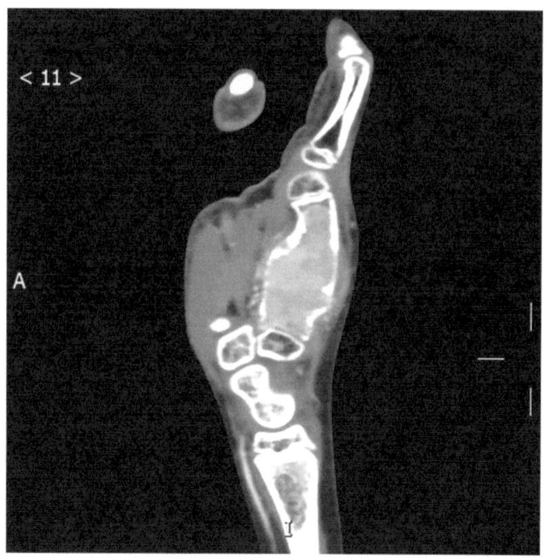

Fig. 12.9 Sagittal post-contrast CT image of the left hand in soft tissue window

12.4 Description and Discussion from Residents

There were expansile, lytic bony destructive changes of the left second metacarpal with thin bony shell without sclerosis or internal calcification. Focal area was noted of cortical break with soft tissue mass. Avid enhancement was noted. The above findings are consistent with giant cell tumor of bone. However, patient's age is too young. Differential diagnoses include enchondroma and tumors-like giant cell tumor of bone (such as solitary plasmacytoma). However, internal calcified matrix is common in enchondroma and the latter one usually affects old populations, not consistent with the current case.

12.5 Analysis and Comments from Professor Cheng Xiao-Guang

The patient is an adolescent girl. Radiographs demonstrated expansile, lytic bony destructive changes of the second metacarpal with adjacent soft tissue swelling. Given the location of the lesion, enchondroma can be considered. However, usually there is no associated soft tissue changes with enchondroma. Then, we consider giant cell tumor of bone. However, our patient is younger than the typical age of patients with giant cell tumor of bone. Giant cell tumor of bone usually involves end of the bone, thus, not our top consideration. Other process that can affect metacarpal could be giant cell reparative granuloma (solid aneurysmal bone cyst). Overall, the radiographic findings favor a benign process. Soft tissue breaks the cortex with avid enhancement on CT images noted, could be giant cell tumor of bone in adult patients; it could be giant cell reparative granuloma in pediatric patient.

12.6 Diagnosis

Giant cell tumor of bone.

Suggested Reading

James SLJ, Davies AM. Giant-cell tumours of bone of the hand and wrist: a review of imaging findings and differential diagnoses. Eur Radiol. 2005;15(9):1855–1866.

Mavrogenis AF, Panagopoulos GN, Angelini A, et al. Tumors of the hand. Eur J Orthop Surg Traumatol. 2017;27(6):747–762.

13 Non-Hodgkin Lymphoma of Bone: Case 13

13.1 Medical History

Patient is a 14-year-old boy. He presented with persistent, severe pain around the left clavicle without inciting event. There was no fever or night sweats. Pain and swelling around the left first metacarpal-phalangeal joint with restricted motion of the left thumb developed later.

13.2 Physical Examination

Left axilla enlarged lymph nodes.

13.3 Imaging Findings

13.3.1 CT Imaging (Figs. 13.1, 13.2, 13.3, 13.4, 13.5, 13.6, 13.7, 13.8, and 13.9)

CT images demonstrated bony destructive changes of the left first metacarpal and proximal left clavicle. There was cortex disruption with periosteal reaction with soft tissue mass. Avid enhancement was noted.

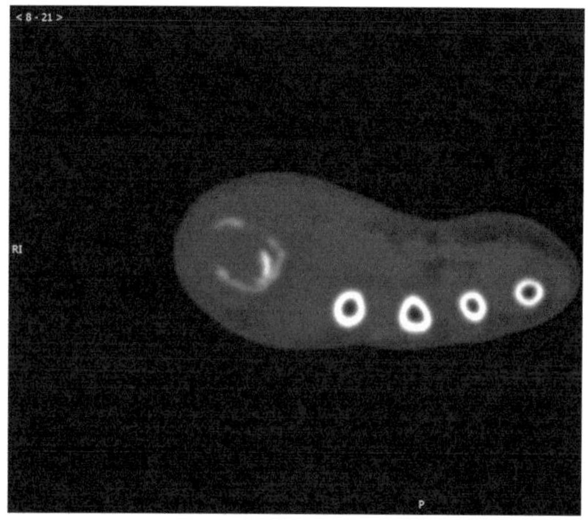

Fig. 13.1 Axial CT image of the left hand in bone window

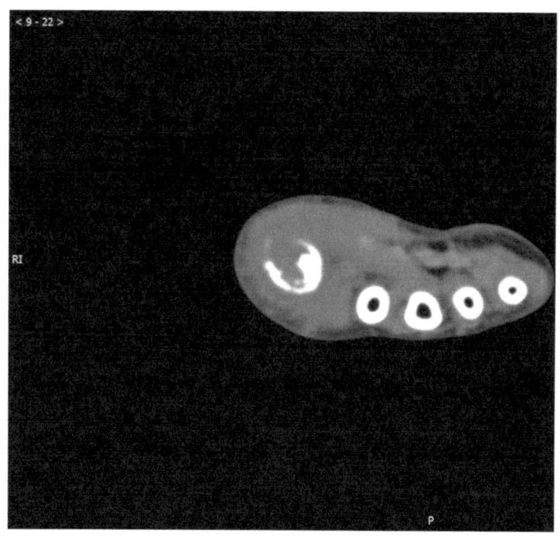

Fig. 13.2 Axial CT image of the left hand in soft tissue window

X. Cheng et al., *Imaging of Bone Tumors in Wrist, Hand, Ankle and Foot*,
https://doi.org/10.1007/978-981-99-6407-9_13

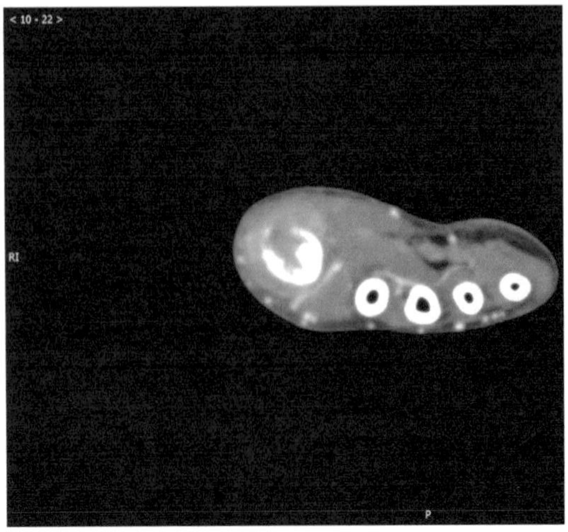

Fig. 13.3 Axial post-contrast CT image of the left hand in soft tissue window

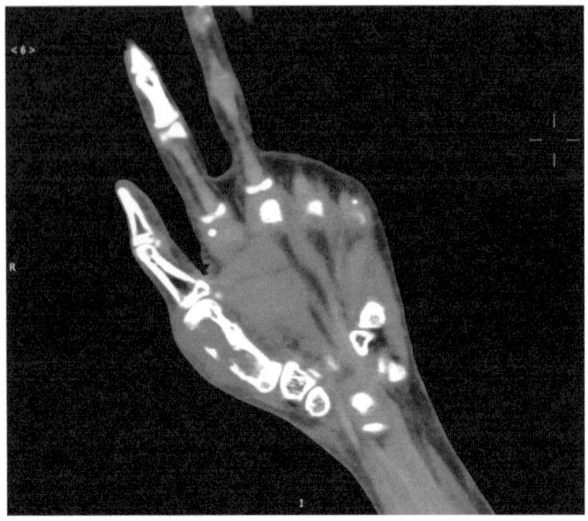

Fig. 13.5 Coronal CT image of the left hand in soft tissue window

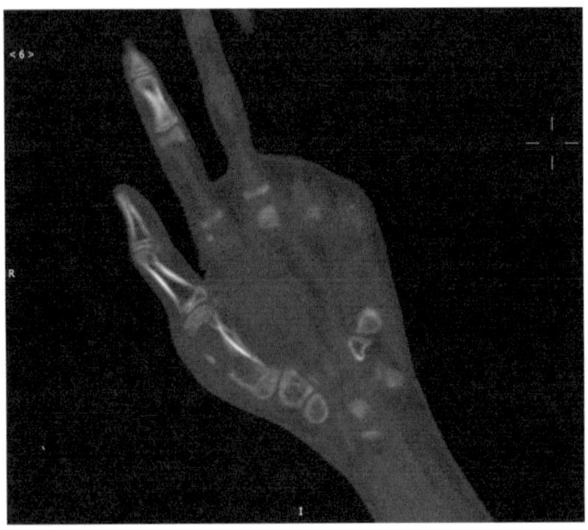

Fig. 13.4 Coronal CT image of the left hand in bone window

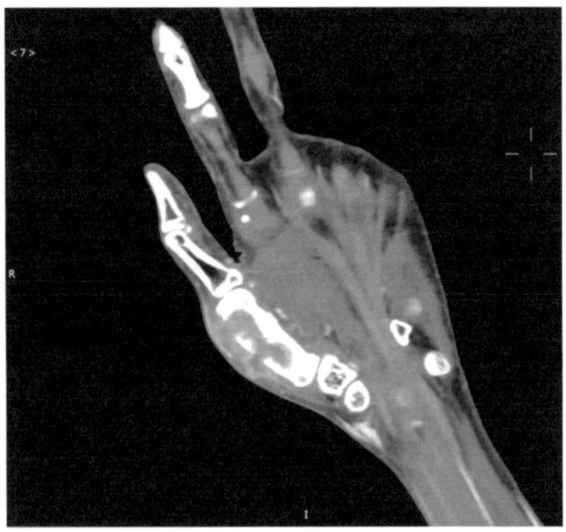

Fig. 13.6 Coronal post-contrast CT image of the left hand in soft tissue window

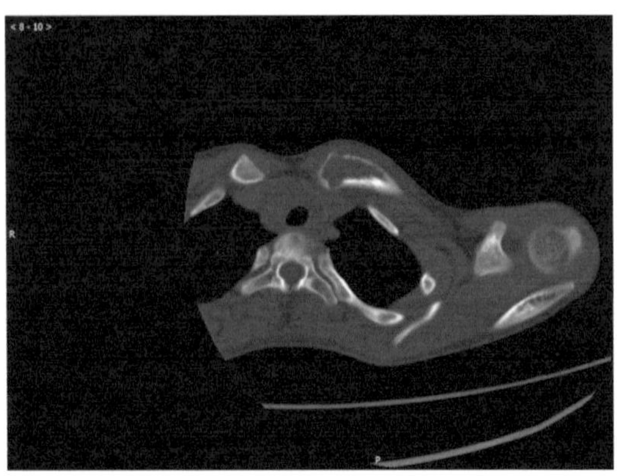

Fig. 13.7 Axial CT image of the left clavicle in bone window

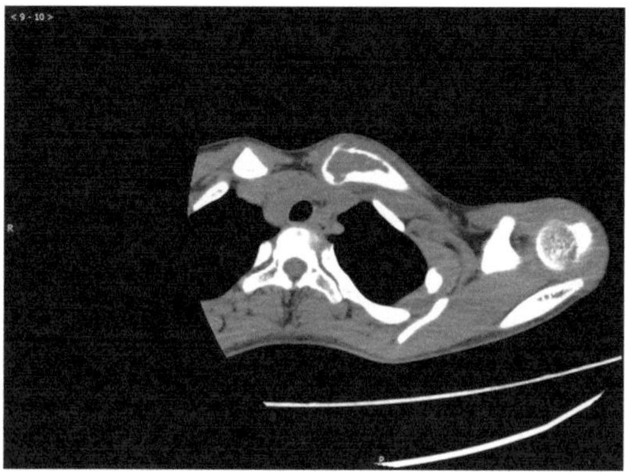

Fig. 13.8 Axial CT image of the left clavicle in soft tissue window

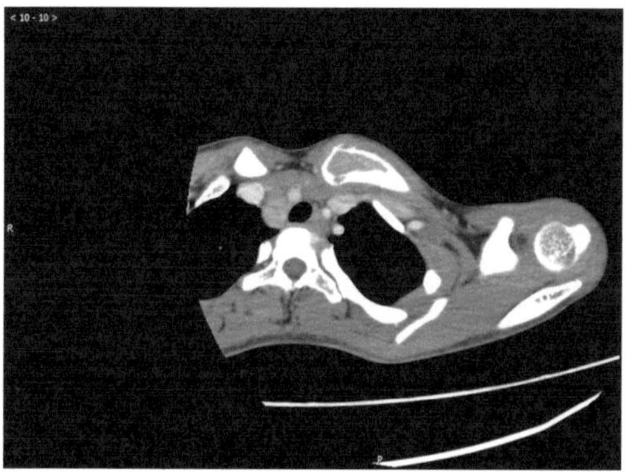

Fig. 13.9 Axial post-contrast CT image of the left clavicle in soft tissue window

13.4 Description and Discussion from Residents

There was mild expansile bony destruction of the left first metacarpal and proximal left clavicle. Apparent destruction of the cortex of the metacarpal with periosteal reaction was noted and soft tissue mass extruded beyond the cortex with avid enhancement. With multiple bone destructive lesions in pediatric patients, we first consider eosinophilic granuloma (Langerhans cell histiocytosis), in keeping with enlarged lymph nodes seen with the patient. However, there was extensive bony destruction with soft tissue mass and avid enhancement, suggesting aggressive nature of the process and malignancy need to be considered. Ewing sarcoma is a common malignancy in pediatric patients, but multiple bone involvements are rare. Additionally, the pattern of bone destruction and soft tissue mass morphology are not consistent with Ewing sarcoma. Given the presence of periosteal reaction and enhancement of the soft tissue component, we favor malignant vascular tumor.

13.5 Analysis and Comments from Professor Cheng Xiao-Guang

There was bony destruction of the left first metacarpal with focal disruption of the cortex and normal density of the remaining bone cortex. Periosteal reaction was noted with avid enhancement of the soft tissue mass. Similar changes were noted in the clavicle. Differential diagnoses include: (1) eosinophilic granuloma: common in pediatric patients with imaging features of neoplasm and inflammation. There were multiple bone involvements of the current case. Patient's history, bone destructive pattern and enhancement are suggestive of inflammatory process, could be put first at the differential diagnosis. (2) Ewing sarcoma: most common bone malignancy in younger kids and intramedullary origin tumor, the periosteal reaction not like the current case. Involvement of multiple bone is rare, thus, very unlikely. (3) Hematological tumor.

13.6 Diagnosis

Non-Hodgkin lymphoma of bone.

Suggested Reading

Krishnan A, Shirkhoda A, Tehranzadeh J, et al. Primary bone lymphoma: radiographic-MR imaging correlation. Radiographics. 2003-Dec;23(6):1371–83; discussion 1384–7.

Ruzek KA, Wenger DE. The multiple faces of lymphoma of the musculoskeletal system. Skeletal Radiol. 2004;33(1):1–8.

Melorheostosis: Case 14

14

14.1 Medical History

Patient is a 5-year-old girl. She presented post-operative of focal release after contracture around the joints in multiple fingers of the left hand for more than 5 years.

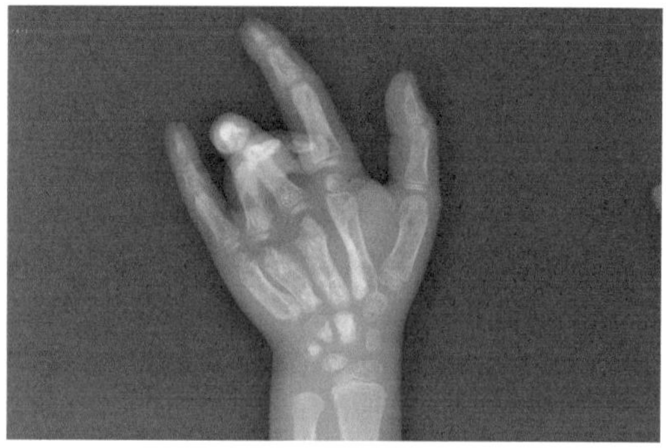

Fig. 14.1 Frontal view of the left hand

14.2 Physical Examination

Flexion contracture of the left third, fourth, and fifth fingers with restricted motion. Post-operative scars noted around the palm side of the hand. Left thumb and second finger with normal range of motion.

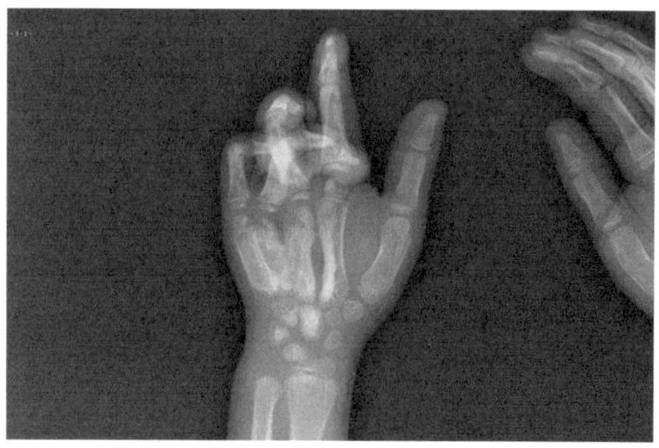

Fig. 14.2 Oblique view of the left hand

14.3 Imaging Findings

14.3.1 Radiograph (Figs. 14.1, 14.2, and 14.3)

Radiographs of the left hand demonstrated flexion deformity of the middle, fourth, and fifth fingers of the left hand. There was tubular cortical thickening of multiple metacarpals with linear high density and multiple carpal bones demonstrated increased bone densities.

X. Cheng et al., *Imaging of Bone Tumors in Wrist, Hand, Ankle and Foot*,
https://doi.org/10.1007/978-981-99-6407-9_14

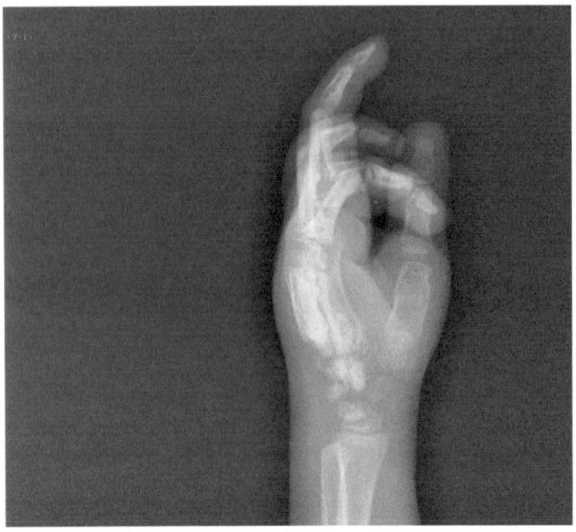

Fig. 14.3 Lateral view of the left hand

14.4 Description and Discussion from Residents

Flexion contracture was noted of right third and fourth fingers. There were cortical sclerosis and thickening of multiple bones. Mild expansile changes noted of third to fifth metacarpals with abnormal epiphysis, and multiple carpal bones showed ivory changes. Overall, multiple bone abnormalities in unilateral limb in a pediatric patient with sclerosis, melorheostosis is the top consideration. Differential diagnoses include osteopoikilosis, osteopetrosis, and chronic sclerosing osteomyelitis.

14.5 Analysis and Comments from Professor Cheng Xiao-Guang

The patient is a female child presented with contracture deformities of the left middle and fourth finger with cortical thickening of multiple bones and increased cortical densities and top consideration is congenital abnormalities.

14.6 Diagnosis

Melorheostosis.

Suggested Reading

Judkiewicz AM, Murphey MD, Resnik CS, et al. Advanced imaging of melorheostosis with emphasis on MRI. Skeletal Radiol. 2001;30(8):447–53.

Suresh S, Muthukumar T, Saifuddin A. Classical and unusual imaging appearances of melorheostosis. Clin Radiol. 2010;65(8):593–600.

15 Epithelioid Hemangioma of Bone: Case 15

15.1 Medical History

Patient is a 37-year-old male. He presented with a mass at the dorsal right wrist about 1 year ago without incentive. The mass was size of a bean, hard, nonmobile with mild point tenderness, and without redness or swelling. It was excised at local hospital about 9 months ago and the wound healed well. However, mass recured at dorsal right wrist about 5 months ago.

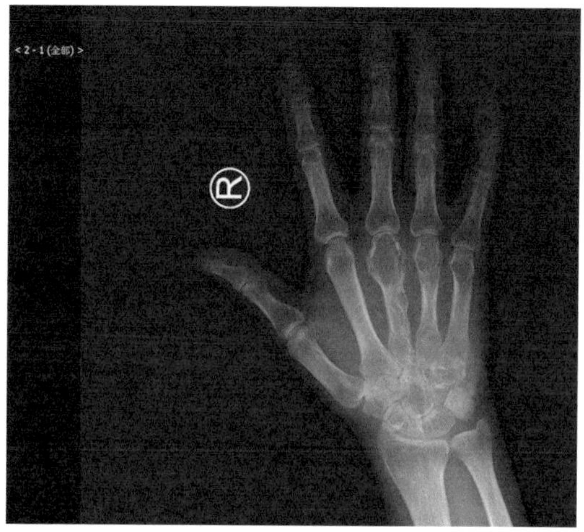

Fig. 15.1 Frontal view of the right hand

15.2 Physical Examination

The size of the mass was about 3 cm × 0.5 cm, hard, without point tenderness and no redness or swelling of surrounding skin.

15.3 Imaging Findings

15.3.1 Radiograph (Figs. 15.1 and 15.2)

Radiographs of the right hand demonstrated irregular shape of the third metacarpal with bony destruction at the head and ulnar side of the shaft. There was decreased bone densities of the fourth metacarpal, capitate, and hamate.

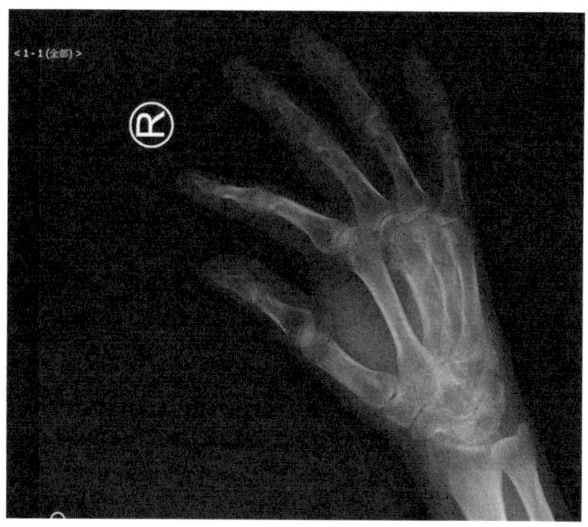

Fig. 15.2 Oblique view of the right hand

X. Cheng et al., *Imaging of Bone Tumors in Wrist, Hand, Ankle and Foot*,
https://doi.org/10.1007/978-981-99-6407-9_15

15.3.2 CT Imaging (Figs. 15.3, 15.4, 15.5, 15.6, 15.7, and 15.8)

CT images of the right hand demonstrated multiple areas of lytic changes of capitate, hamate and third, fourth metacarpals with cortical thinning and focal disruption. There was multiple area of bone destruction of the third metacarpal involving the cortex and medullary cavity with surrounding soft tissue swelling.

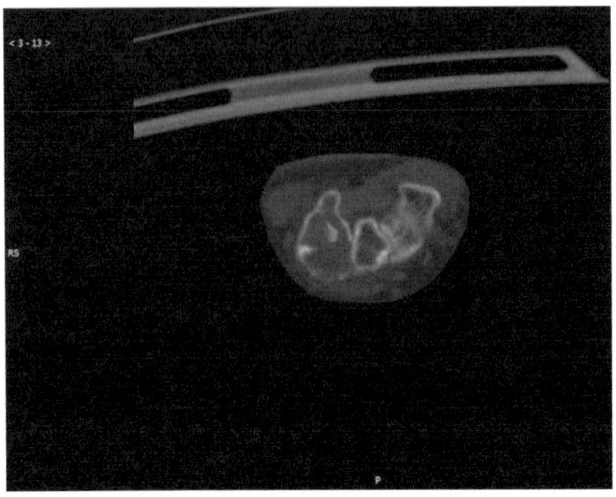

Fig. 15.3 Axial CT image of the right hand in bone window (wrist level)

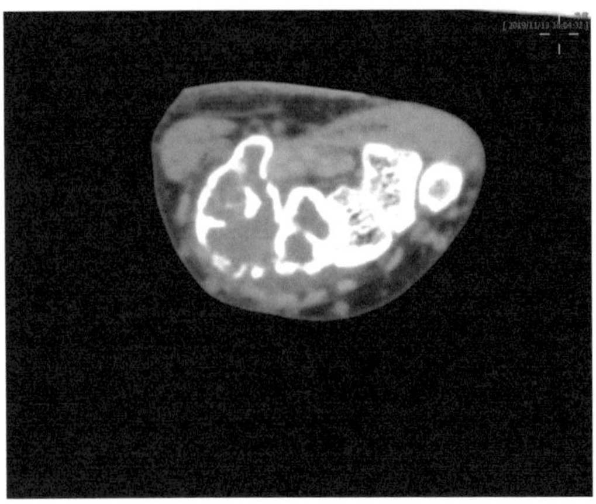

Fig. 15.4 Axial CT image of the right hand in soft tissue window (wrist level)

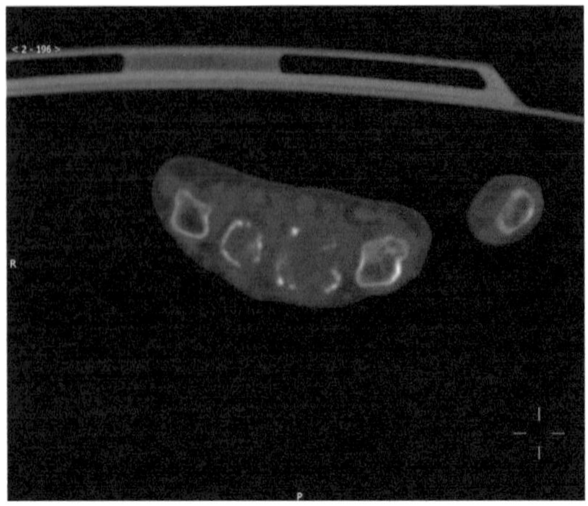

Fig. 15.5 Axial CT image of the right hand in bone window (metacarpal level)

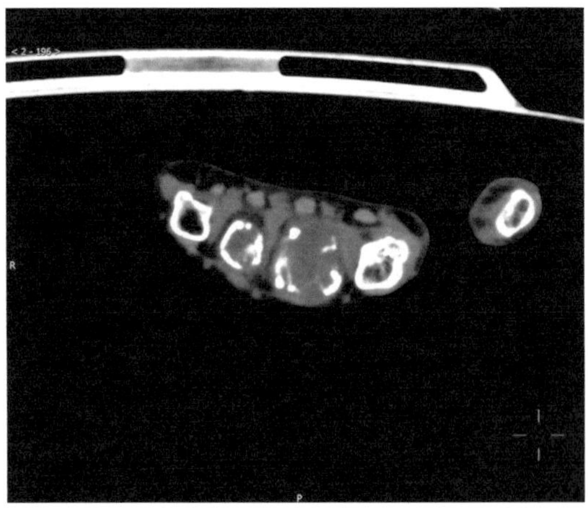

Fig. 15.6 Axial CT image of the right hand in soft tissue window (metacarpal level)

15.3.3 Description and Discussion from Residents

Radiographs demonstrated irregular shape of the right third metacarpal with expansile lytic changes at the head with irregular cortical thinning, and internal bone crest. There was heterogenous bone densities of the shaft and proximal

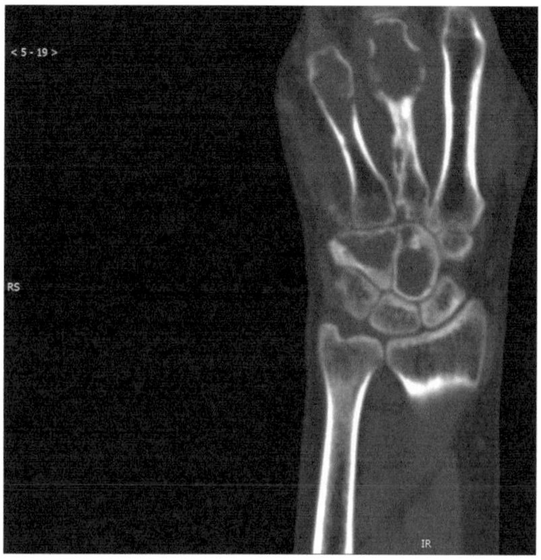

Fig. 15.7 Coronal CT image of the right hand in bone window

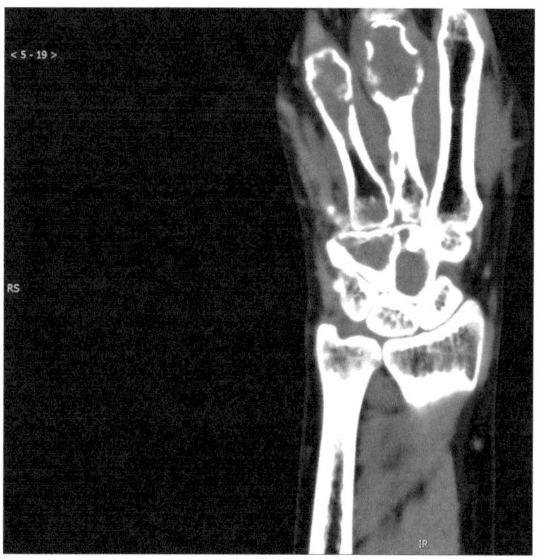

Fig. 15.8 Coronal CT image of the right hand in soft tissue window

third metacarpal. Bone destruction also noted at head, and shaft of the fourth metacarpal, capitate, hamate with decreased densities. CT images demonstrated cortical break of the above-described areas with soft tissue mass, suggesting aggressive nature of the lesion. Heterogenous densities noted in some foci with patchy high densities could be calcifications. Thus, our consideration is chondrogenic tumor, such as multiple enchondromas with hemangioma (Maffucci Syndrome). Differential diagnoses include giant cell tumor of the tendon sheath.

15.3.4 Analysis and Comments from Professor Cheng Xiao-Guang

The patient is a 37-year-old male with relative long history. Multiple bone destruction involving right third, fourth metacarpals, capitate, and hamate with irregular margin and decreased densities, but no joint involvement. Thus, we could exclude infection and consider neoplasms that can affect multiple bones with invasive imaging features. Given patient's age, first consideration is hematological tumor, such as lymphoma. There was osteopenia noted of this case, so brown tumors from hyperparathyroidism cannot be entirely excluded. The residents mentioned multiple enchondromas in the differential diagnoses, even though, this is a common lesion in the hand, the imaging findings are not consistent with the current case. Overall, there are difficulties on diagnose based on imaging alone, given extensive bone destruction, we favor malignancy.

15.3.5 Diagnosis

Epithelioid hemangioma of bone.

Suggested Reading

Fairfax A, Dey CB, Shaves S. Multifocal epithelioid hemangioma of the metacarpal bones: A case report. Radiol Case Rep. 2019;14(12):1467–1472.

Ramkumar S. Epithelioid haemangioma of bone: a case series and comprehensive literature review reappraising the diagnostic classification of all epithelioid vascular neoplasms of bone. Cureus. 2021;13(6):e15371.

16 Fibrous Dysplasia: Case 16

16.1 Medical History

Patient is a 43-year-old female. She presented with right hand swelling with periodic tingling pain about 5 years ago and followed by two resections with bone graft with recurrence of symptoms about 1 week ago.

16.2 Physical Examination

Not done.

16.3 Imaging Findings

16.3.1 Radiograph (Fig. 16.1 and 16.2)

Radiographs of the right thumb demonstrated ground glass like changes of the bones of the thumb with expansive deformity of the first metacarpal and decreased bone density of the trapezium.

16.3.2 CT Imaging (Figs. 16.3, 16.4, and 16.5)

CT images of the right thumb demonstrated heterogeneous densities of the first metacarpal and phalanges with focal ground glass changes. Expansile deformity was noted of the first metacarpal. Focal decreased densities were noted of base of the first metacarpal and trapezium with clear margin and peripheral sclerosis. No enhancement was seen.

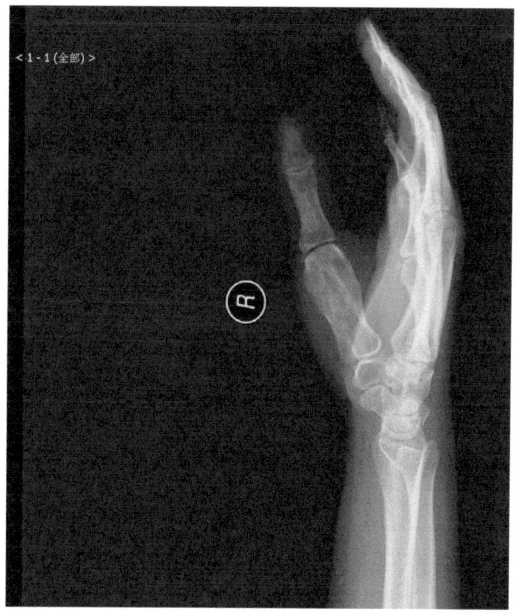

Fig. 16.1 Frontal view of the right thumb

X. Cheng et al., *Imaging of Bone Tumors in Wrist, Hand, Ankle and Foot*,
https://doi.org/10.1007/978-981-99-6407-9_16

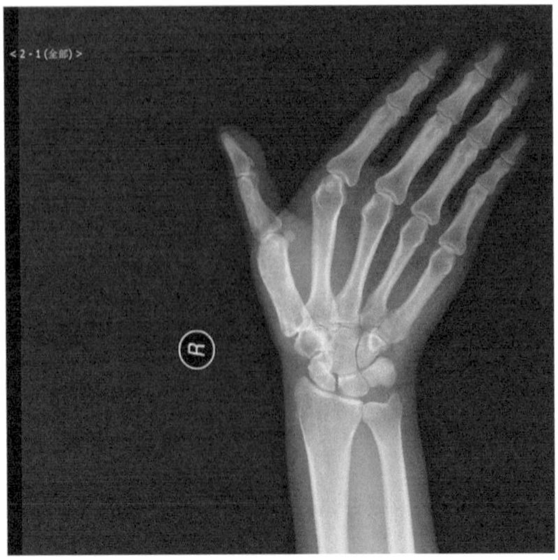

Fig. 16.2 Lateral view of the right thumb

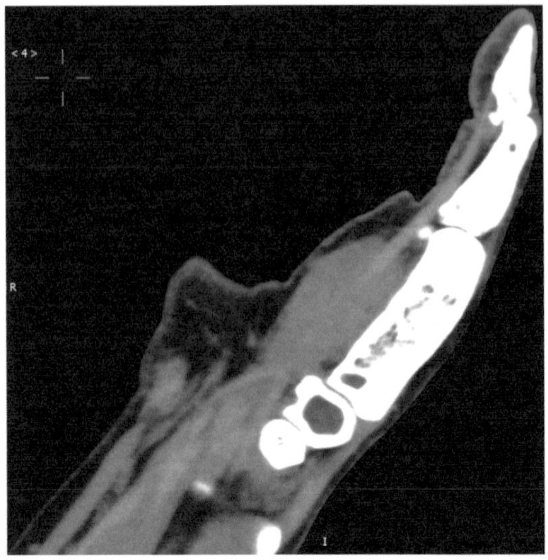

Fig. 16.4 Coronal CT image of the right thumb in soft tissue window

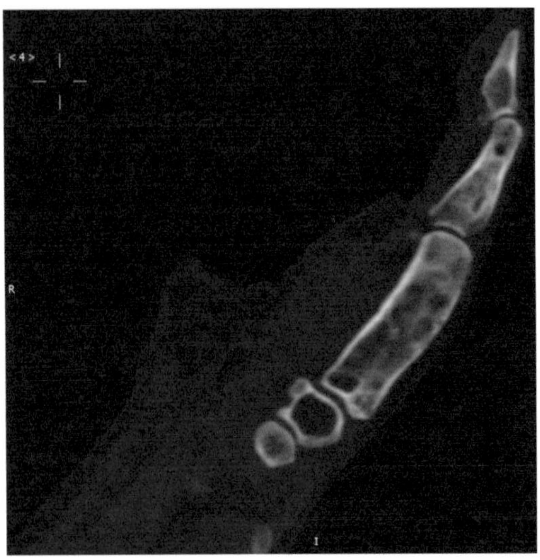

Fig. 16.3 Coronal CT image of the right thumb in bone window

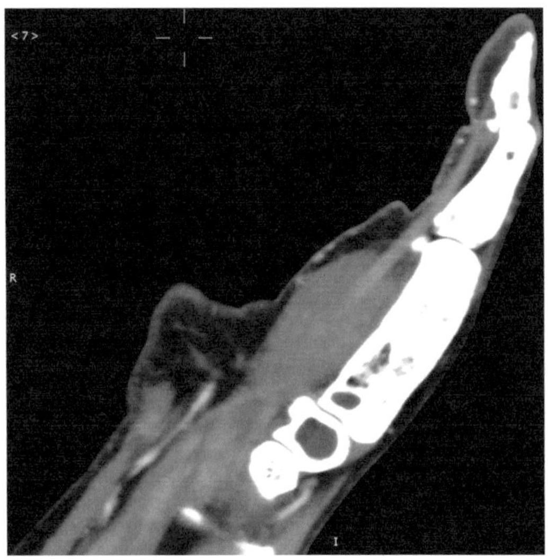

Fig. 16.5 Coronal post-contrast CT image of the right thumb in soft tissue window

16.4 Description and Discussion from Residents

There was expansile deformity of the right first metacarpal with geographic grand glass changes. Imaging evaluation was difficult, complicated by history of surgery. Our top consideration is fibrous dysplasia with Paget's disease in the differential diagnosis. Cystic changes noted at the base of the first metacarpal and most of trapezium, thus suggesting reactive arthropathy.

16.5 Analysis and Comments from Professor Cheng Xiao-Guang

Grand glass changes of right first metacarpal and phalanges with expansile deformity of the first metacarpal with narrowing of the medullary cavity and destruction of the trapezium with clear margin, indicating benign process that affects multiple bones and top consideration is fibrous dysplasia. Coarsening trabeculae and thickening of the cortex are usually seen with Paget's disease, not apparent bone destruction, not consistent with current case.

16.6 Diagnosis

Fibrous dysplasia.

Suggested Reading

Fitzpatrick KA, Taljanovic MS, Speer DP, et al. Imaging findings of fibrous dysplasia with histopathologic and intraoperative correlation. AJR Am J Roentgenol. 2004;182(6):1389–98.

Kinnunen AR, Sironen R, Sipola P. Magnetic resonance imaging characteristics in patients with histopathologically proven fibrous dysplasia-a systematic review. Skeletal Radiol. 2020;49(6):837–845.

Paget Disease: Case 17

17

17.1 Medical History

Patient is a 52-year-old female. She presented with lower back pain without clear causes about 3 years ago and had lumbar spine MRI with diagnose of disc herniation and symptoms improved with physical therapy. Symptoms returned and increased about half a year ago with neck, pelvis pain and soreness, not severe and self-described right shoulder drop and up tilting of the right pelvis.

17.2 Physical Examination

Not done.

17.3 Imaging Findings

17.3.1 Radiograph (Fig. 17.1)

Radiograph of both hands demonstrated bone mineral density decrease in both hands. Coarse trabeculae of right distal radius and focal decreased densities of the right second proximal phalanx were noted.

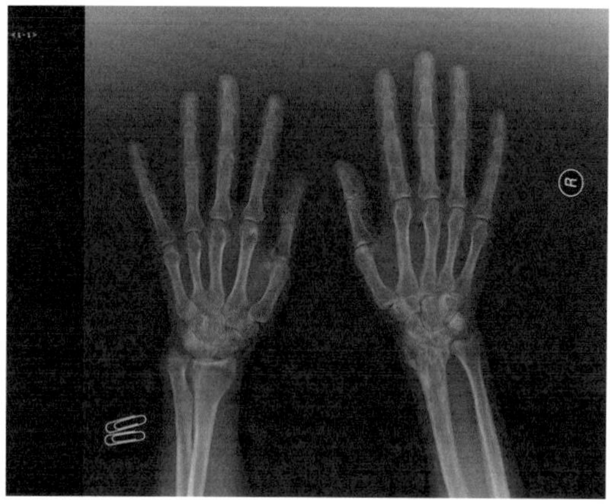

Fig. 17.1 Frontal view of both hands

17.4 Description and Discussion from Residents

There was osteopenia in both hands with cortical architectural distortion, coarsening of the trabeculae, irregular cortex, and no surrounding soft tissue mass. Cystic bony destructive changes with peripheral sclerosis noted around the right second proximal phalanx without soft tissue mass. Given patient's age and multiple bone involvement, we first consider metabolic bone disease,

X. Cheng et al., *Imaging of Bone Tumors in Wrist, Hand, Ankle and Foot*,
https://doi.org/10.1007/978-981-99-6407-9_17

such as hyperparathyroidism, Paget's disease. Bone destruction is the major finding with hyperparathyroidism, but there were destructive changes with productive, reparative, and remodeling process at the distal radius resulting in architectural distortion, not consistent with hyperparathyroidism. We favor Paget's disease as the diagnoses.

17.5 Analysis and Comments from Professor Cheng Xiao-Guang

The patient is a middle-aged female. The bone mineralization on radiograph is consistent with this age group and sex, not necessarily from reactive changes. Coarsening of the trabeculae with deformity of the right distal radius and bone destruction of the second proximal phalanx are noted. Given patient's history, first consideration is metabolic bone disease, such as Paget's disease. We can make the diagnoses with further imaging and combining with lab results. For example, we can see coarsening of the trabeculae with disorganization but preserved normal yellow marrow signal on MRI in stable phase of Paget's disease, characteristic of Paget's disease and can exclude neoplasm.

17.6 Diagnosis

Paget disease.

Suggested Reading

Lalam RK, Cassar-Pullicino VN, Winn N. Paget disease of bone. Semin Musculoskelet Radiol. 2016;20(3):287–299.

Theodorou DJ, Theodorou SJ, Kakitsubata Y, et al. Imaging of Paget disease of bone and its musculoskeletal complications: review. AJR Am J Roentgenol. 2011;196(6 Suppl):S64–75.

18 Rheumatoid Arthritis: Case 18

18.1 Medical History

Patient is a 43-year-old male. He presented with multiple arthralgia with morning stiffness for 6 years and worsened in the past 1 year.

18.2 Physical Examination

Not done.

18.3 Imaging Findings

18.3.1 Radiograph (Fig. 18.1)

Radiograph of both hands demonstrated multiple joint space narrowing of carpometacarpal, intercarpal, distal radioulnar joints. There are indistinct borders of the carpal bones, cystic changes noted at distal radius abutting the articular surface with peripheral sclerosis.

18.3.2 CT Imaging (Figs. 18.2 and 18.3)

CT images of the right wrist demonstrated multiple joint space narrowing, involving carpometacarpal, inter-carpal, and radiocarpal joints and multiple small cystic marginal erosions with

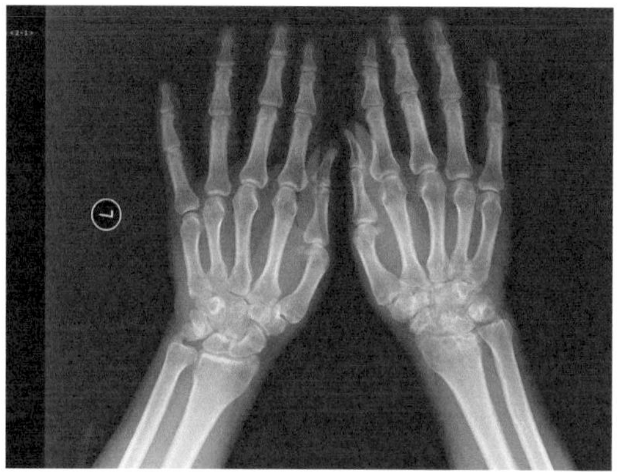

Fig. 18.1 Frontal view of both hands

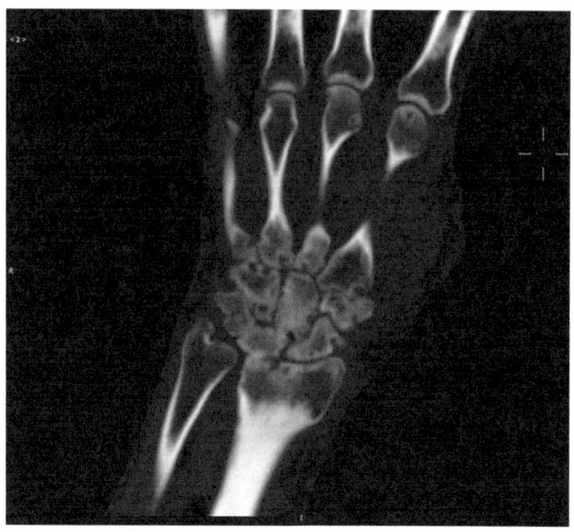

Fig. 18.2 Coronal CT image of the right wrist in bone window

X. Cheng et al., *Imaging of Bone Tumors in Wrist, Hand, Ankle and Foot*,
https://doi.org/10.1007/978-981-99-6407-9_18

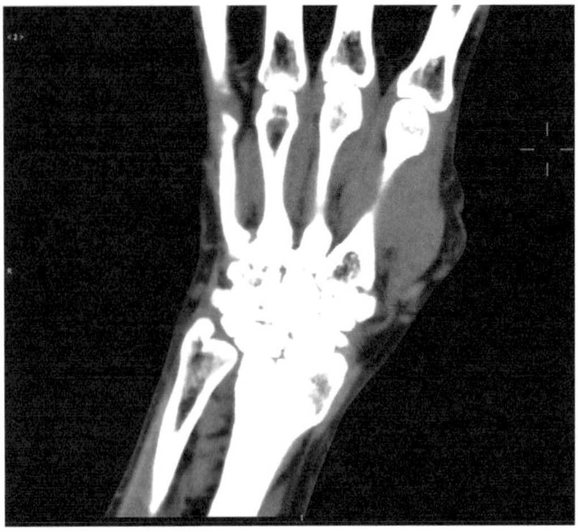

Fig. 18.3 Coronal CT image of the right wrist in soft tissue window

peripheral sclerosis. Small cystic changes were also noted of the second and third metacarpal heads.

18.3.3 MR Imaging(Figs. 18.4, 18.5, 18.6, and 18.7)

MR images of the right wrist demonstrated diffuse synovitis with erosions of multiple bones and extensive marrow edema.

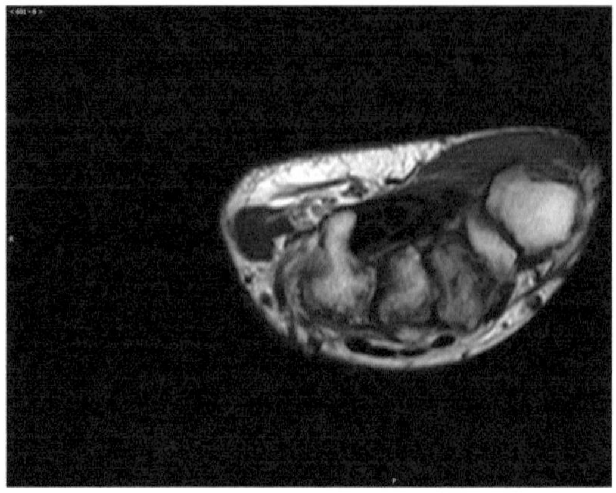

Fig. 18.4 Axial T1-weighted MR image of the right wrist

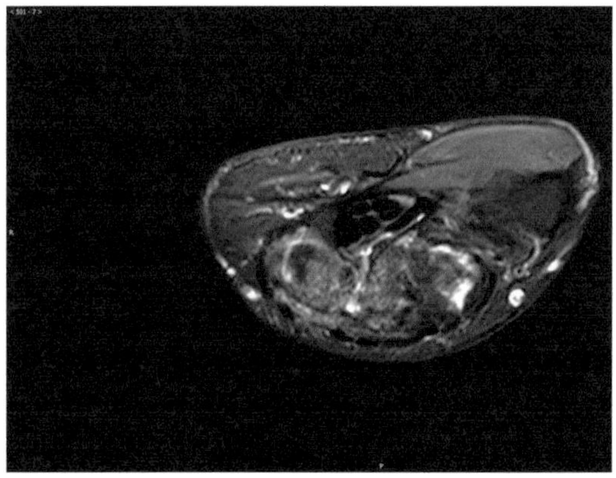

Fig. 18.5 Axial fat-suppressed proton density weighted MR image of the right wrist

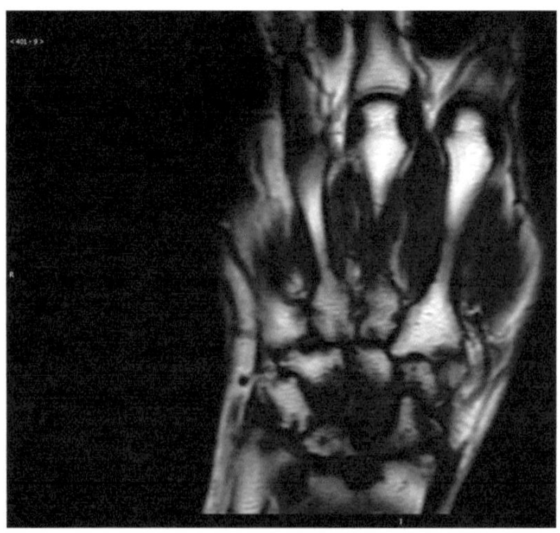

Fig. 18.6 Coronal T1-weighted MR image of the right wrist

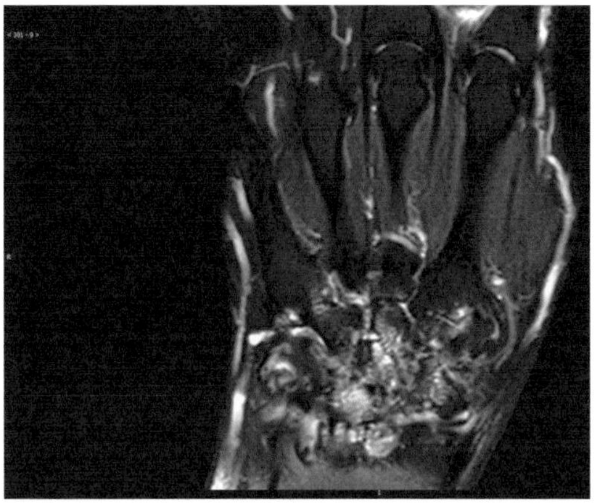

Fig. 18.7 Coronal fat-suppressed proton density weighted MR image of the right wrist

18.4 Description and Discussion from Residents

Radiograph and CT images both demonstrated diffuse osteopenia, joint space narrowing of the carpometacarpal, inter-carpal, and radiocarpal joints with multiple erosions along the articular surface with peripheral sclerosis. There were relatively preserved joint spaces of the interphalangeal and metacarpophalangeal joints. Diffuse synovitis with extensive marrow edema was seen on MR images. The clinical presentation and imaging findings are consistent with rheumatoid arthritis. However, patient is a middle-aged man with unilateral limb involvement, and reactive arthropathy needs to be excluded.

18.5 Analysis and Comments from Professor Cheng Xiao-Guang

The patient is a middle-aged male. No obvious osteopenia of both hands and the lesions focused on right wrist with synovitis, multiple small erosions along the carpal bones with peripheral sclerosis, joint space loss, irregularity, most suggestive of arthritis such as rheumatoid arthritis, TB, or gout. Bilateral symmetrical involvement with multiple joints involved is typical of rheumatoid arthritis with osteopenia. The current case is not typical for rheumatoid arthritis with unilateral involvement and combining lab results, clinical symptom and treatment information would be helpful.

18.6 Diagnosis

Rheumatoid arthritis.

Suggested Reading

Narváez JA, Narváez J, Lama ED, et al. MR imaging of early rheumatoid arthritis. Radiographics. 2010;30(1):143–63; discussion 163–5.

Sommer OJ, Kladosek A, Weiler V, et al. Rheumatoid arthritis: a practical guide to state-of-the-art imaging, image interpretation, and clinical implications. Radiographics. 2005;25(2):381–98.

19 Osteosarcoma: Case 19

19.1 Medical History

Patient is a 20-year-old male. He presented with left wrist pain with restricted range of motion for over 3 months. The pain was sharp and more intense in the morning and can be alleviated by rest. He is status post needle and open biopsy.

19.2 Physical Examination

Apparent swelling at the distal left forearm.

19.3 Imaging Findings

19.3.1 Radiograph (Figs. 19.1 and 19.2)

Radiographs of left hand demonstrated ivory like bone formation around distal radius with spiculated periosteal reaction and Codman's triangle.

19.3.2 CT Imaging (Figs. 19.3, 19.4, 19.5, 19.6, and 19.7)

CT images of the left wrist demonstrated ivory like bone formation at distal radius with spiculated periosteal reaction and associated soft tissue mass with predominant bone matrix.

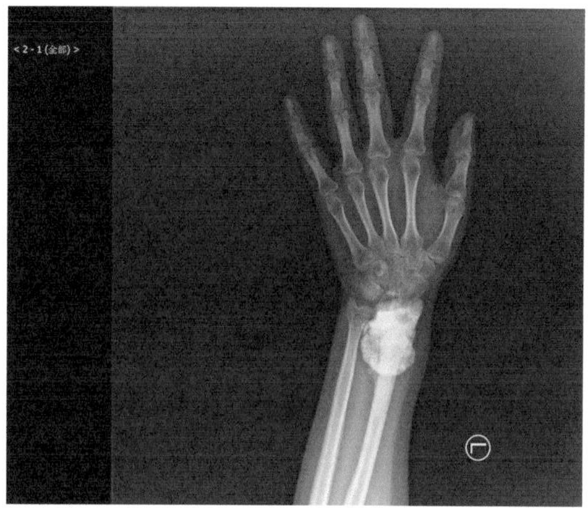

Fig. 19.1 Frontal view of left hand

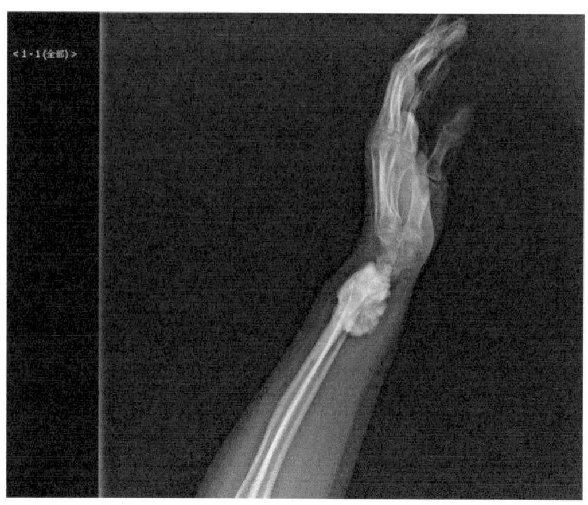

Fig. 19.2 Lateral view of left hand

X. Cheng et al., *Imaging of Bone Tumors in Wrist, Hand, Ankle and Foot*,
https://doi.org/10.1007/978-981-99-6407-9_19

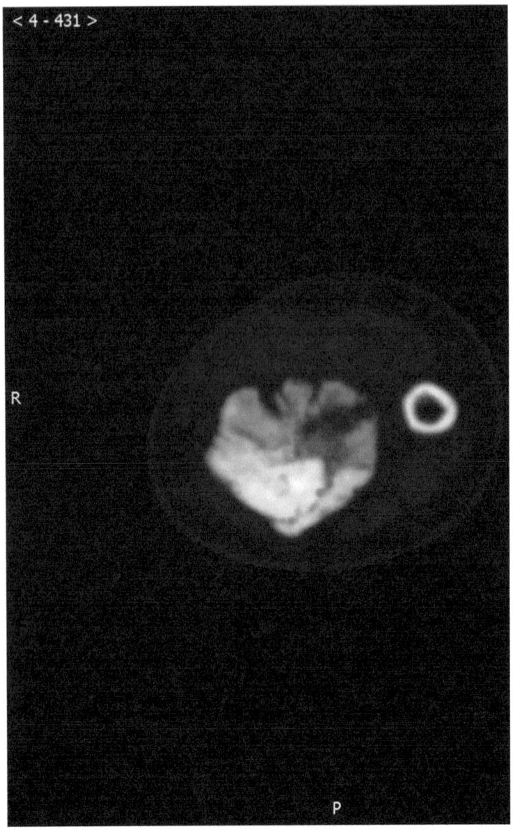

Fig. 19.3 Axial CT image of the left wrist in bone window

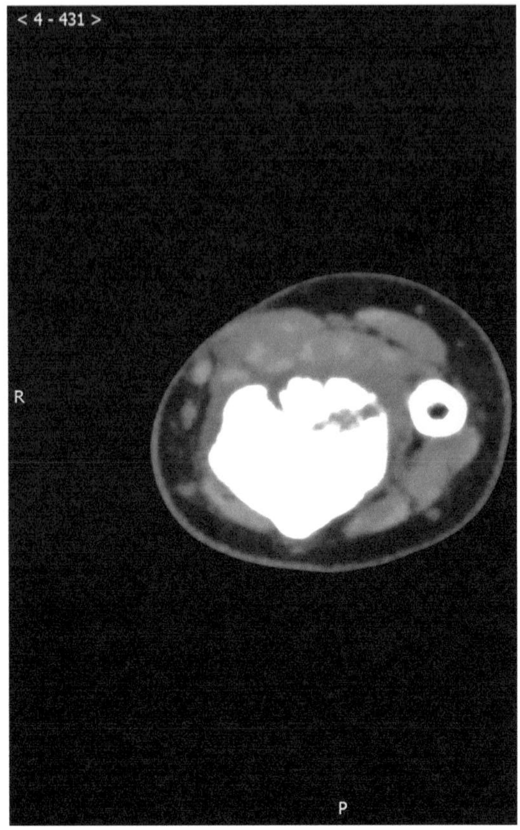

Fig. 19.4 Axial CT image of the left wrist in soft tissue window

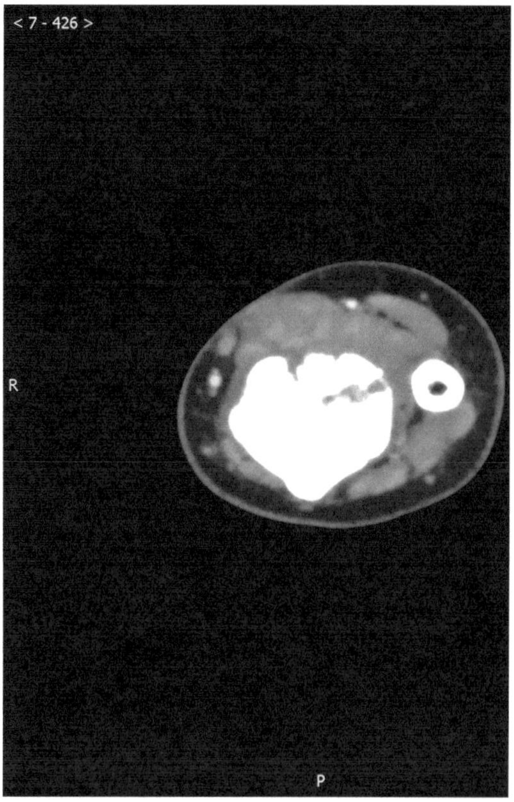

Fig. 19.5 Axial post-contrast CT image of the left wrist in soft tissue window

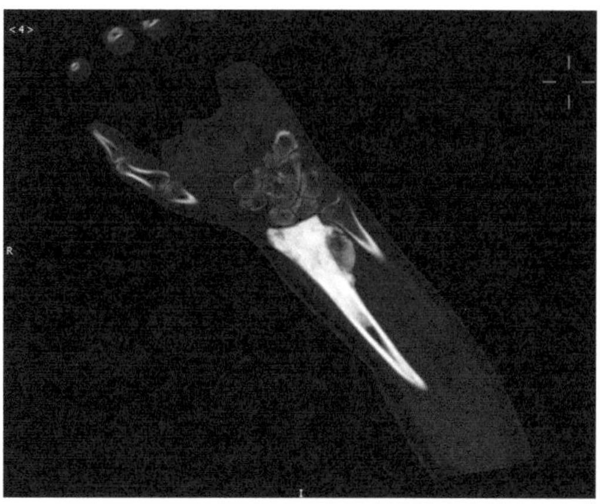

Fig. 19.6 Coronal CT image of the left wrist in bone window

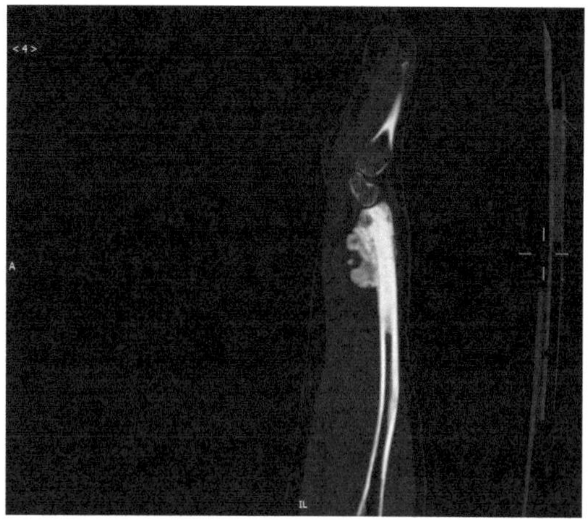

Fig. 19.7 Sagittal CT image of the left wrist in bone window

19.3.3 MR Imaging (Figs. 19.8, 19.9, 19.10, 19.11, 19.12, and 19.13)

MR images of the left wrist demonstrated heterogeneous low signal on all sequences at distal left radius with soft tissue mass. Enhancement was noted in portion of the mass on a background of diffuse soft tissue swelling.

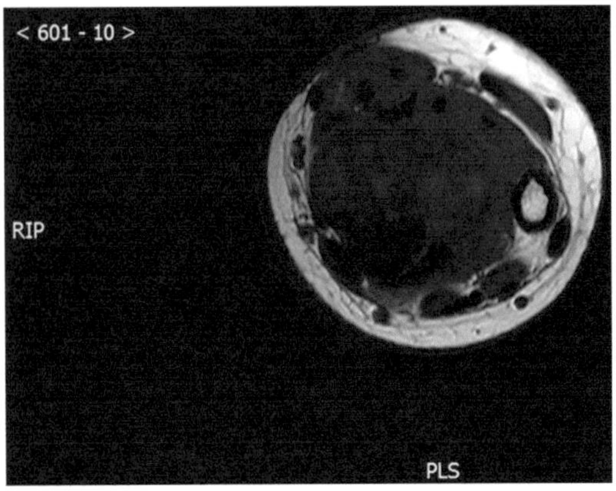

Fig. 19.8 Axial T1-weighted MR image of the left wrist

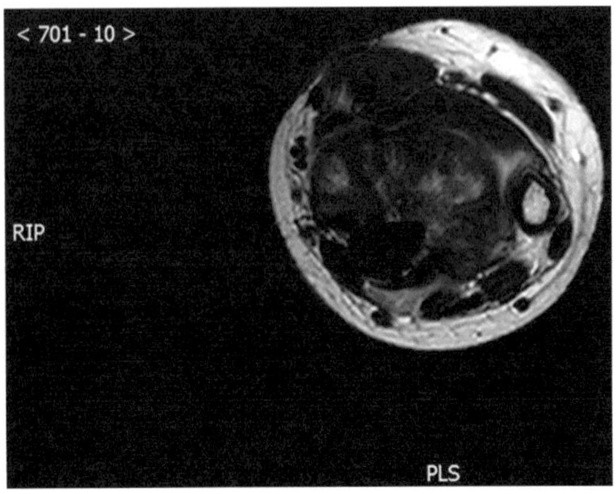

Fig. 19.9 Axial T2-weighted MR image of the left wrist

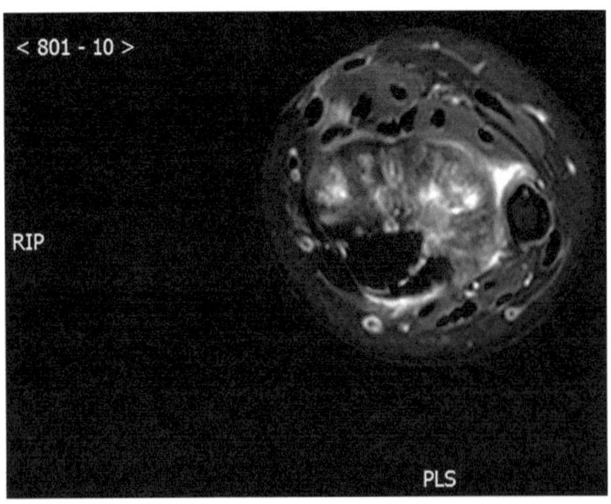

Fig. 19.10 Axial fat-suppressed T2-weighted MR image of the left wrist

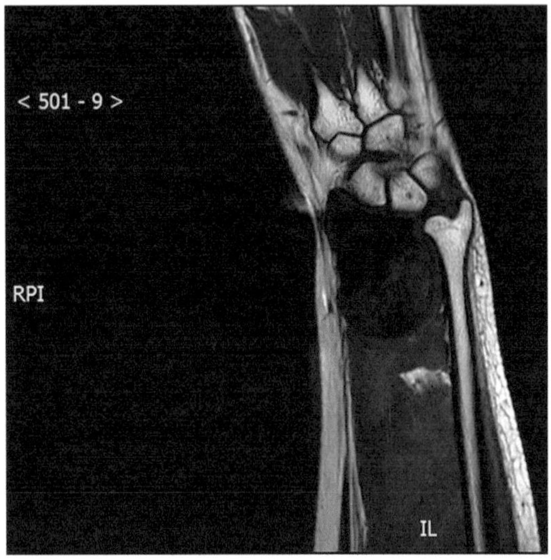

Fig. 19.11 Coronal T1-weighted MR image of the left wrist

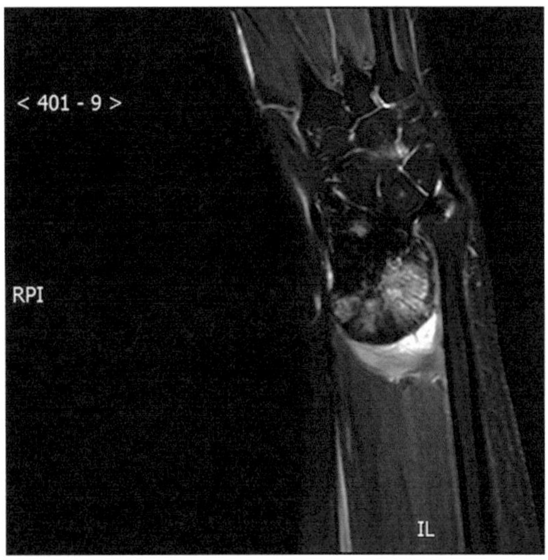

Fig. 19.12 Coronal fat-suppressed T2-weighted MR image of the left wrist

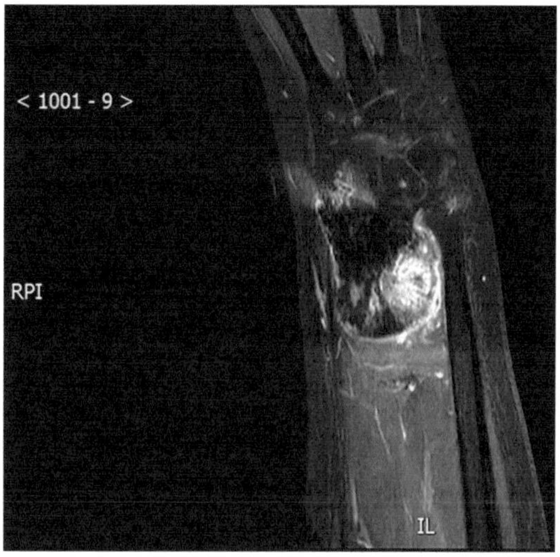

Fig. 19.13 Coronal post-contrast fat-suppressed T1-weighted MR image of the left wrist

19.4 Description and Discussion from Residents

There was tumoral bone formation at distal radius with disappearance of the normal intramedullary cavity and no apparent lytic change. Needle-like radiating periosteal reaction was present. No avid enhancement was seen on CT images. Surrounding soft tissue with high fluid signal is noted on MR images, indicating congestive and edematous reaction. Overall, our consideration is sclerosing osteosarcoma.

19.5 Analysis and Comments from Professor Cheng Xiao-Guang

The patient is a young male in his twenties. Osteogenic changes, noted at left distal radius with invasion into the medullary cavity, are characteristic of osteosarcoma on imaging. High T2 signal was noted on fat-suppressed T2-weighted sequence on MR images of the lesion, suggesting the presence of chondroid matrix.

19.6 Diagnosis

Osteosarcoma.

Suggested Reading

Murphey MD, Robbin MR, McRae GA, et al. The many faces of osteosarcoma. Radiographics. 1997;17(5):1205–31.

Yarmish G, Klein MJ, Landa J, et al. Imaging characteristics of primary osteosarcoma: nonconventional subtypes. Radiographics. 2010;30(6):1653–72.

20 Loose Bodies After Wrist Injury: Case 20

20.1 Medical History

Patient is a 37-year-old male. He fell with outstretched right hand on the ground about 3 months ago while working. The right wrist pain subsided without treatment. However, he started to experience increasing right wrist pain about 2 months ago.

20.2 Physical Examination

There is mild swelling about the right wrist, more in the ulnar aspect. Point tenderness elicited around the scapholunate interval, triangular fibrocartilage complex (TFCC), and proximal extensor tendons around the right wrist. There is preserved flexion and dorsiflexion of the right wrist with positive ulnar wrist pressure test.

20.3 Imaging Findings

20.3.1 Radiograph (Figs. 20.1 and 20.2)

Radiographs of right wrist demonstrated multiple loose nodular bone densities around the distal ulnar.

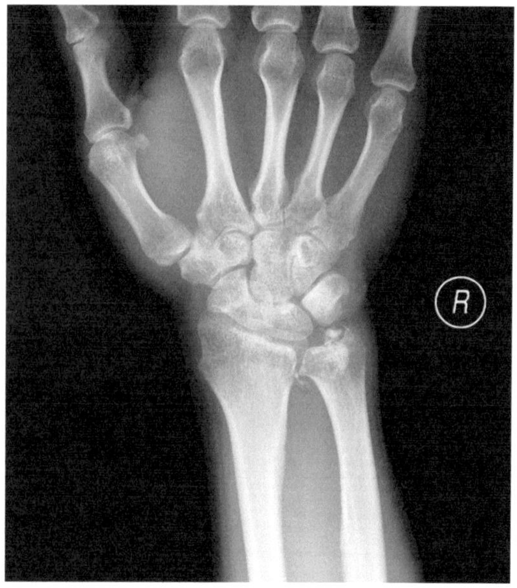

Fig. 20.1 Frontal view of right wrist

20.3.2 CT Imaging (Figs. 20.3, 20.4, 20.5, and 20.6)

CT images of the right wrist demonstrated multiple loose bone densities at the distal ulna in the surrounding soft tissues with irregular shapes.

X. Cheng et al., *Imaging of Bone Tumors in Wrist, Hand, Ankle and Foot*,
https://doi.org/10.1007/978-981-99-6407-9_20

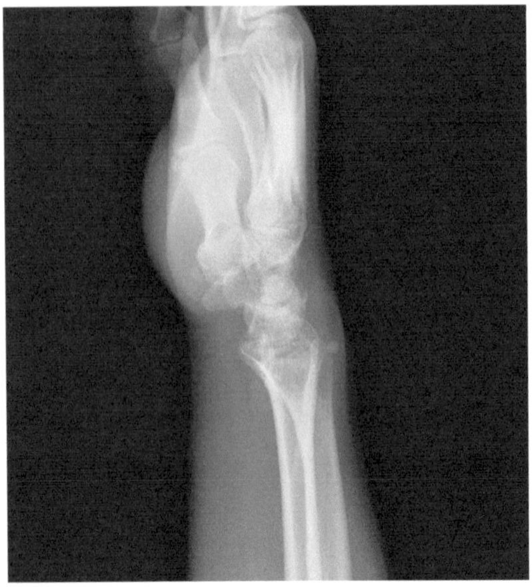

Fig. 20.2 Lateral view of right wrist

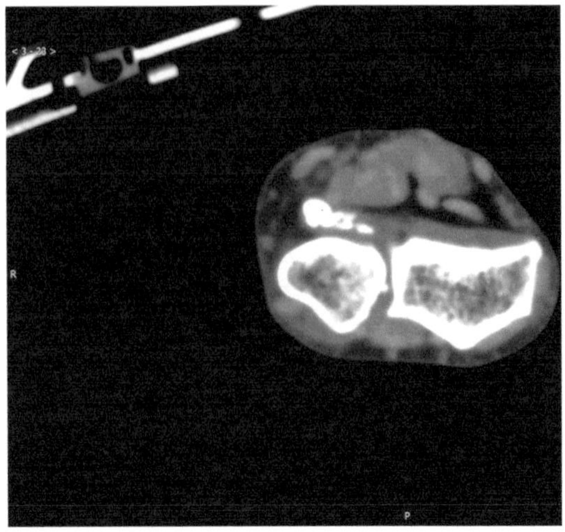

Fig. 20.4 Axial CT image of the right wrist in soft tissue window

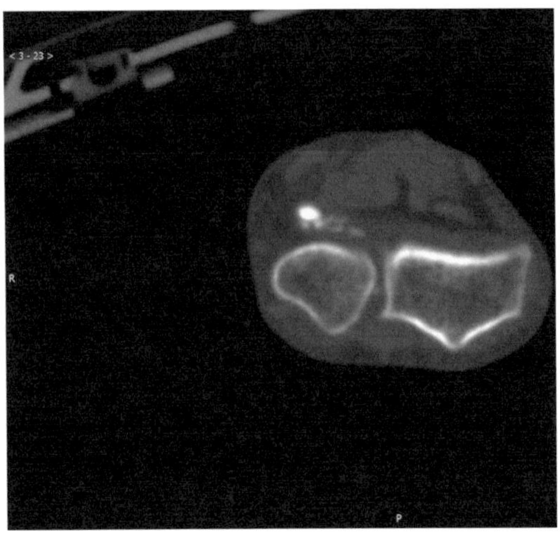

Fig. 20.3 Axial CT image of the right wrist in bone window

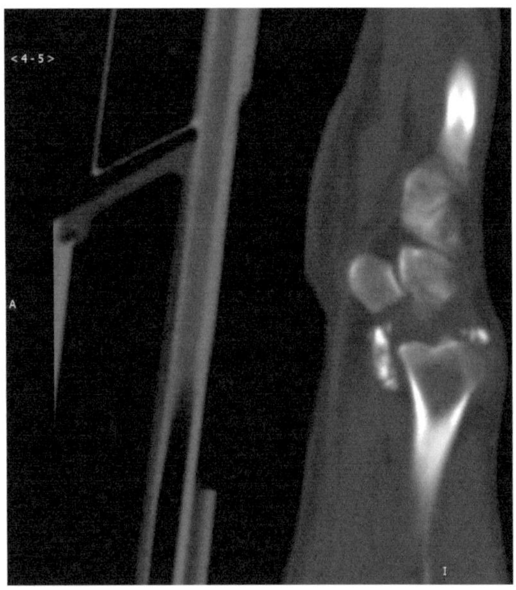

Fig. 20.5 Sagittal CT image of the right wrist in bone window

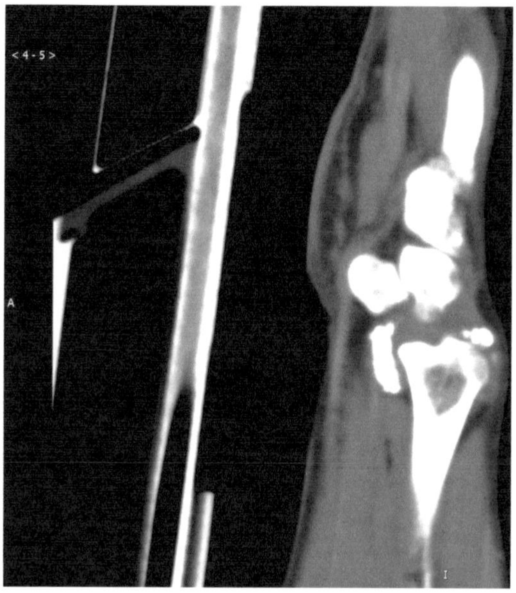

Fig. 20.6 Sagittal CT image of the right wrist in soft tissue window

20.4 Description and Discussion from Residents

There are multiple loose bone densities around the distal ulna in the surrounding soft tissues and no other abnormalities noted. Given patient's history of trauma, our top consideration is sequela of prior osteochondral injury with hemorrhage leading to heterotopic ossifications. Synovial osteochondromatosis is in the differential diagnosis, however, there is no association with history of injury for this entity and the ossifications commonly seen with synovial osteochondromatosis tend to be relatively more in number with rather uniformed size.

20.5 Analysis and Comments from Professor Cheng Xiao-Guang

Given multiple loose bone densities around the right distal ulna with intact underlying osseous structures, the differential diagnosis includes synovial osteochondromatosis, crystal deposition disorder. However, there is no other specific findings to narrow down the diagnosis, just manifestation of intra-articular bodies.

20.6 Diagnosis

Loose bodies after wrist injury.

Suggested Reading

Koh S, Nakamura R, Horii E, et al. Loose body in the wrist: diagnosis and treatment. Arthroscopy. 2003;19(8):820–4.

Woon CYL, Phoon ES, Lee JYL, et al. Rice bodies, millet seeds, and melon seeds in tuberculous tenosynovitis of the hand and wrist. Ann Plast Surg. 2011;66(6):610–7.

21 Tuberculous Dactylitis: Case 21

21.1 Medical History

Patient is a 15-year-old male. He presented with swelling and pain of the left ring finger at the outpatient clinic.

21.2 Physical Examination

Not done.

21.3 Imaging Findings

21.3.1 Radiograph (Figs. 21.1 and 21.2)

Radiographs of the left hand demonstrated osseous destructive changes of the proximal fourth phalanx with relative continuous periosteal reaction and adjacent soft tissue swelling.

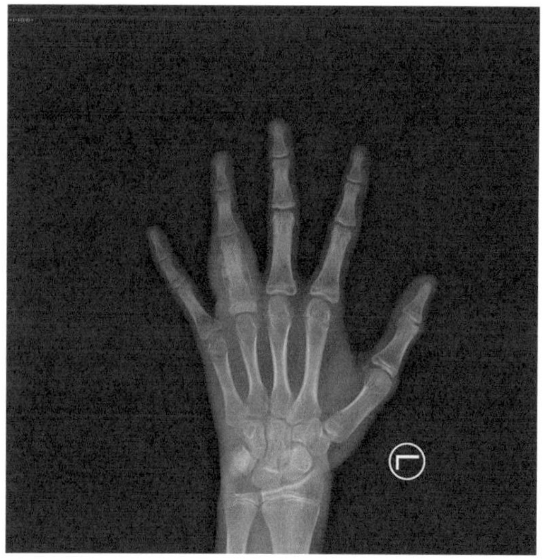

Fig. 21.1 Frontal view of the left hand

21.3.2 CT Imaging (Figs. 21.3, 21.4, 21.5, 21.6, 21.7, 21.8, and 21.9)

CT images of the left hand demonstrated cortical destruction with irregular margin of the left fourth proximal phalanx with extensive layering periosteal reaction and apparent adjacent soft tissue swelling. Majority of the lesion demonstrated avid enhancement with irregular margin and internal small foci of non-enhancement. Chest CT images showed opacities in the left upper lobe with lymphadenopathy in the mediastinum.

X. Cheng et al., *Imaging of Bone Tumors in Wrist, Hand, Ankle and Foot*,
https://doi.org/10.1007/978-981-99-6407-9_21

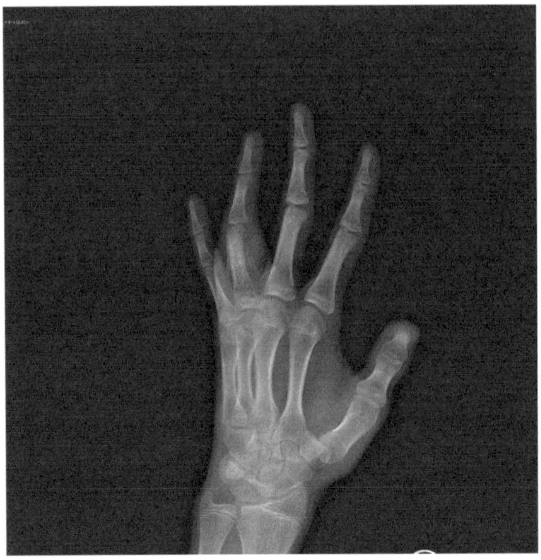

Fig. 21.2 Oblique view of the left hand

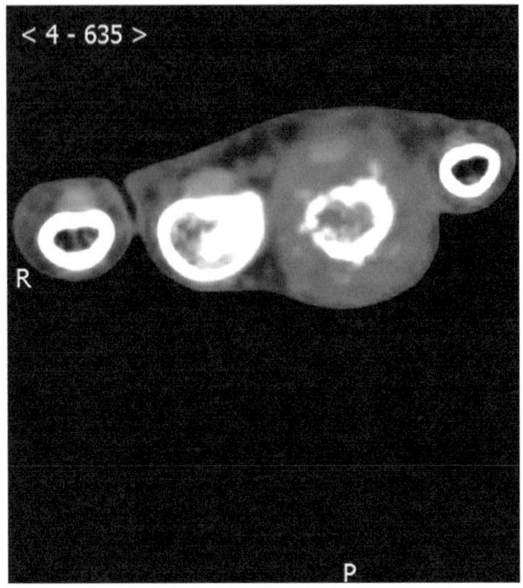

Fig. 21.4 Axial CT image of the left hand in soft tissue window

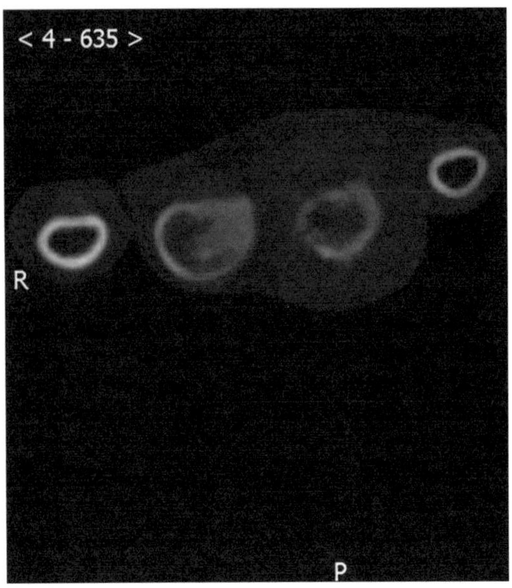

Fig. 21.3 Axial CT image of the left hand in bone window

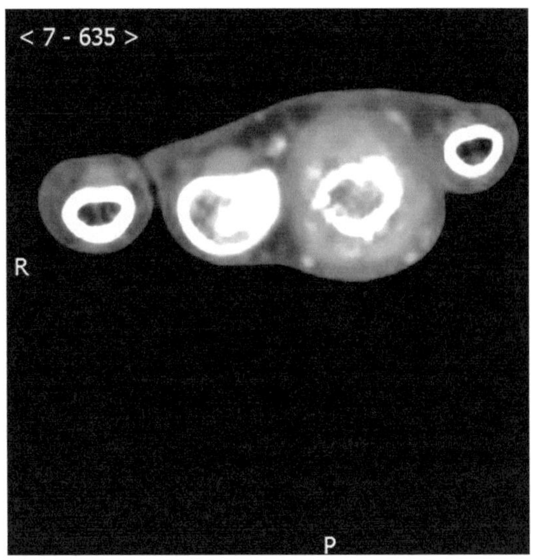

Fig. 21.5 Axial post-contrast CT image of the left hand in soft tissue window

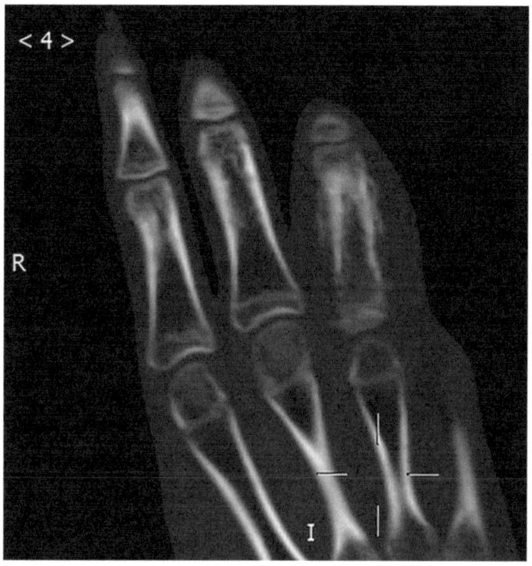

Fig. 21.6 Coronal CT image of the left hand in bone window

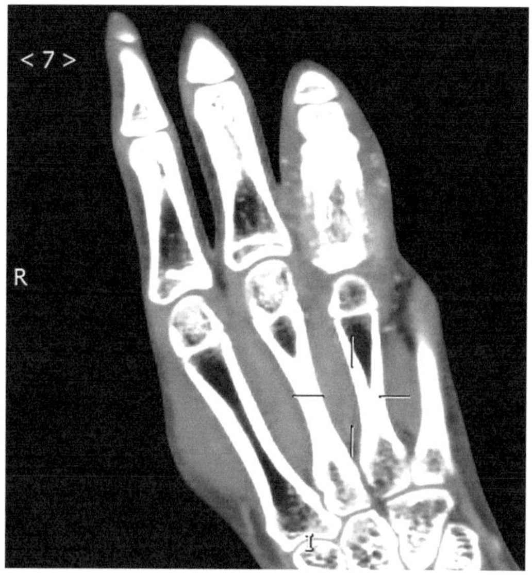

Fig. 21.8 Coronal post-contrast CT image of the left hand in soft tissue window

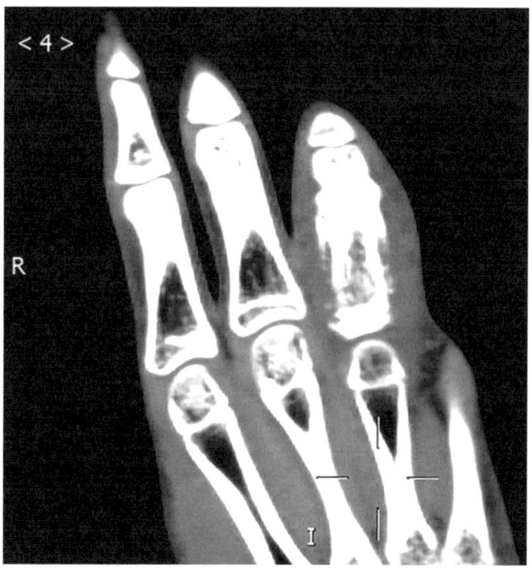

Fig. 21.7 Coronal CT image of the left hand in soft tissue window

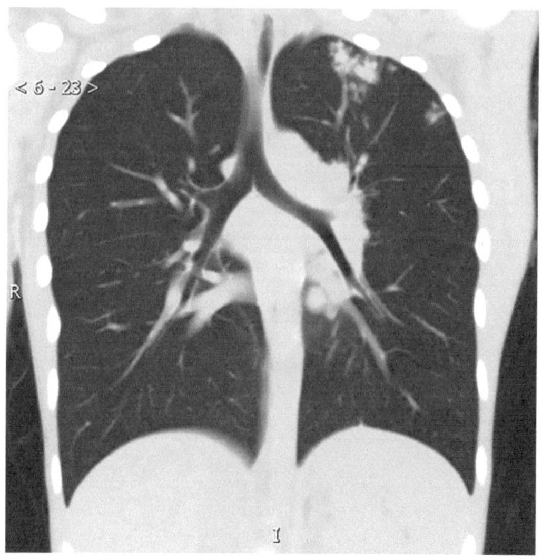

Fig. 21.9 Coronal chest CT image in lung window (additional scan obtained later)

21.4 Description and Discussion from Residents

Bone destruction observed of the left fourth proximal phalanx with focal permeative cortical destruction and periosteal reaction with soft tissue swelling. Avid enhancement is noted of the soft tissues. Our top consideration is malignant tumor, such as Ewing sarcoma.

21.5 Analysis and Comments from Professor Cheng Xiao-Guang

Radiographs demonstrated that bone destruction around the fourth proximal phalanx mainly affects the diaphysis with periosteal reaction and soft tissue swelling. These findings in young adolescent patients are commonly seen with Ewing sarcoma or infection. CT images demonstrated apparent soft tissue swelling including the flexor tendon with focal discontinuous periosteal reaction and majority avid enhancement of the lesion. The above constellation of findings again point to Ewing sarcoma or infection. However, there is normal marrow in the affected region, not consistent with Ewing sarcoma and infection cannot be excluded. Chest CT obtained later showed patchy and linear opacities in the left upper lobe, suspicious for tuberculosis. Thus, the lesion in the phalanx is most likely related to tuberculosis. Overall, this case is not typical of tuberculous dactylitis (spina ventosa), but there are features of infection, such as soft tissue sausage-like swelling, involvement of the flexor tendon and normal marrow.

21.6 Diagnosis

Tuberculous dactylitis.

Suggested Reading

Sahli H, Roueched L, Sbai MA, et al. The epidemiology of tuberculous dactylitis: A case report and review of literature. Int J Mycobacteriol. 2017;6(4):333–335.

Saibaba B, Gopinathan NR, Santhanam SS, et al. Tubercular dactylitis in children. J Pediatr Orthop B. 2017;26(3):261–265.

Infection: Case 22

22

22.1 Medical History

Patient is a 29-year-old male. He was injured about fourth month ago with right scaphoid fracture and lunate dislocation and treated at local hospital with surgery.

22.2 Physical Examination

There is stiffness of right wrist with focal skin scar and contracture, and no flexion or dorsiflexion. Right fourth finger and fifth fingers demonstrated restricted flexion.

22.3 Imaging Findings

22.3.1 Radiograph (Figs. 22.1 and 22.2)

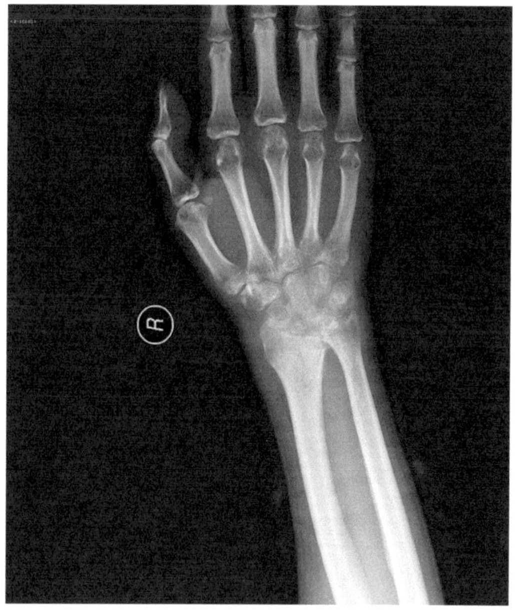

Fig. 22.1 Frontal view of the right wrist

Radiographs of the right wrist demonstrated diffuse decreased bone densities of the right carpal bones with generalized mal-alignment and decreased inter-carpal joint spaces.

22.3.2 CT Imaging (Figs. 22.3, 22.4, 22.5, 22.6, 22.7, and 22.8)

CT images of the right wrist demonstrated destruction along the articular surface of multiple carpal bones with focal sclerosis and decreased joint spaces. No normal lunate was seen with focal sand-like high densities in the region noted.

X. Cheng et al., *Imaging of Bone Tumors in Wrist, Hand, Ankle and Foot*,
https://doi.org/10.1007/978-981-99-6407-9_22

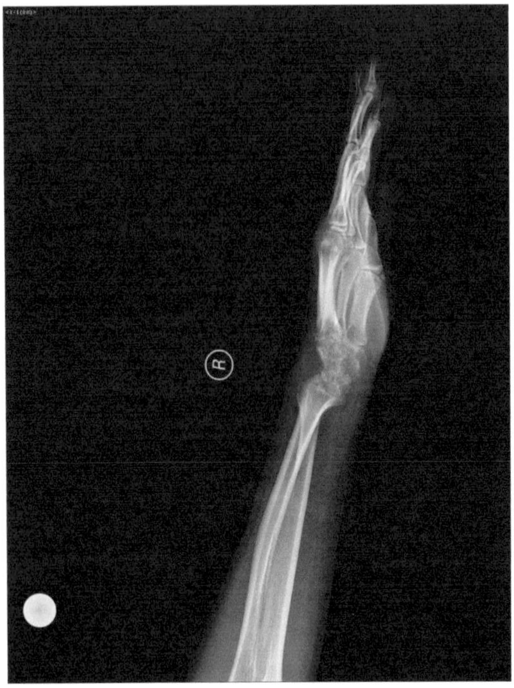

Fig. 22.2 Lateral view of the right wrist

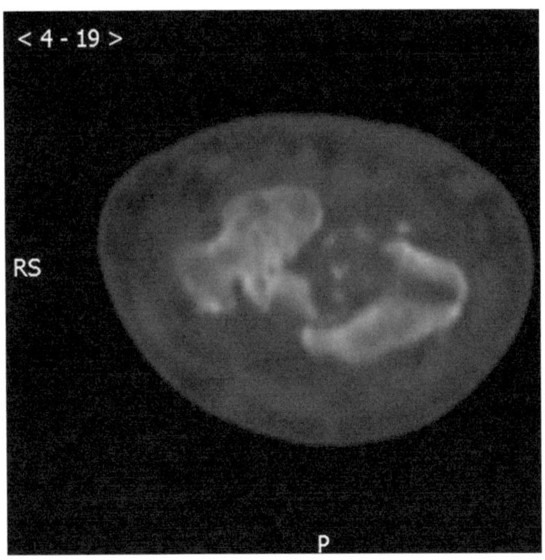

Fig. 22.3 Axial CT image of the right wrist in bone window

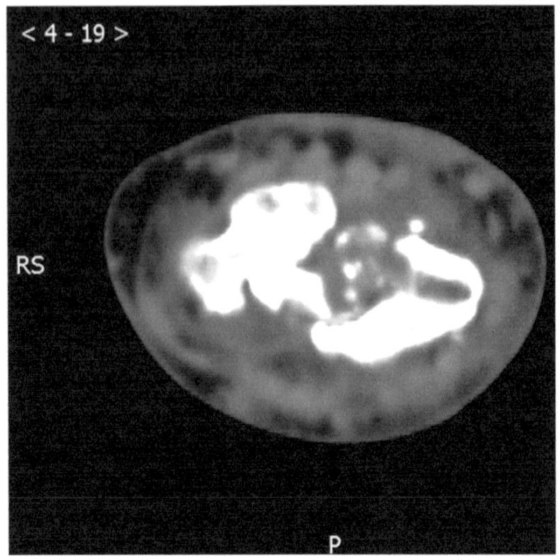

Fig. 22.4 Axial CT image of the right wrist in soft tissue window

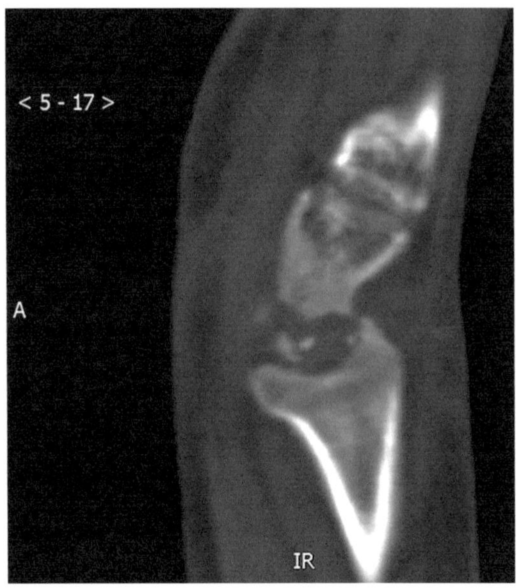

Fig. 22.5 Sagittal CT image of the right wrist in bone window

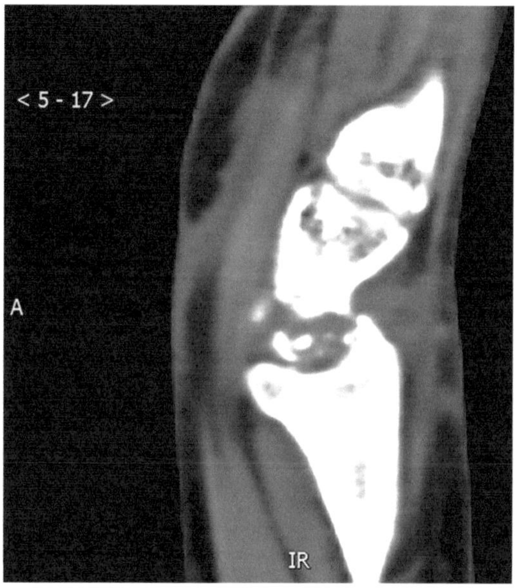

Fig. 22.6 Sagittal CT image of the right wrist in soft tissue window

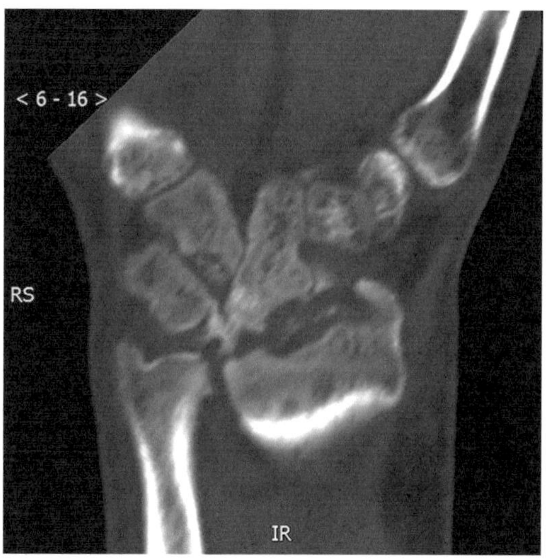

Fig. 22.7 Coronal CT image of the right wrist in bone window

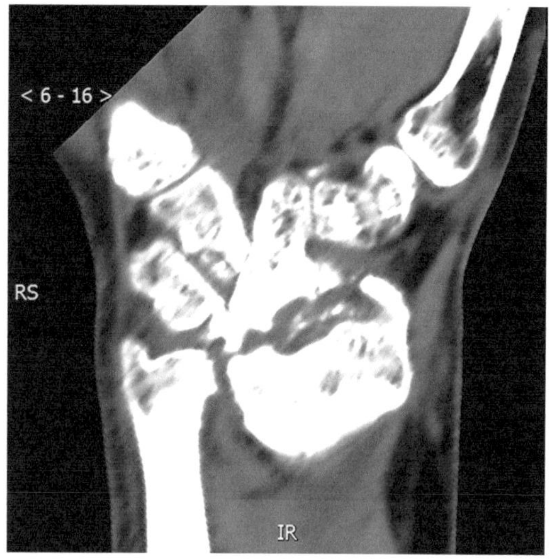

Fig. 22.8 Coronal CT image of the right wrist in soft tissue window

22.4 Description and Discussion from Residents

The radiographs demonstrated mal-alignment of the right carpal bones with abnormal lunate. There is decreased radial inclination, likely with scaphoid and lunate articular surface collapse after trauma. However, there is diffuse osteopenia of the right wrist with decreased joint spaces, raising concern for superimposed infection, such as tuberculosis. CT images demonstrated articular surface erosions of the distal radioulnar and radiocarpal joints and several smaller joints with bony ankylosis of several carpal bones and sand-like high densities in the joint space (could be sequestrum) and synovial hypertrophy on the soft tissue windows with soft tissue swelling, most suggestive of infectious etiology, such as tuberculosis.

22.5 Analysis and Comments from Professor Cheng Xiao-Guang

The patient presented with long medical history and clear history of trauma. Scaphoid and lunate were not well seen on the radiographs with indistinct and narrowed joint spaces of the distal radioulnar and inter-carpal joints. Sand-like high densities were noted on the CT images in the joint spaces. Overall, there were destructions of multiple bones with suggestion of sequestrum formation and joint space narrowing, all suggestive of infection and tuberculosis is the top consideration. However, osteopenia is commonly seen with tuberculosis, not typical in the current case.

22.6 Diagnosis

Infection.

Suggested Reading

Hsu CY, Lu HC, Shih TTF. Tuberculous infection of the wrist: MRI features. AJR Am J Roentgenol. 2004;183(3):623–8.

Jennings JD, Ilyas AM. Septic arthritis of the wrist. J Am Acad Orthop Surg. 2018;26(4):109–115.

Tenosynovial Giant Cell Tumor: Case 23

23

23.1 Medical History

Patient is a 38-year-old male. He presented with mass around his left wrist about 7 years ago. The mass was resected at a local hospital with pathology as giant cell tumor of bone. He is about 2 years postoperative and mass reappeared around the surgical bed and enlarging.

23.2 Physical Examination

Not done.

23.3 Imaging Findings

23.3.1 Radiograph (Figs. 23.1 and 23.2)

Radiographs of the left hand demonstrated soft tissue protuberance around the dorsum of the left wrist, and cystic changes around the scaphoid, capitate, and triquetrum.

23.3.1.1 CT Imaging (Figs. 23.3, 23.4, 23.5, 23.6, 23.7, and 23.8)

CT images of the left wrist demonstrated dorsal soft tissue mass with compression and invasion to multiple carpal bones. Avid enhancement is noted.

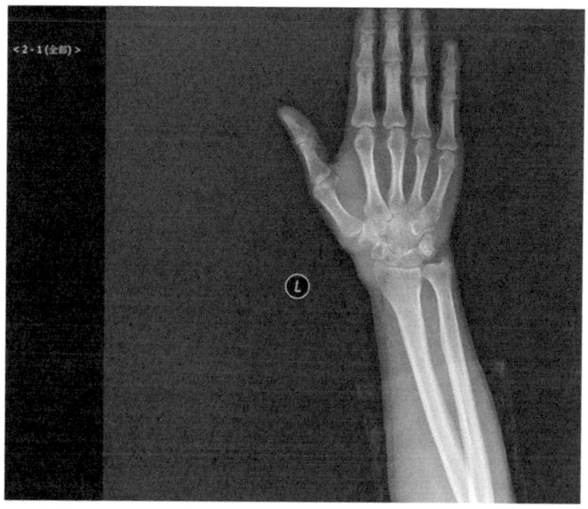

Fig. 23.1 Frontal view of the left hand

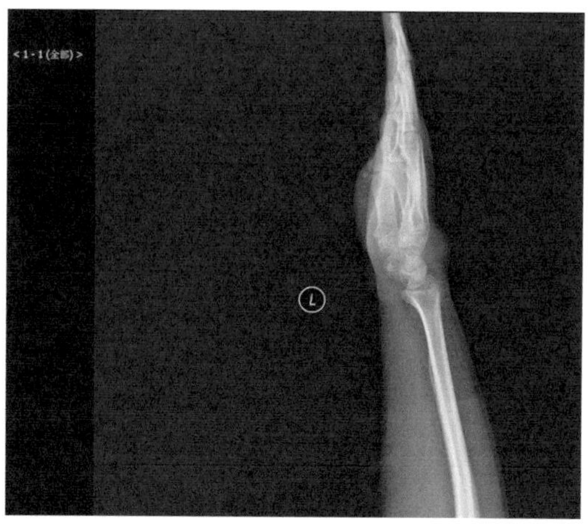

Fig. 23.2 Lateral view of the left hand

X. Cheng et al., *Imaging of Bone Tumors in Wrist, Hand, Ankle and Foot*,
https://doi.org/10.1007/978-981-99-6407-9_23

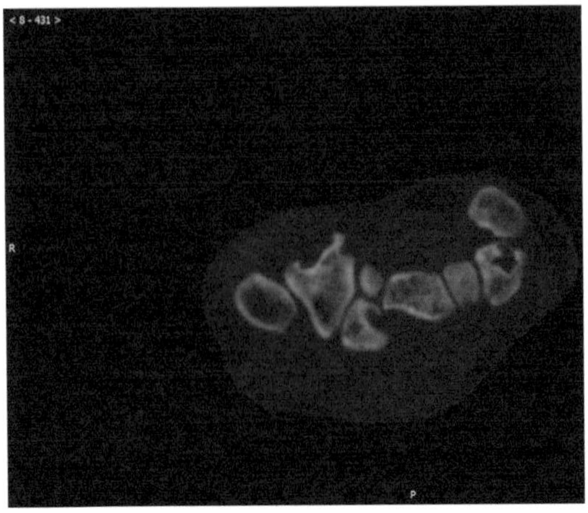

Fig. 23.3 Axial CT image of the left wrist in bone window

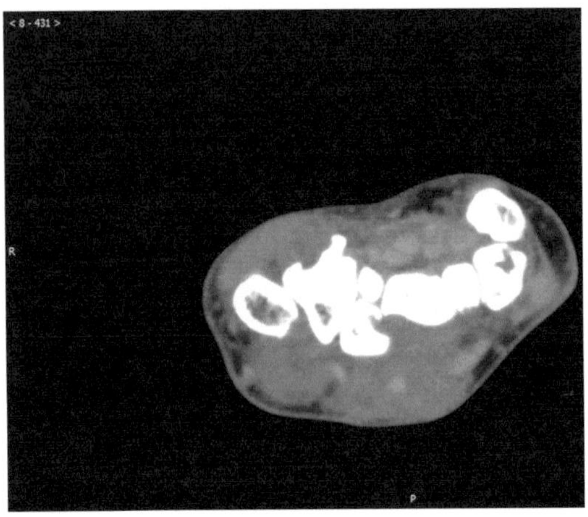

Fig. 23.4 Axial CT image of the left wrist in soft tissue window

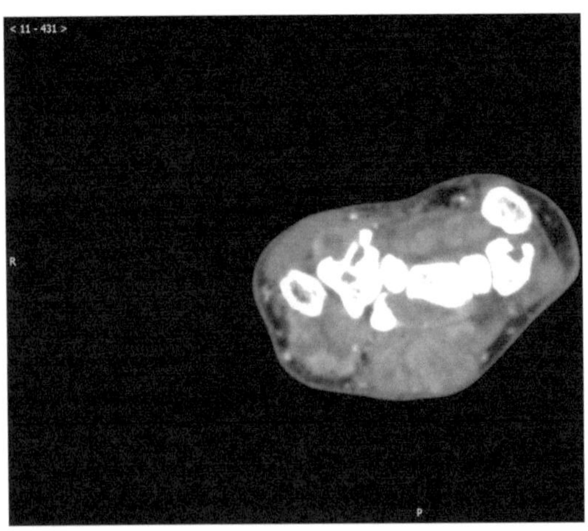

Fig. 23.5 Axial post-contrast CT image of the left wrist in soft tissue window

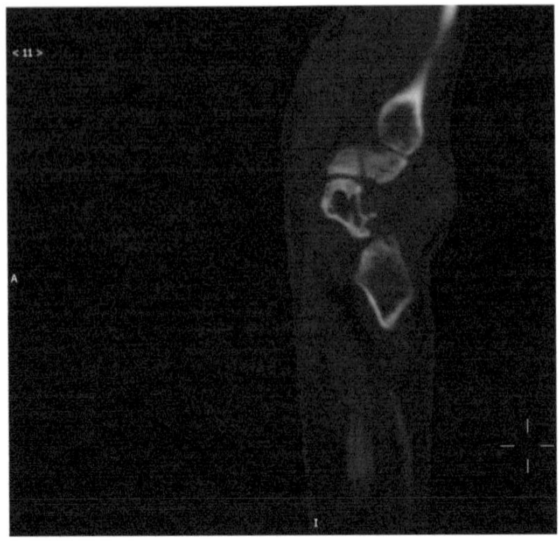

Fig. 23.6 Sagittal CT image of the left wrist in bone window

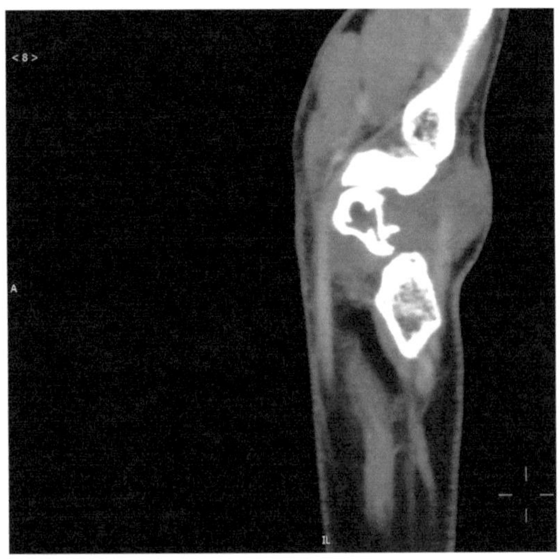

Fig. 23.7 Sagittal CT image of the left wrist in soft tissue window

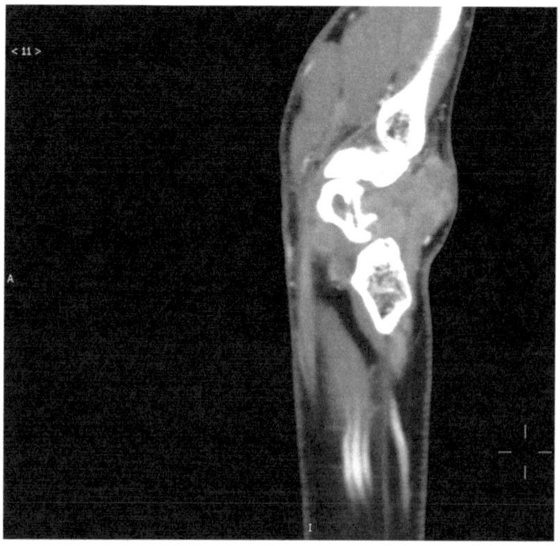

Fig. 23.8 Sagittal post-contrast CT image of the left wrist in soft tissue window

23.4 Description and Discussion from Residents

Mild osteopenia is noted of the left wrist on radiographs. Scaphoid, capitate, and hamate showed signs of compressive changes with clear margin and sclerosis and overlying soft tissue protuberance. Left wrist dorsal lumpy soft tissue mass is seen on CT images with nodular enhancement. Multiple cystic compressive changes are noted of scaphoid, triquetrum, capitate, and distal radius. Among the process of peri-articular soft tissue lesions invading the bone, pigmented villonodular synovitis (PVNS) is the most common one and also known as diffuse type of giant cell tumor of the tendon sheath, with same pathology findings.

23.5 Analysis and Comments from Professor Cheng Xiao-Guang

Patient had protracted medical history including surgery. Radiographs showed scaphoid and capitate bone destruction with clear margin and adjacent soft tissue swelling with increased density. However, the joint spaces are preserved. Right dorsal soft tissue mass with compressive bone destruction of multiple carpal bones is demonstrated on the CT images with avid enhancement. Most common condition that can cause these changes is PVNS. This is not an aggressive lesion on pathology but can be challenging for clinical management for it is difficult to achieve complete resection. However, this disease usually does not affect patient function with the characteristics as severe imaging findings with mild clinical symptoms. And no osteoporosis or joint space narrowing usually seen in this disease.

23.6 Diagnosis

Tenosynovial giant cell tumor (currently pigmented villonodular synovitis and giant cell tumor of the tendon sheath are all called tenosynovial giant cell tumor).

Suggested Reading

Cheng XG, You YH, Liu W, et al. MRI features of pigmented villonodular synovitis (PVNS). Clin Rheumatol. 2004;23(1):31–4.

Crim J, Dyroff SL, Stensby JD, et al. Limited usefulness of classic MR findings in the diagnosis of tenosynovial giant cell tumor. Skeletal Radiol. 2021;50(8):1585–1591.

24 Non-specific Synovitis: Case 24

24.1 Medical History

Patient is a 52-year-old female. She presented with right wrist pain after wrist sprain with restricted motion for 10 months.

24.2 Physical Examination

Range of motion of the right wrist: flexion, dorsiflexion, radial deviation, and ulnar deviation all 10°, muscle strength level 4.

24.3 Imaging Findings

24.3.1 Radiograph (Figs. 24.1 and 24.2)

Radiographs of the right wrist demonstrated low-density lucency at the distal radius with decreased joint space at radiocarpal joint.

24.3.2 CT Imaging (Figs. 24.3, 24.4, and 24.5)

CT images of the right wrist demonstrated diffuse soft tissue swelling with focal erosions at the distal ulna, distal radius, and triquetrum. Avid soft tissue enhancement was noted.

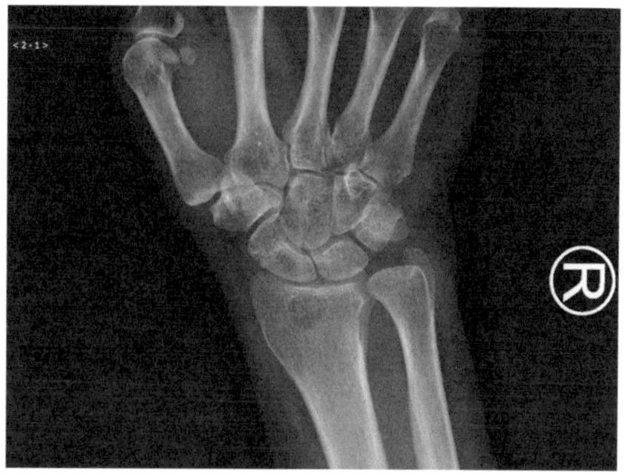

Fig. 24.1 Frontal view of the right wrist

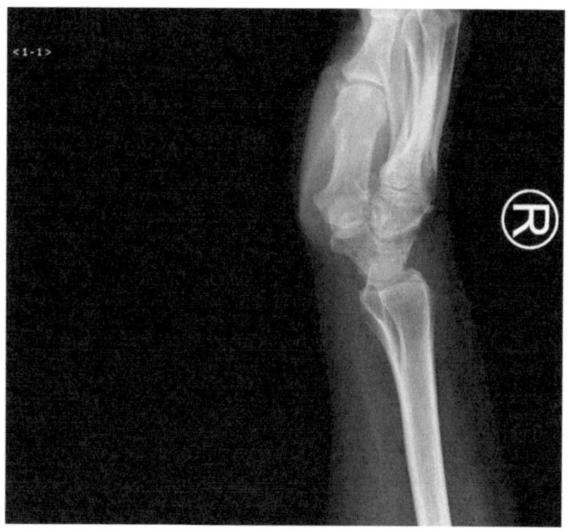

Fig. 24.2 Lateral view of the right wrist

X. Cheng et al., *Imaging of Bone Tumors in Wrist, Hand, Ankle and Foot*,
https://doi.org/10.1007/978-981-99-6407-9_24

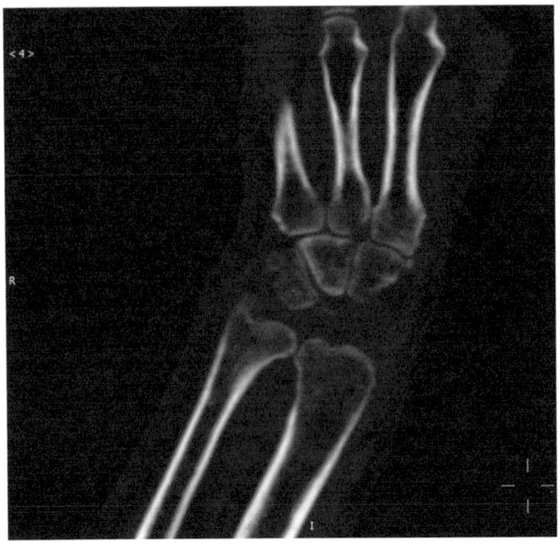

Fig. 24.3 Coronal CT image of the right wrist in bone window

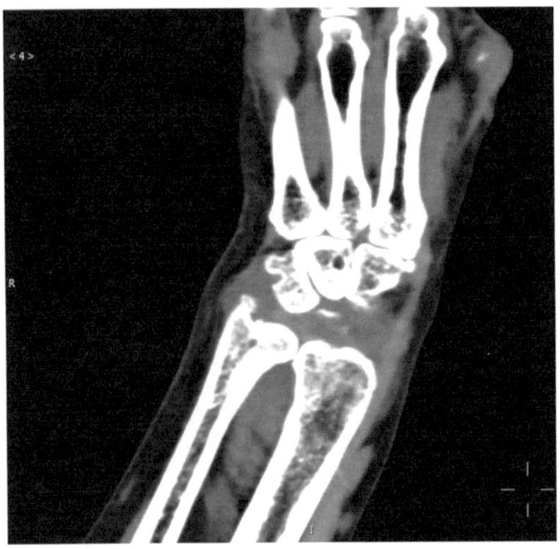

Fig. 24.4 Coronal CT image of the right wrist in soft tissue window

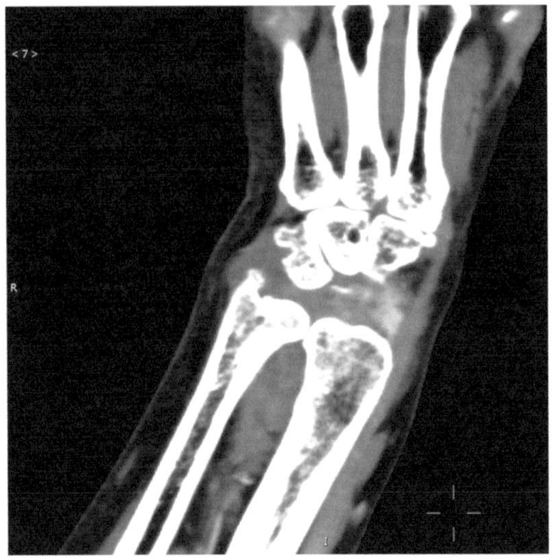

Fig. 24.5 Coronal post-contrast CT image of the right wrist in soft tissue window

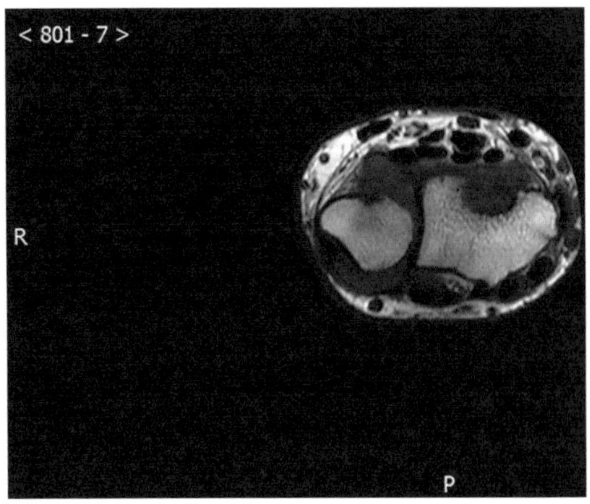

Fig. 24.6 Axial T1-weighted MR image of the right wrist

24.3.3 MR Imaging (Figs. 24.6, 24.7, 24.8, 24.9, 24.10, 24.11, and 24.12)

MR images of the right wrist demonstrated diffuse synovial hypertrophy with joint effusion, and erosions of the distal radius, ulna, scaphoid, lunate, triquetrum and adjacent marrow edema. No low signal focus noted on the gradient echo sequence and avid enhancement in the synovium noted.

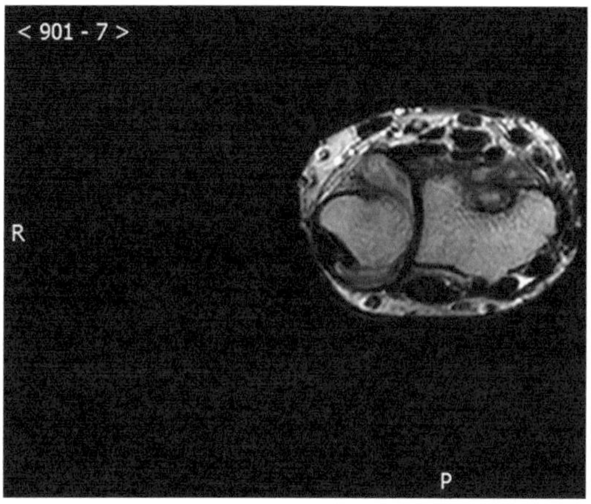

Fig. 24.7 Axial T2-weighted MR image of the right wrist

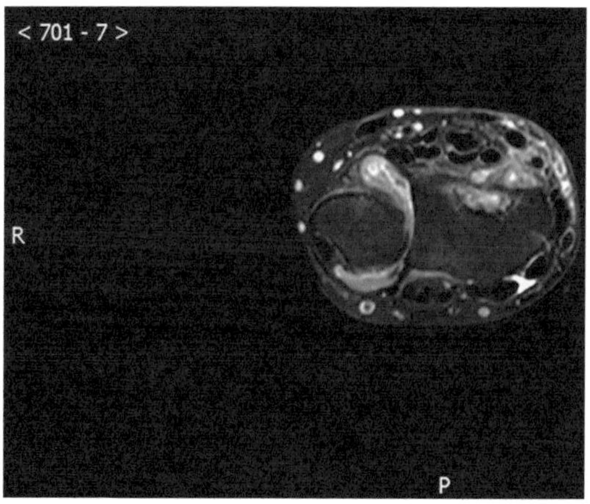

Fig. 24.8 Axial fat-suppressed T2-weighted MR image of the right wrist

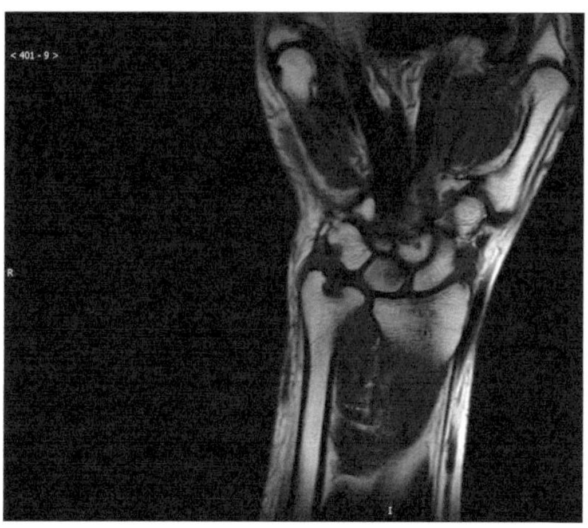

Fig. 24.9 Coronal T1-weighted MR image of the right wrist

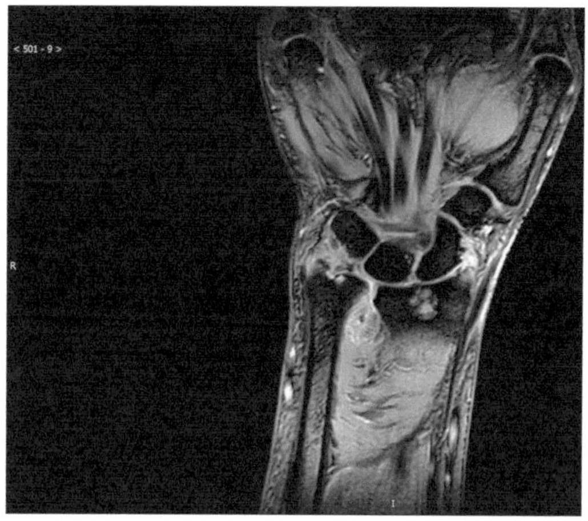

Fig. 24.10 Coronal gradient echo sequence MR image of the right wrist

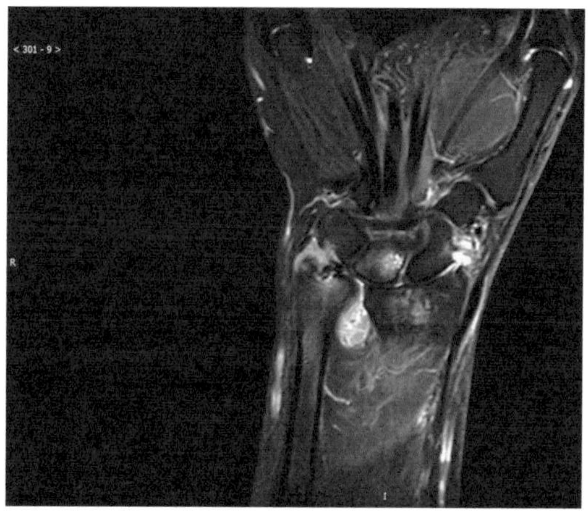

Fig. 24.11 Coronal fat-suppressed T2-weighted MR image of the right wrist

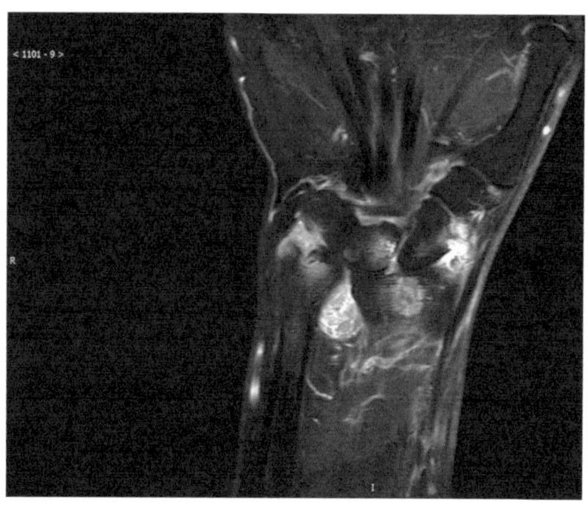

Fig. 24.12 Coronal post-contrast fat-suppressed T1-weighted MR image of the right wrist

24.4 Description and Discussion from Residents

Radiographs show normal alignment at the right wrist with mild osteopenia and narrowing of the radiocarpal joint (could be secondary to loss of the cartilage). Heterogeneous decreased bone densities noted at the distal radius and waist of the scaphoid, could be from tuberculous arthritis or rheumatoid arthritis. Bone destructions at the distal radius and ulna were demonstrated on CT images, as erosions from synovium hypertrophy. A suspected small abscess noted at the anterior distal radius after enhancement, raise the concern for tuberculous arthritis. Diffuse synovial hypertrophy around the distal radioulnar and radiocarpal joints with heterogeneous signal on MRI could be early signs of rice body formation, typical for nonspecific synovitis, rheumatoid arthritis, tuberculous synovitis. There was no enlarged or oval lymph node associated with rheumatoid arthritis. We favor tuberculous arthritis.

24.5 Analysis and Comments from Professor Cheng Xiao-Guang

The bone mineral density of the right wrist on radiographs is consistent with patient's age. Bone destruction along distal radius, normal joint space of the inter-carpal and carpometacarpal joints are not consistent with rheumatoid arthritis. Multiple bone destruction and soft tissue thickening with avid enhancement are most suggestive of diffuse synovial process. MR images further demonstrated the above findings. Multiple scattered non-enhancing foci could be rice bodies. The differential diagnosis includes rheumatoid arthritis, tuberculous arthritis, PVNS, etc. Overall, this is a chronic synovial process, without specific imaging features, the diagnose need to be combined with clinical findings and pathology.

24.6 Diagnosis

Non-specific synovitis.

Suggested Reading

Barakat MS, Schweitzer ME, Morisson WB, et al. Reactive carpal synovitis: initial experience with MR imaging. Radiology. 2005;236(1):231–6.

Rubin DA. MRI and ultrasound of the hands and wrists in rheumatoid arthritis. I. Imaging findings. Skeletal Radiol. 2019;48(5):677–695.

Lipomatosis of Nerve: Case 25

25

25.1 Medical History

Patient is a 19-year-old male who presented with large deformity around the right thumb and index fingers and additional mass at the right wrist since birth and enlarging with repeated episodes of right wrist pain for 3 years.

25.2 Physical Examination

Swelling and unsymmetrical enlargement of the right thumb and index fingers noted when comparing to the left side. Ulnar deviation noted around the distal interphalangeal joint of the right index finger. Enlargement of the radial aspect of the right palm is noted. There is a 4.0 cm mass at the palmer aspect of the right wrist, soft with clear margin and non-mobile with point tenderness. Increased palmer tenderness and pressure can be elicited by wrist dorsiflexion and decreased by wrist flexion. Severe numbness around the right middle finger present with restricted motion of the joints of the thumb and index finger with normal range of motion of the joints of the middle, ring and fifth fingers.

25.3 Imaging Findings

25.3.1 Radiograph (Figs. 25.1 and 25.2)

Radiographs of the right hand demonstrated deformities of the right thumb and index finger with macrodactyly and increased soft tissue thickness in the palmer aspect. Ulnar deviation is noted at the distal index finger. No bony destruction is noted.

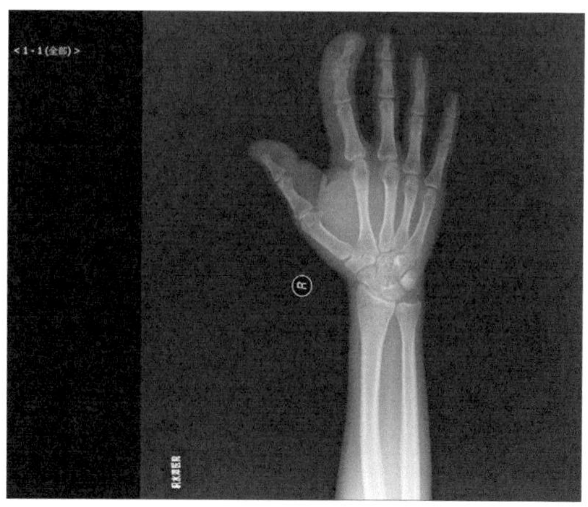

Fig. 25.1 Frontal view of the right hand

X. Cheng et al., *Imaging of Bone Tumors in Wrist, Hand, Ankle and Foot*,
https://doi.org/10.1007/978-981-99-6407-9_25

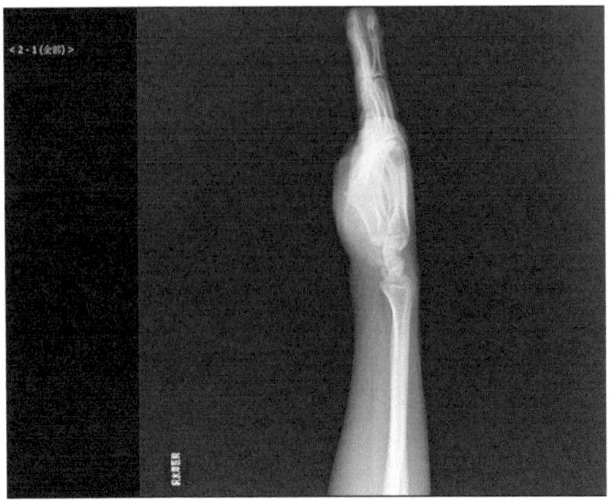

Fig. 25.2 Lateral view of the right hand

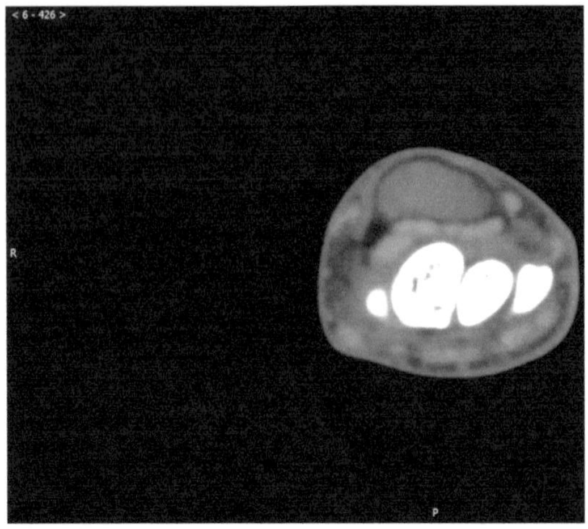

Fig. 25.3 Axial CT image of the right wrist in soft window

25.3.2 CT Imaging (Figs. 25.3, 25.4, 25.5, and 25.6)

CT images of the right wrist demonstrated soft tissue mass at the palmer aspect of the distal right forearm and wrist with clear margin and along the course of the median nerve. Fat densities are noted within the lesion. There is mild heterogeneous enhancement.

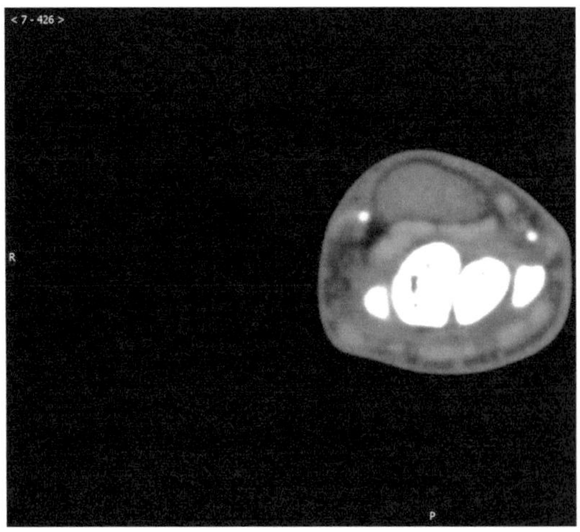

Fig. 25.4 Axial post-contrast CT image of the right wrist in soft window

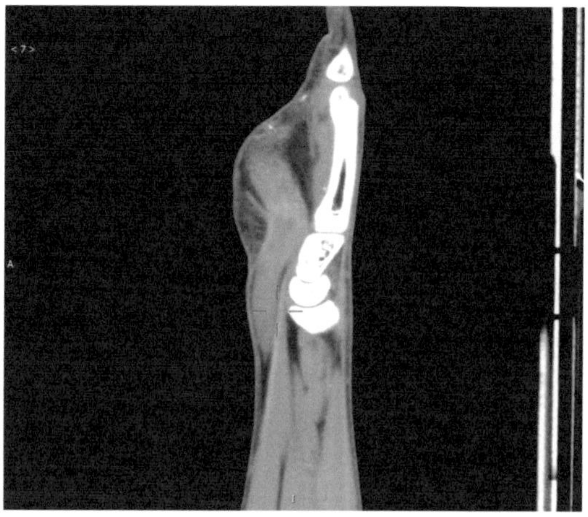

Fig. 25.5 Sagittal CT image of the right wrist in soft tissue window

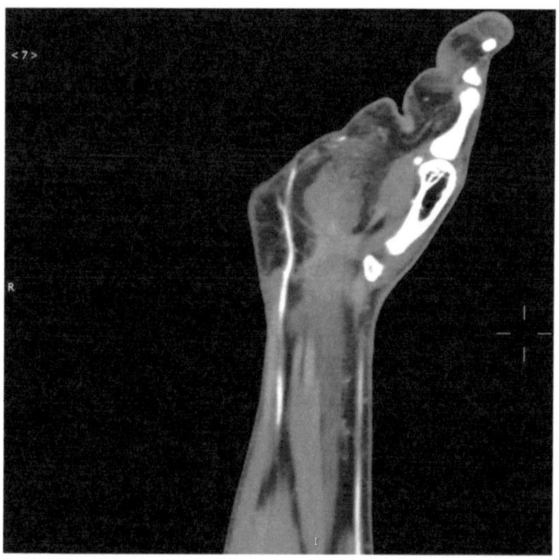

Fig. 25.6 Coronal post-contrast CT image of the right wrist in soft tissue window

25.4 Description and Discussion from Residents

Radiographs show ulnar deviation of the index finger with bowing but no apparent bone destruction. Soft tissue mass is noted between the first and second metacarpals with relatively homogenous density. Soft tissue mass at palmer aspect of the distal right forearm, and right wrist is seen on the CT scan with extended long axis and clear margin. Fat inter-space with adjacent tissue is noted. Mass effect upon adjacent tendon is also seen. The lesion located in the wrist is with intimate relationship with the tendons. There may be vessels within the lesion on the post-contrast images. The CT value measured around soft tissue density and we could exclude ganglion cyst. Overall, our consideration is benign neurovascular lesion.

25.5 Analysis and Comments from Professor Cheng Xiao-Guang

Typical macrodactyly is noted on the radiographs with hypertrophy of the bone and soft tissues of the thumb and index fingers. Lesion extending along the median nerve is noted on the CT scan with focal enclosed high density of flexor retinaculum (transverse carpal ligament). This is a case of dysplasia of the median nerve and disperses from one nerve to the others with lots of fat and fibrous tissue in between.

25.6 Diagnosis

Lipomatosis of nerve.

Suggested Reading

Ahlawat S, Chhabra A, Blakely J. Magnetic resonance neurography of peripheral nerve tumors and tumorlike conditions. Neuroimaging Clin N Am. 2014;24(1):171–92.

Marek T, Amrami KK, Spinner RJ, et al. MR spectroscopy differences between lipomatosis of nerve and neuromuscular choristoma: a potential adjunctive diagnostic tool. Skeletal Radiol. 2020;49(12):2051–2057.

Part II

Ankle

26 Periosteal Chondrosarcoma: Case 1

26.1 Medical History

Patient is a 37-year-old male. He presented with right ankle pain and swelling after exercise about 10 years ago and symptoms usually relieved by cold compress. He did not seek medical attention for this. The symptoms recur about 4 months ago, and radiographs show a lesion at the distal right tibia.

26.2 Physical Examination

Nothing abnormal.

26.3 Imaging Findings

26.3.1 Radiograph

Radiographs of the right ankle demonstrated bone destruction with protuberance at the anterior distal tibia with anterior soft tissue thickening (Figs. 26.1 and 26.2).

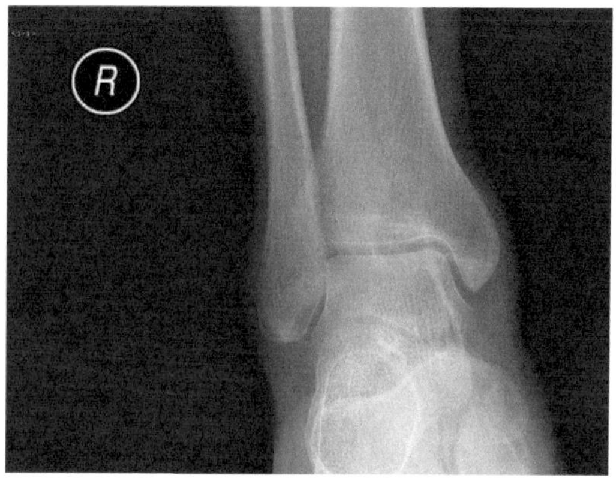

Fig. 26.1 Frontal view of the right ankle

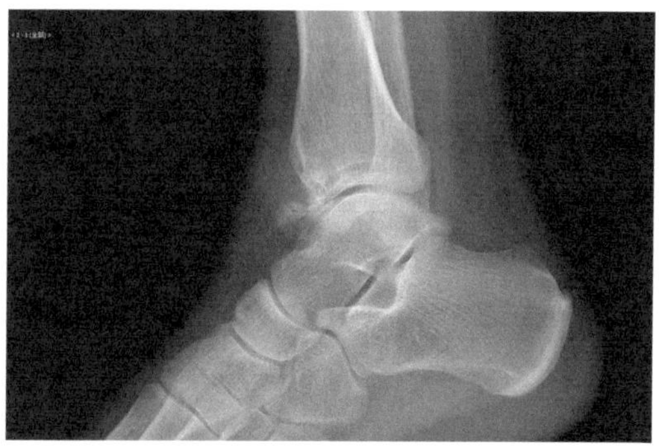

Fig. 26.2 Lateral view of the right ankle

26.3.2 CT Imaging

CT images of the right ankle demonstrated bone destruction along the anterior distal tibia with clear margin and sclerosis with anterior soft tissue mass. There were several internal patchy high densities and peripheral mild enhancement noted (Figs. 26.3, 26.4, 26.5, 26.6, 26.7, and 26.8).

X. Cheng et al., *Imaging of Bone Tumors in Wrist, Hand, Ankle and Foot*,
https://doi.org/10.1007/978-981-99-6407-9_26

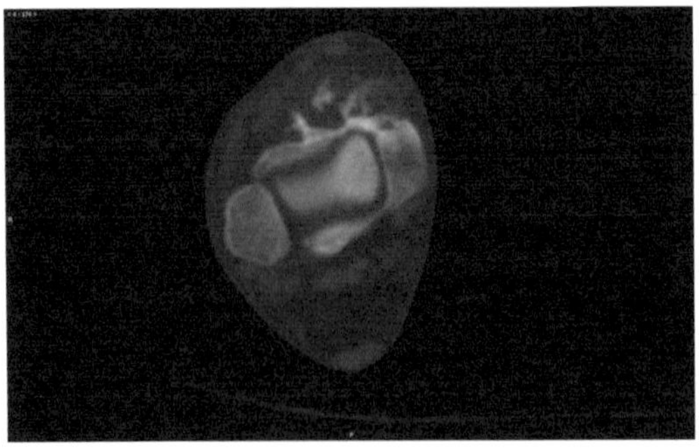

Fig. 26.3 Axial CT image of the right ankle in bone window

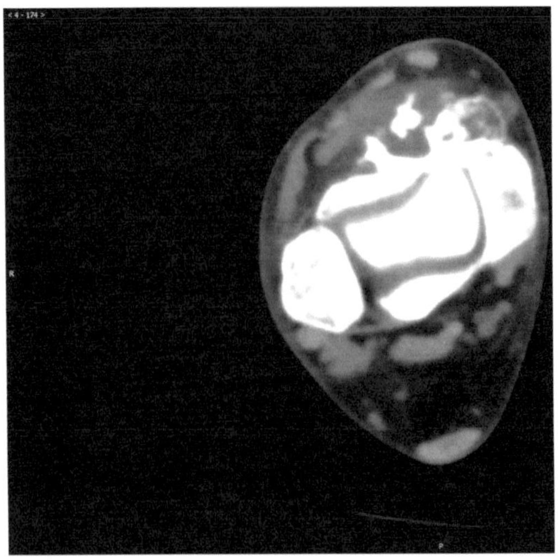

Fig. 26.4 Axial CT image of the right ankle in soft tissue window

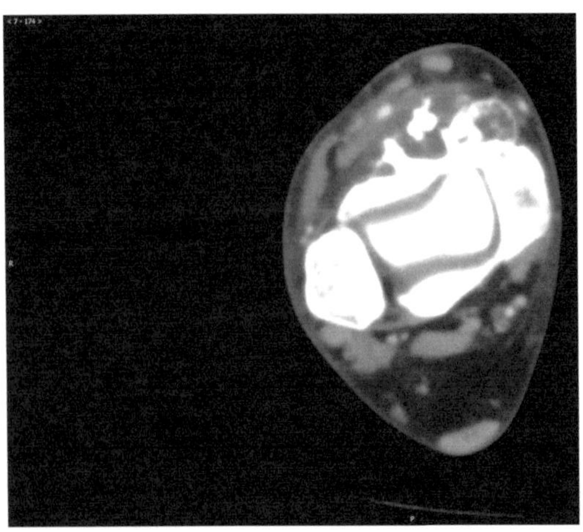

Fig. 26.5 Axial post-contrast CT image of the right ankle in soft tissue window

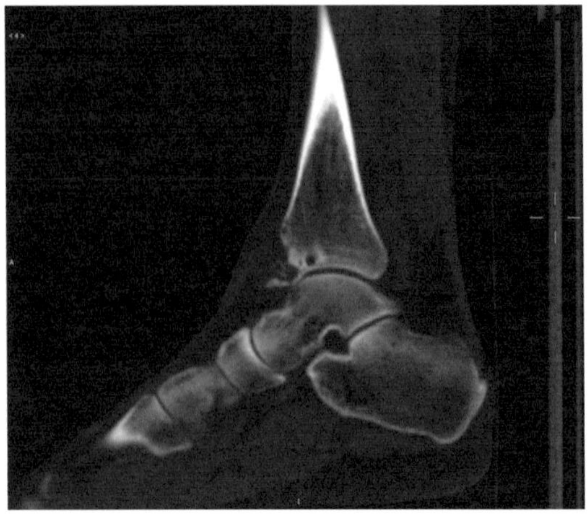

Fig. 26.6 Sagittal CT image of the right ankle in bone window

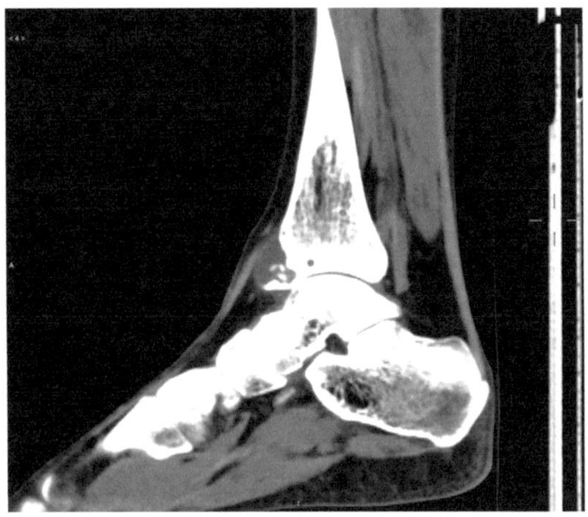

Fig. 26.7 Sagittal CT image of the right ankle in soft tissue window

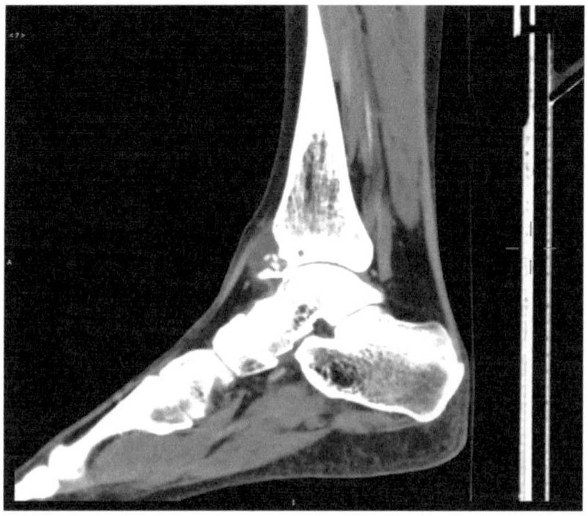

Fig. 26.8 Sagittal post-contrast CT image of the right ankle in soft tissue window

26.4 Description and Discussion from Residents

Radiographs show bony protuberance along the right anterior distal tibia along the articular surface with heterogeneous density and associated soft tissue mass. Expansile bone destruction is noted at the distal anterior tibia on the CT images with lifting of the focal cortex and relative low density soft tissue mass with punctate high densities and no clear enhancement. Given patient's prolonged history, we favor benign process, likely of chondroid lesion. However, giant cell tumor of bone and aneurysmal bone cyst are in the differential diagnoses.

26.5 Analysis and Comments from Professor Cheng Xiao-Guang

Patient is a young male with prolonged clinical history. Imaging shows bone destruction with soft tissue mass at anterior distal tibia, and solid portion of the mass shows relative low density with internal punctate calcification/ossification and no clear enhancement. Given the history, I favor benign or low-grade malignant lesion, such as chondroma or chondrosarcoma originating from the periosteum. Based on the location of the lesion, gout and giant cell tumor of bone are in the differential diagnoses.

26.6 Diagnosis

Periosteal chondrosarcoma.

Suggested Reading

Chaabane S, Bouaziz MC, Drissi C, et al. Periosteal chondrosarcoma. AJR Am J Roentgenol. 2009;192(1):W1–6.

Tilden W, Andrei V, O'Donnell P, et al. Peripheral and periosteal chondrosarcoma: MRI-pathological correlation in 58 cases. Skeletal Radiol. 2022;51(6):1189–1199.

27 Dysplasia Epiphysealis Hemimelica: Case 2

27.1 Medical History

Patient is a 3-year-old boy. His parents noticed him limping on the right lower extremity about 1 year ago. Radiographs at the time showed no abnormality. Follow-up exam 1 month ago showed mass around the right ankle.

27.2 Physical Examination

Limping of the right lower extremity and restricted right ankle eversion.

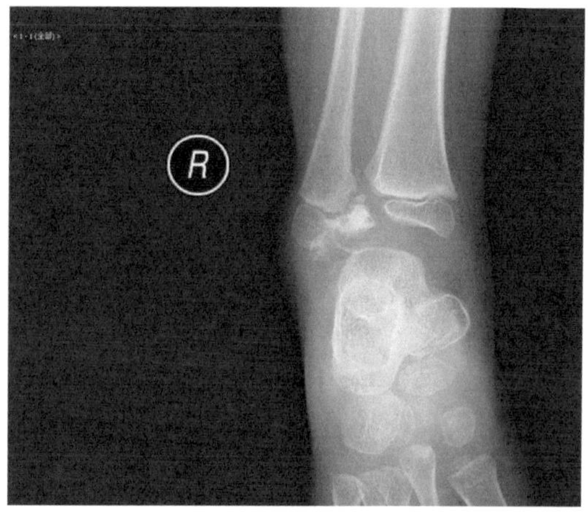

Fig. 27.1 Frontal view of the right ankle

27.3 Imaging Findings

27.3.1 Radiograph

Radiographs of the right ankle demonstrated enlarging epiphysis of the right distal fibula with irregular shape. Irregular high densities are noted along the bulging medial and anterior aspect of the epiphysis (Figs. 27.1 and 27.2).

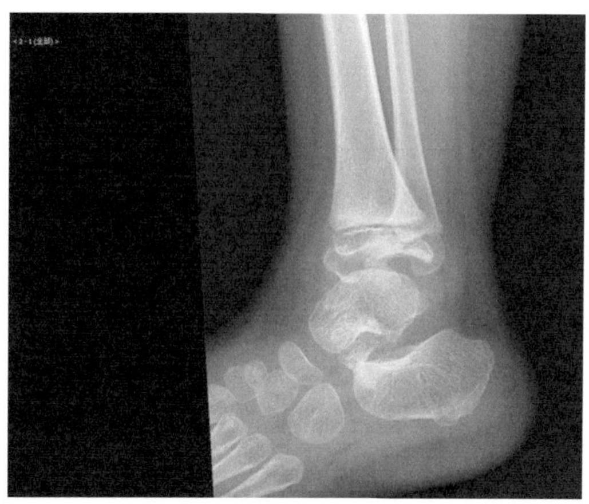

Fig. 27.2 Lateral view of the right ankle

27.3.2 CT Imaging

CT images of the right ankle demonstrated enlarging and irregular epiphysis of the right distal fibula. There is bony bulging at the medial and

X. Cheng et al., *Imaging of Bone Tumors in Wrist, Hand, Ankle and Foot*,
https://doi.org/10.1007/978-981-99-6407-9_27

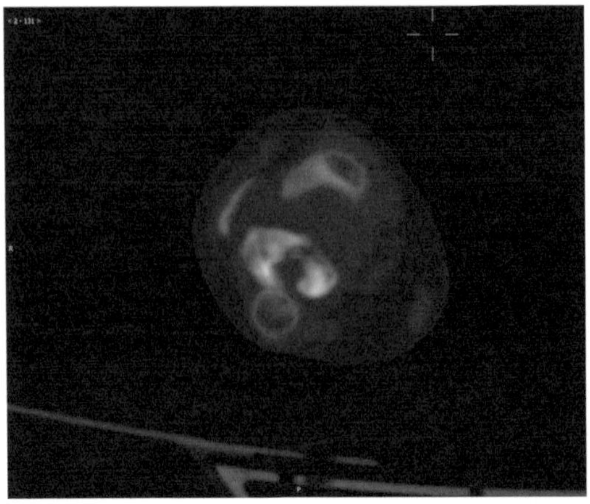

Fig. 27.3 Axial CT image of the right ankle in bone window

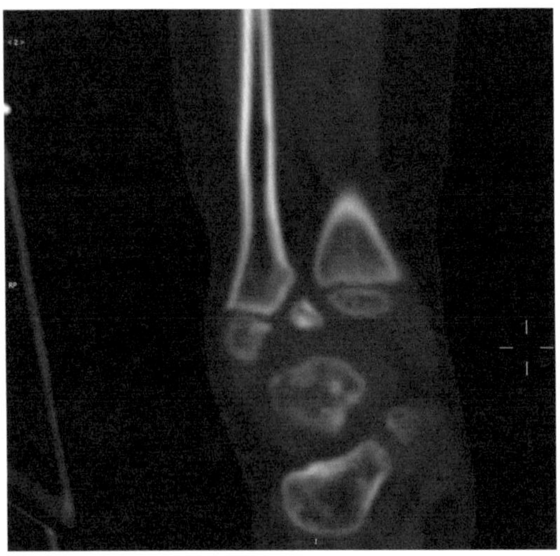

Fig. 27.4 Coronal CT image of the right ankle in bone window

anterior aspect with focal mature bone formation (Figs. 27.3, 27.4, 27.5, and 27.6).

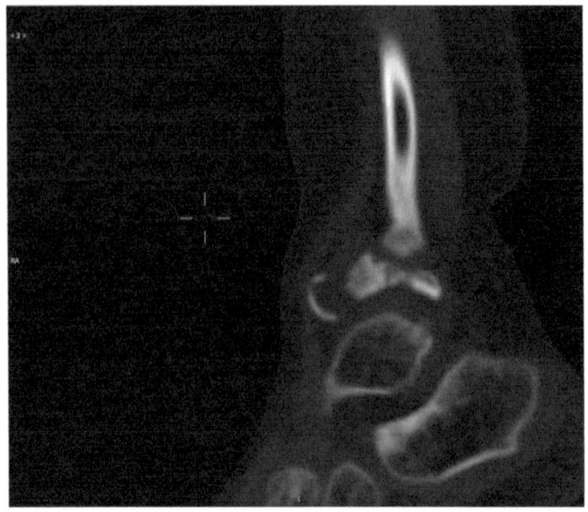

Fig. 27.5 Sagittal CT image of the right ankle in bone window

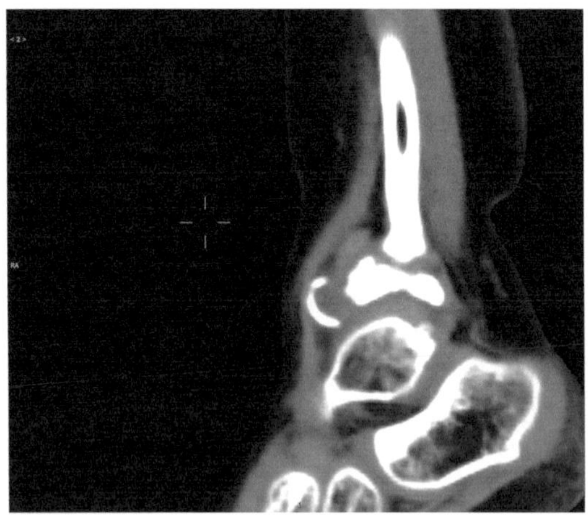

Fig. 27.6 Sagittal CT image of the right ankle in soft tissue window

27.3.3 MR Imaging

MR images of the right ankle showed bulging of the medial right distal fibula epiphysis with internal chondral osteogenesis and joint effusion (Figs. 27.7, 27.8, and 27.9).

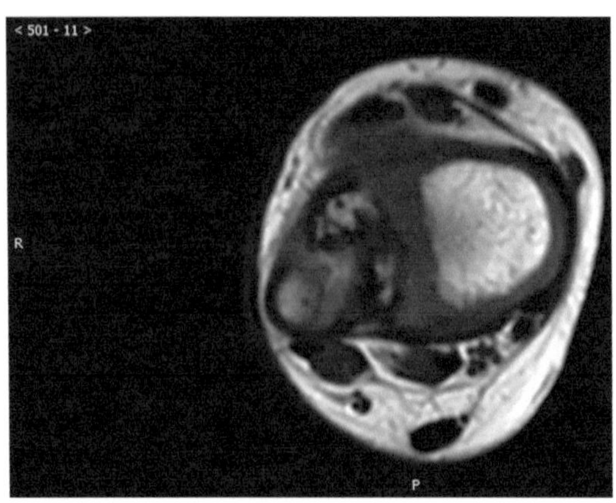

Fig. 27.7 Axial T1-weighted image of the right ankle

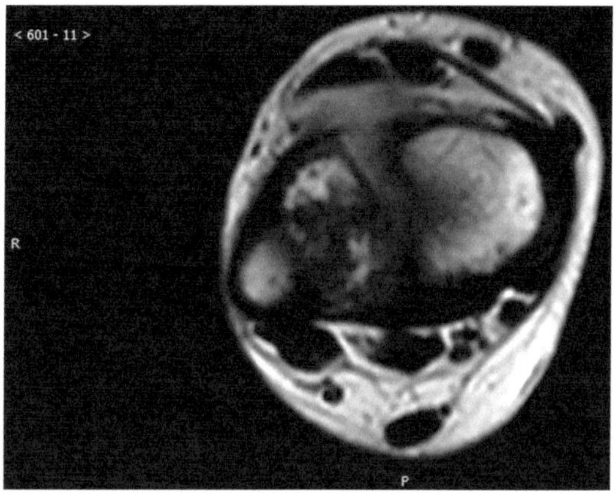

Fig. 27.8 Axial T2-weighted image of the right ankle

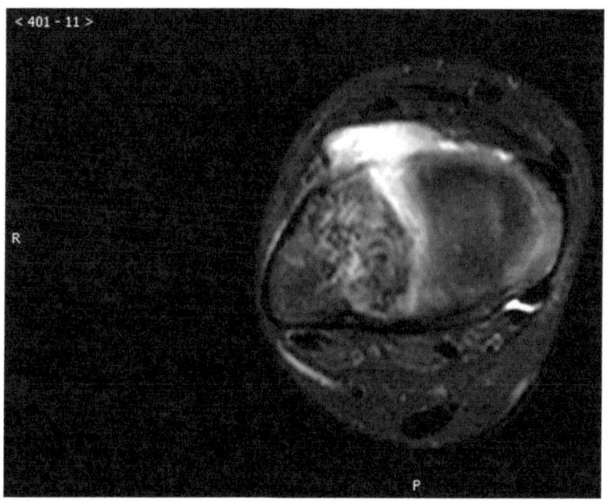

Fig. 27.9 Axial fat-suppressed T2-weighted image of the right ankle

27.4 Description and Discussion from Residents

Radiographs show irregular epiphysis of the right distal fibula and irregular high densities in the distal tibia and fibula interval. CT images demonstrated bony protuberance along the medial distal fibula epiphysis. The internal signal of the bony protuberance is similar to the normal bone on the MR images. In pediatric patient with bony protuberance of epiphysis, our first consideration is epiphyseal osteochondroma, also known as dysplasia epiphysealis hemimelica.

27.5 Analysis and Comments from Professor Cheng Xiao-Guang

Patient is a boy with prolonged clinical history. There was irregular bone protuberance along the medial distal fibula epiphysis. MRI images demonstrated connection between the bony protuberance and the fibula epiphysis, consistent with epiphyseal osteochondroma, also known as dysplasia epiphysealis hemimelica.

27.6 Diagnosis

Dysplasia epiphysealis hemimelica (Trevor disease).

Suggested Reading

Celıkyay RY, Celikyay F, Bilgic E, et al. Dysplasia epiphysealis hemimelica of the lower limb. Skeletal Radiol. 2017;46(1):111–115.

Degnan AJ, Ho-Fung VM. More than epiphyseal osteochondromas: updated understanding of imaging findings in dysplasia epiphysealis hemimelica (Trevor disease).

28 Chondroblastoma: Case 3

28.1 Medical History

Patient is a 29-year-old female. She developed right ankle pain about 6 months ago without clear inciting event. The pain was episodic and worsened with running, going up and down the stairs, and relieved with rest. She did not seek medical treatment then. The symptoms worsened about 2 months ago, and she underwent needle biopsy about 2 weeks ago.

28.2 Physical Examination

Apparent focal point tenderness around the right ankle.

28.3 Imaging Findings

28.3.1 Radiograph

Radiographs of the right ankle demonstrated lytic osseous destruction around the medial aspect of the talus with clear margin and enlarged medial tubercle (Figs. 28.1 and 28.2).

28.3.2 CT Imaging

CT images of the right ankle demonstrated lytic bone destruction around the medial talus with

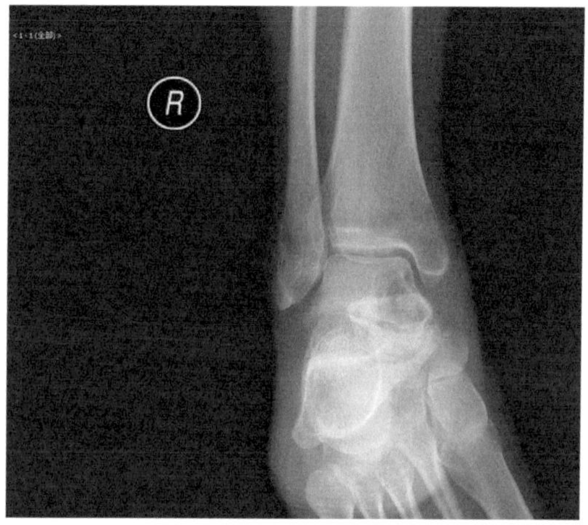

Fig. 28.1 Frontal view of the right ankle

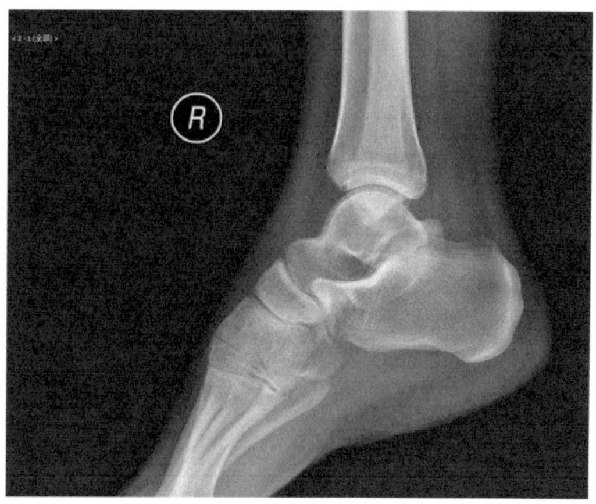

Fig. 28.2 Lateral view of the right ankle

X. Cheng et al., *Imaging of Bone Tumors in Wrist, Hand, Ankle and Foot*,
https://doi.org/10.1007/978-981-99-6407-9_28

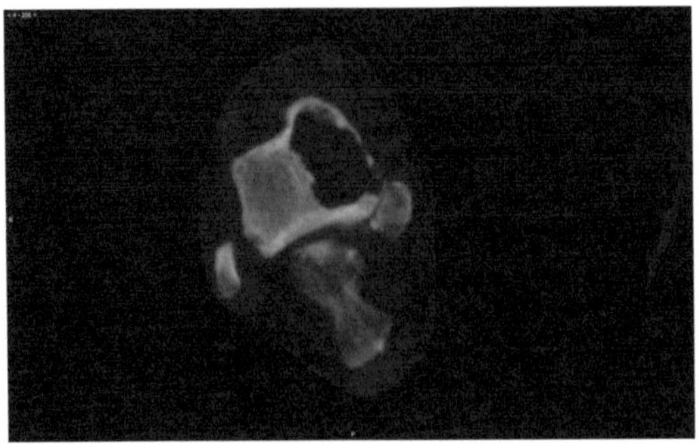

Fig. 28.3 Axial CT image of the right ankle in bone window

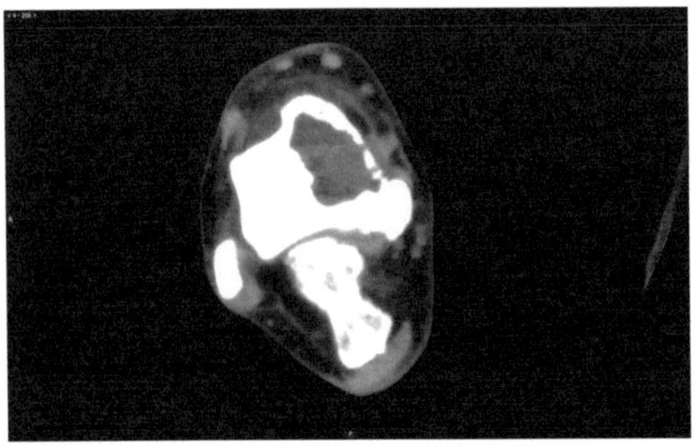

Fig. 28.4 Axial CT image of the right ankle in soft window

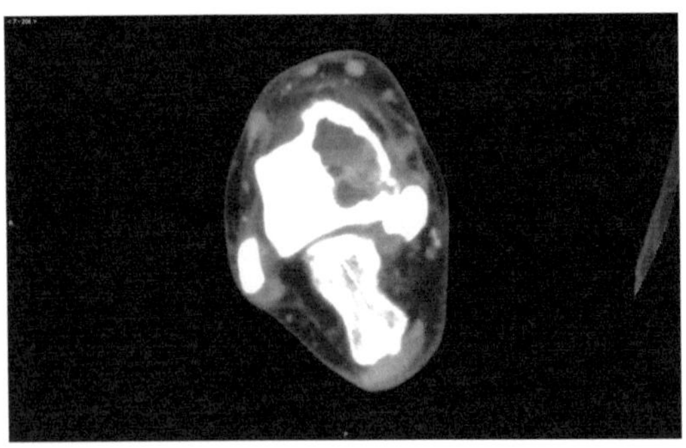

Fig. 28.5 Axial post-contrast CT image of the right ankle in soft window

internal heterogeneous densities and fluid-fluid levels. There are focal dis-continuous cortex and adjacent soft tissue swelling. Solid portion of the lesion shows avid enhancement (Figs. 28.3, 28.4, 28.5, 28.6, 28.7, 28.8, and 28.9).

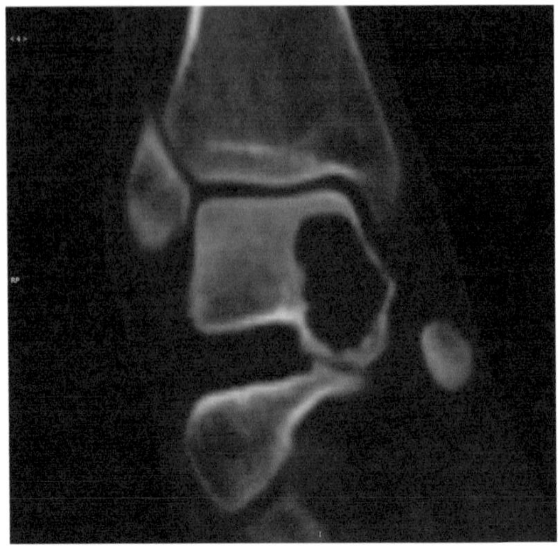

Fig. 28.6 Coronal CT image of the right ankle in bone window

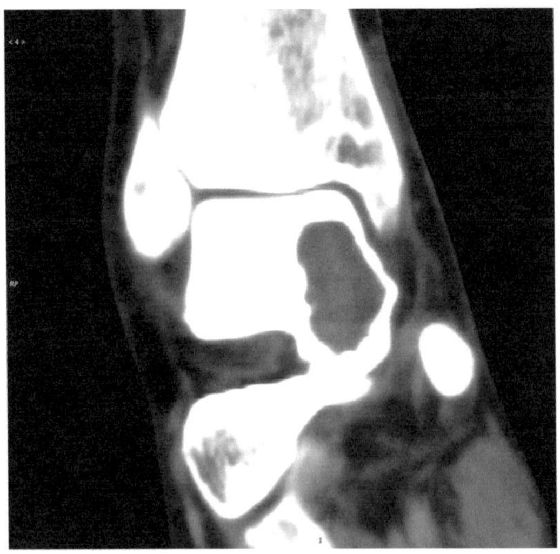

Fig. 28.7 Coronal CT image of the right ankle in soft tissue window

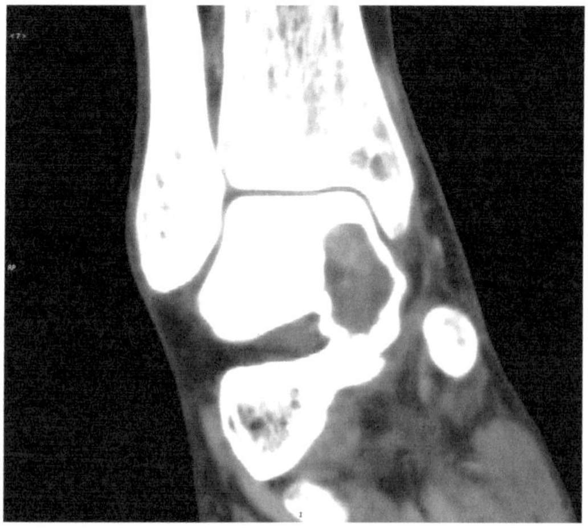

Fig. 28.8 Coronal post-contrast CT image of the right ankle in soft tissue window

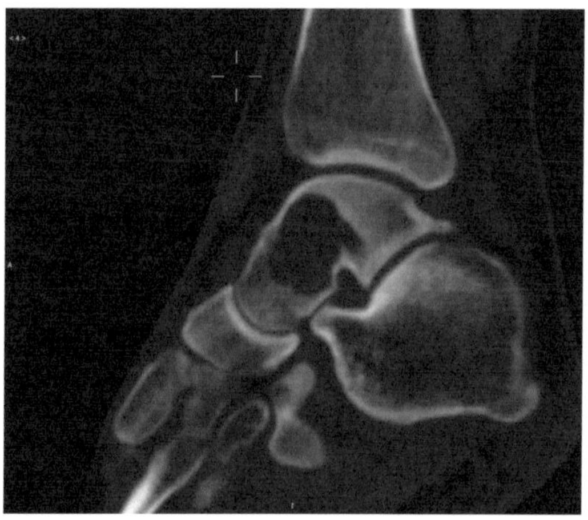

Fig. 28.9 Sagittal CT image of the right ankle in bone window

28.4 Description and Discussion from Residents

Radiographs demonstrated lytic bone destruction with clear margin and no peripheral sclerosis with smooth articular surface. CT images show focal cortical disruption and internal heterogeneous densities and avid enhancement of the solid portion with fluid-fluid levels. Based on the location and imaging findings, our top consideration is giant cell tumor of bone with chondroid lesion in the differential diagnoses.

28.5 Analysis and Comments from Professor Cheng Xiao-Guang

The patient is a young female. The radiographs showed lytic bone destruction of the medial talus with clear margin and no adjacent soft tissue abnormalities, favoring benign process. CT images demonstrated internal heterogeneous densities with fluid-fluid level and no calcification with heterogeneous enhancement of focal avid enhancement. Given the above findings, my top consideration is chondroblastoma with giant cell tumor and aneurysmal bone cyst in the differential diagnoses. In most cases, giant cell tumor of bone would show more apparent enhancements in the solid portion on CT images. If there was non-solid component, I would favor aneurysmal bone cyst.

28.6 Diagnosis

Chondroblastoma.

Suggested Reading

Angelini A, Arguedas F, Varela A, et al. Chondroblastoma of the foot: 40 cases from a single institution. J Foot Ankle Surg. 2018;57(6):1105–1109.

Boo SI, Saad A, Murphy J, et al. Tumours of the talus - A pictorial review. J Clin Orthop Trauma. 2020;11(3):410–416.

Subchondral Cyst: Case 4

29

29.1 Medical History

Patient is a 15-year-old girl. She sprained her right ankle about 5 months ago with dull pain, episodic and worsened with walking and mildly relieved with rest. She did not seek medical treatment. The symptoms worsened about 1 month ago.

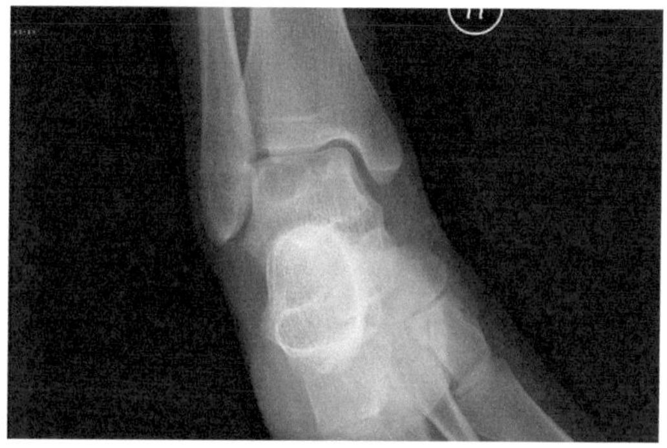

Fig. 29.1 Frontal view of the right ankle

29.2 Physical Examination

Mild swelling about the right ankle with palpable mass, of indistinct border and point tenderness.

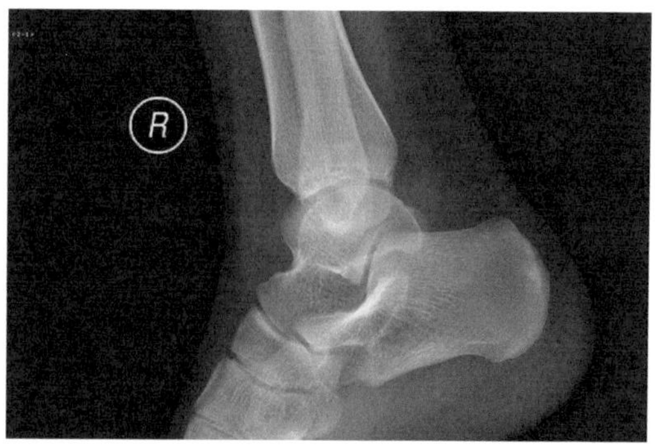

Fig. 29.2 Lateral view of the right ankle

29.3 Imaging Findings

29.3.1 Radiograph

Radiographs of the right ankle demonstrated lytic bone destruction of the talus with peripheral sclerosis and clear margin (Figs. 29.1 and 29.2).

29.3.2 CT Imaging

CT images of the right ankle demonstrated lytic bone destruction of the talus with peripheral sclerosis. The lesion showed intermediate density without enhancement. There was mild collapse of the articular surface of the talar dome with mild soft tissue swelling (Figs. 29.3, 29.4, 29.5, 29.6, and 29.7).

X. Cheng et al., *Imaging of Bone Tumors in Wrist, Hand, Ankle and Foot*,
https://doi.org/10.1007/978-981-99-6407-9_29

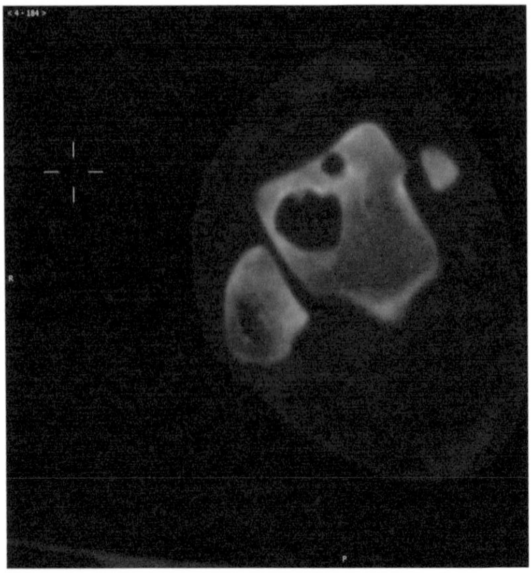

Fig. 29.3 Axial CT image of the right ankle in bone window

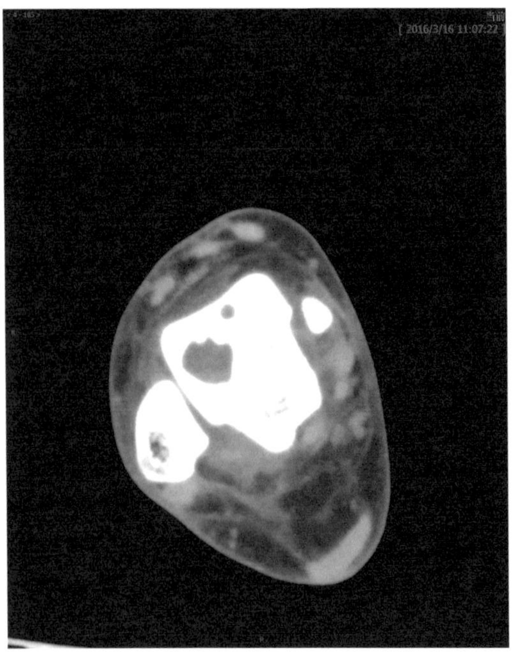

Fig. 29.4 Axial CT image of the right ankle in soft tissue window

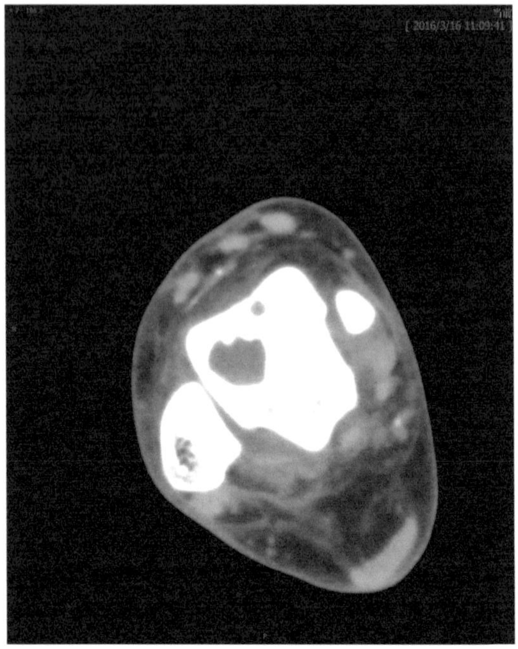

Fig. 29.5 Axial post-contrast CT image of the right ankle in soft tissue window

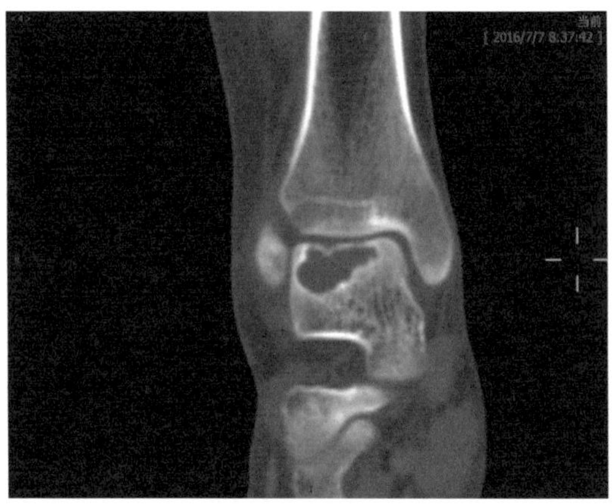

Fig. 29.6 Coronal CT image of the right ankle in bone window

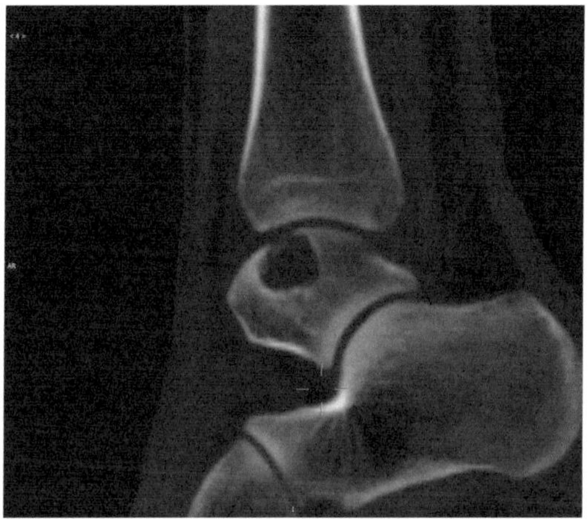

Fig. 29.7 Sagittal CT image of the right ankle in bone window

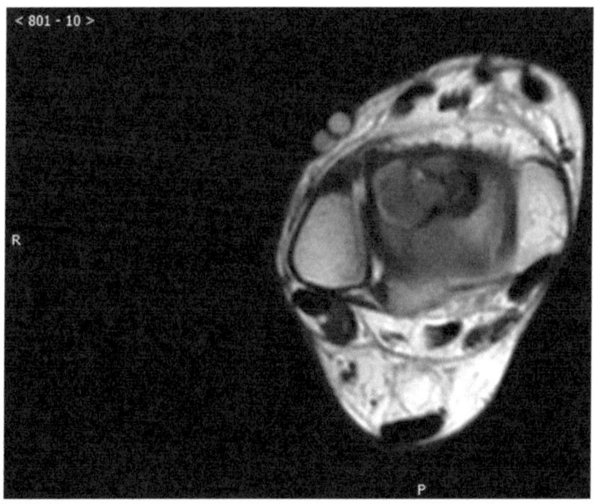

Fig. 29.8 Axial T1-weighted image of the right ankle

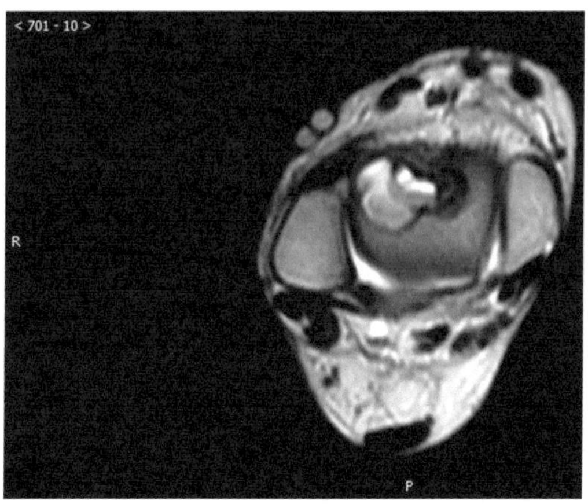

Fig. 29.9 Axial T2-weighted image of the right ankle

29.3.3 MR Imaging

MR images of the right ankle showed focal destruction below the articular surface of the talar dome with irregular shape. The lesion demonstrated predominant intermediate T1, high T2 signal and multiple septations with fluid-fluid levels. There was peripheral and septation enhancement. Small nodular enhancement was noted at the medial aspect of the lesion (Figs. 29.8, 29.9, 29.10, and 29.11).

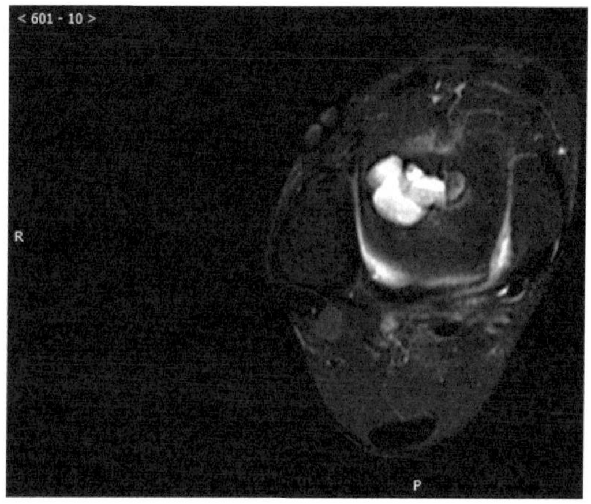

Fig. 29.10 Axial fat-suppressed T2-weighted image of the right ankle

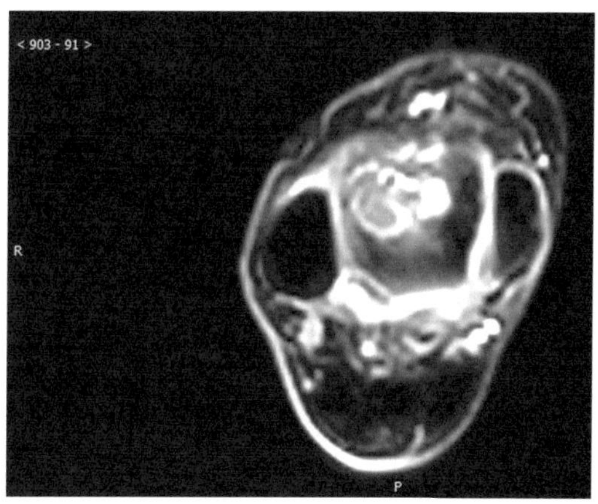

Fig. 29.11 Axial post-contrast fat-suppressed T1-weighted image of the right ankle

29.4 Description and Discussion from Residents

Radiographs show lytic bone destruction below the talar dome articular surface with clear margin, and sclerosis. The overall articular surface contour was preserved. CT images show cystic bone destruction below the talar dome articular surface with internal heterogeneous density and small patchy high density with septations and no enhancement. Cystic lesions below the talar dome articular surface with multiple septations and fluid-fluid levels were noted on the MRI images. Avid enhancement was noted around the septations and no enhancement in the center of the lesion. The above findings are consistent with benign process and given patient's age and duration of the disease, our top consideration is chondroblastoma, with simple bone cyst and giant cell tumor of bone in the differential diagnoses.

29.5 Analysis and Comments from Professor Cheng Xiao-Guang

Patient is an adolescent girl. Radiographs show the lesion at the talus with clear margin, smooth articular surface, and normal distal tibiofibular interval. CT images show internal heterogeneous density within the lesion and floating high density which could be calcification. Subtle articular surface collapse was noted on the coronal and sagittal reformatted images. There were joint effusion and no enhancement. The lesion appeared to be cystic on MR images with multiple septations and fluid-fluid levels internally. Small area of solid component was noted medially. There were adjacent soft tissue swelling and enhancement of the septations. Given patient's age, my top consideration is chondroblastoma, with simple bone cyst in the differential diagnose. There is usually symmetrical expansion with simple bone cyst and internal septations are rare, thus, not my top consideration.

29.6 Diagnosis

Subchondral cyst.

Suggested Reading

Williams HJ, Davies AM, Allen G, et al. Imaging features of intraosseous ganglia: a report of 45 cases. Eur Radiol. 2004;14(10):1761–9.

Reilingh ML, Blankevoort L, Eekeren ICM, et al. Morphological analysis of subchondral talar cysts on microCT. Knee Surg Sports Traumatol Arthrosc. 2013;21(6):1409–17.

30 Osteomyelitis: Case 5

30.1 Medical History

Patient is a 1-year-old infant boy. He presented with right foot limping with fever about 1 month ago without clear inciting event. His temperature was 40° then and seen at a local hospital with blood work showing elevated white count. He was treated with cooling treatment with relief. His parents noticed apparent right ankle swelling and no weight-bearing about 2 weeks ago.

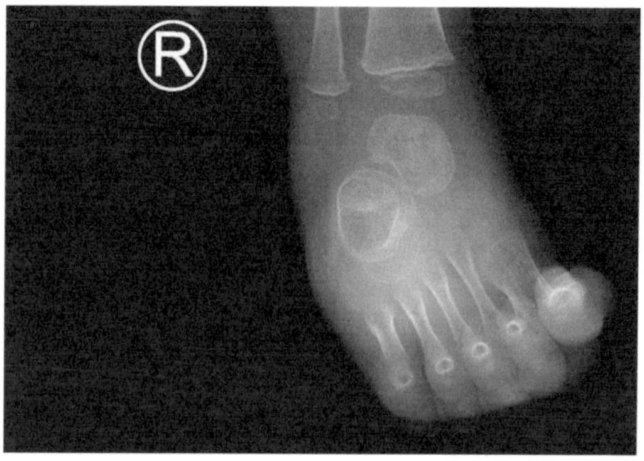

Fig. 30.1 Frontal view of the right ankle

30.2 Physical Examination

Apparent swelling of the right ankle and foot with focal pigmentation. There was mild redness around the ankle with increased warmth around the skin of the right ankle and foot. There was no point tenderness.

30.3 Imaging Findings

30.3.1 Radiograph

Radiographs of the right ankle demonstrated focal decreased bone density around the talus with irregular margin and soft tissue swelling around the ankle (Figs. 30.1 and 30.2).

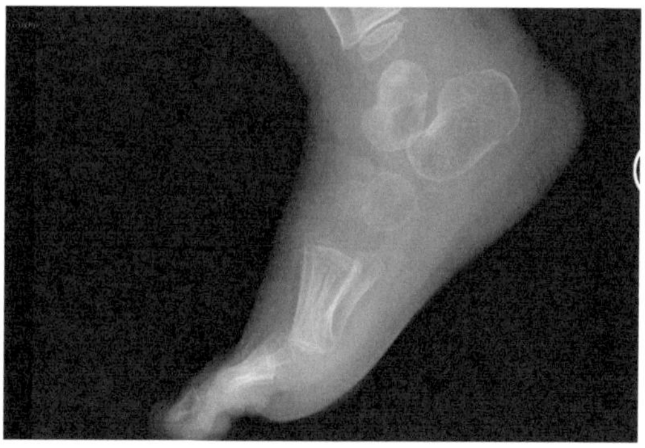

Fig. 30.2 Lateral view of the right ankle

30.3.2 CT Imaging

CT images of the right ankle demonstrated focal bone destruction of the right talus with peripheral reactive sclerosis and internal low density with

X. Cheng et al., *Imaging of Bone Tumors in Wrist, Hand, Ankle and Foot*,
https://doi.org/10.1007/978-981-99-6407-9_30

punctate high densities. There were multiple areas of cortical disruption and communicating with the soft tissues. Right ankle joint effusion was noted with soft tissue swelling (Figs. 30.3, 30.4, 30.5, 30.6, 30.7, and 30.8).

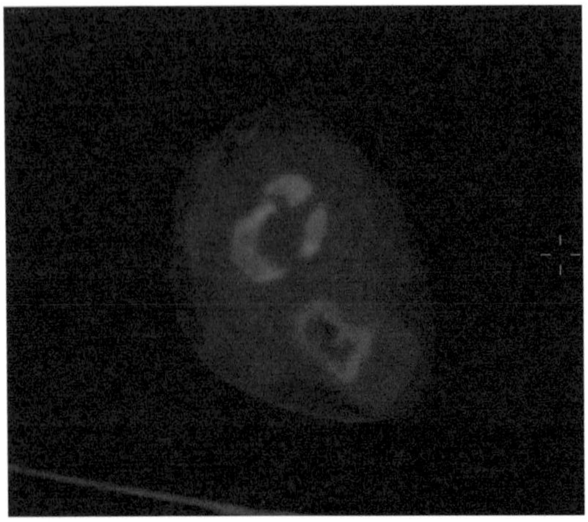

Fig. 30.3 Axial CT image of the right ankle in bone window

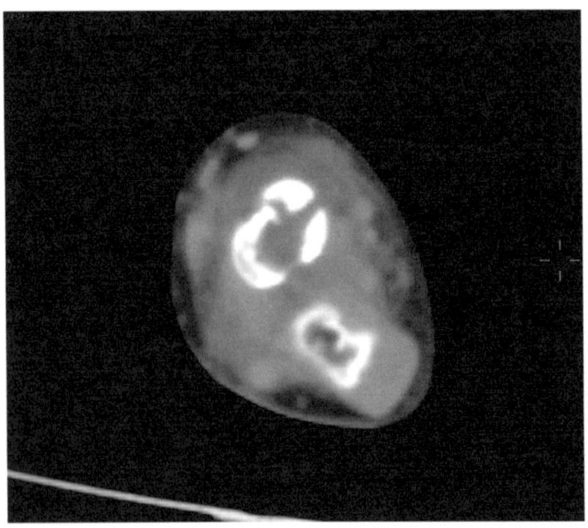

Fig. 30.4 Axial CT image of the right ankle in soft tissue window

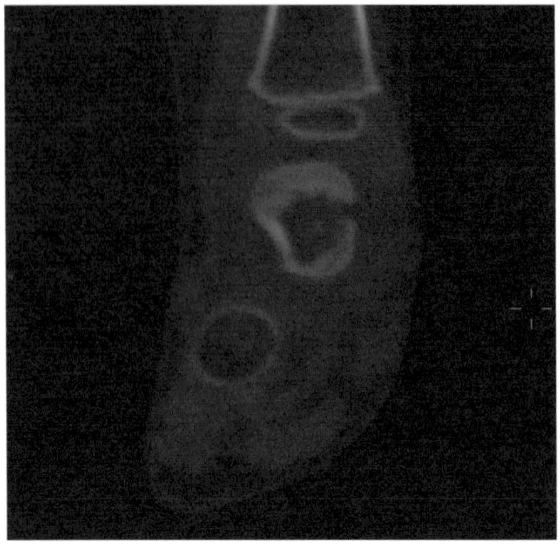

Fig. 30.5 Coronal CT image of the right ankle in bone window

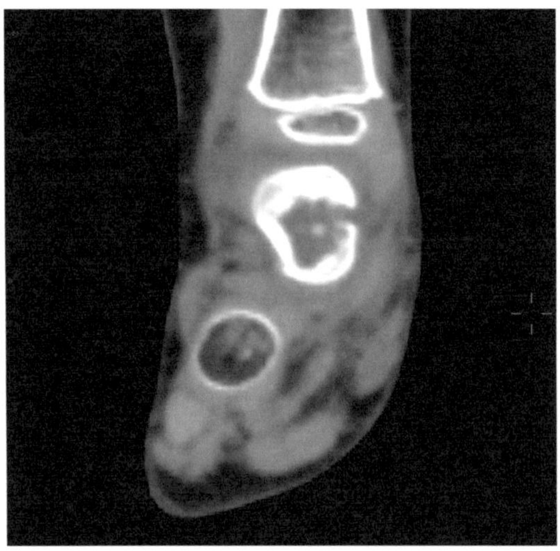

Fig. 30.6 Coronal CT image of the right ankle in soft tissue window

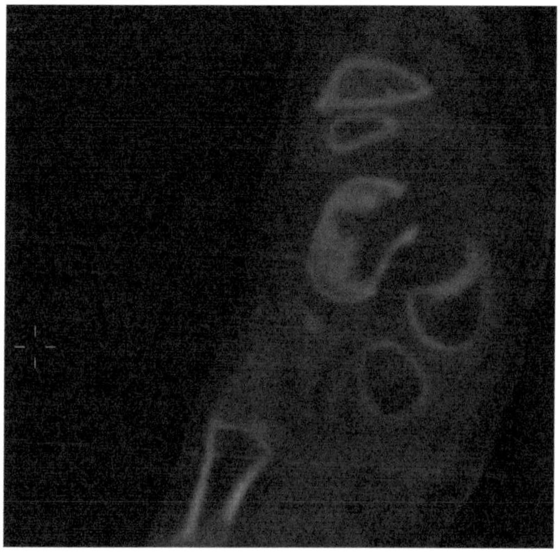

Fig. 30.7 Sagittal CT image of the right ankle in bone window

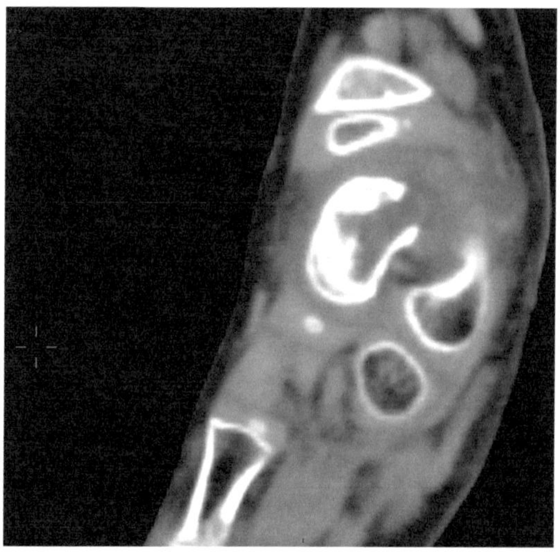

Fig. 30.8 Sagittal CT image of the right ankle in soft tissue window

30.4 Description and Discussion from Residents

Radiographs show bone destruction of the right talus with peripheral sclerosis with sharp margin. Peripheral patchy reparative changes were noted on the CT images with cortical disruption and sinus formation with adjacent soft tissue swelling. Given redness with swelling and pain around the joint clinically, out top consideration is purulent infection. Differential diagnoses would include eosinophilic granuloma if based on imaging findings alone.

30.5 Analysis and Comments from Professor Cheng Xiao-Guang

Patient is an infant. Radiographs show internal heterogeneous density of the right talus with bone destruction. Lesion with sinus tract is seen on CT images with peripheral reactive sclerosis. My top consideration is purulent osteomyelitis with tuberculosis and eosinophilic granuloma in the differential diagnoses. However, the patient's clinical manifestations are not consistent with tuberculosis or eosinophilic granuloma.

30.6 Diagnosis

Osteomyelitis.

Suggested Reading

Pabla R, Tibrewal S, Ramachandran M, et al. Primary subacute osteomyelitis of the talus in children: a case series and review. Acta Orthop Belg. 2011;77(3):294–8.

Stupina TA, Sudnitsyn AS, Subramanyam KN, et al. Applicability of histopathological osteomyelitis evaluation score (HOES) in chronic osteomyelitis of the foot - A feasibility study. Foot Ankle Surg. 2020;26(3):273–279.

31 Giant Cell Tumor of Bone: Case 6

31.1 Medical History

Patient is a 31-year-old male. He injured his left ankle 2 weeks ago and radiographs showed lesion at the talus. He complained of no symptoms before this incident.

31.2 Physical Examination

No abnormality.

31.3 Imaging Findings

31.3.1 Radiograph

Radiographs of the left ankle demonstrated lytic bone destruction of the talus with clear margin and peripheral sclerosis (Figs. 31.1 and 31.2).

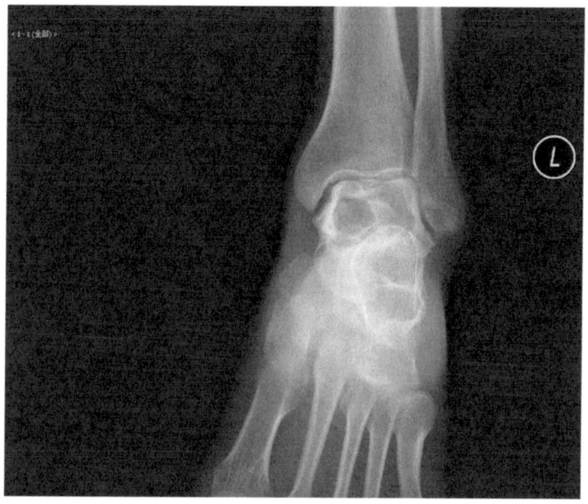

Fig. 31.1 Frontal view of the left ankle

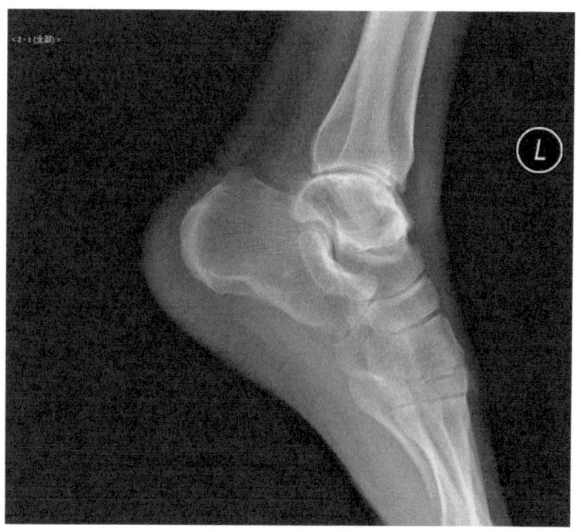

Fig. 31.2 Lateral view of the left ankle

31.3.2 CT Imaging

CT images of the left ankle demonstrated bone destruction of the talus with internal homogenous density and peripheral sclerosis. No mineral density was noted within the lesion. There was some focal cortical thinning without disruption and no adjacent soft tissue mass. The lesion is well circumscribed. There was focal avid

X. Cheng et al., *Imaging of Bone Tumors in Wrist, Hand, Ankle and Foot*,
https://doi.org/10.1007/978-981-99-6407-9_31

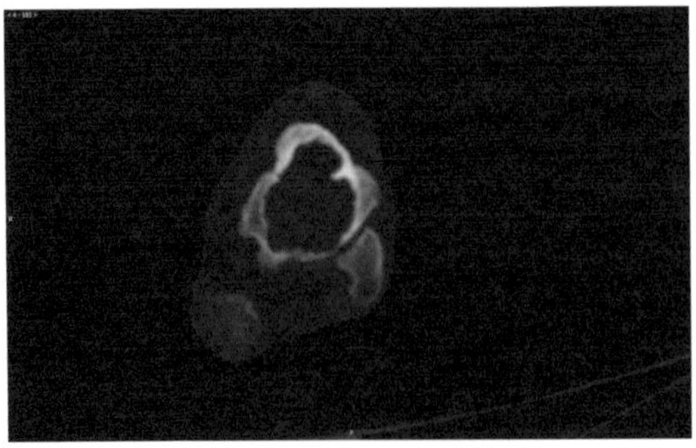

Fig. 31.3 Axial CT image of the left ankle in bone window

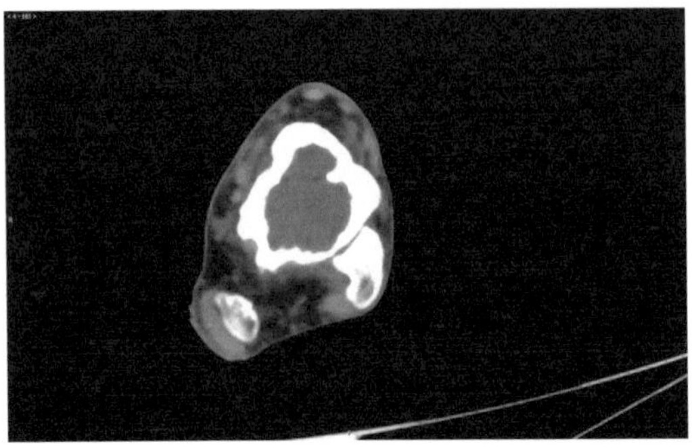

Fig. 31.4 Axial CT image of the left ankle in soft tissue window

enhancement on a background of heterogeneous enhancement (Figs. 31.3, 31.4, 31.5, 31.6, 31.7, 31.8, and 31.9).

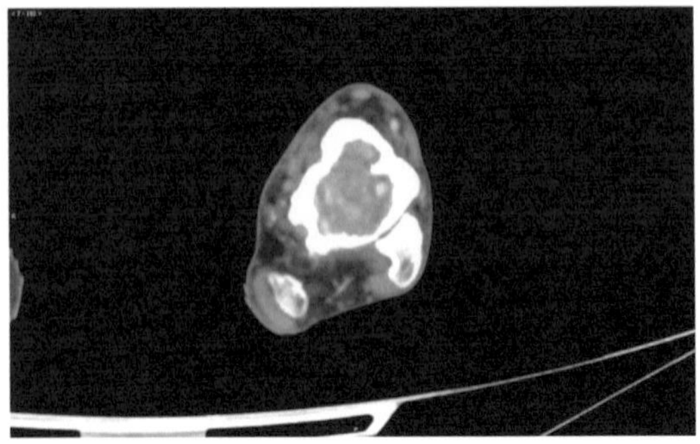

Fig. 31.5 Axial post-contrast CT image of the left ankle in soft tissue window

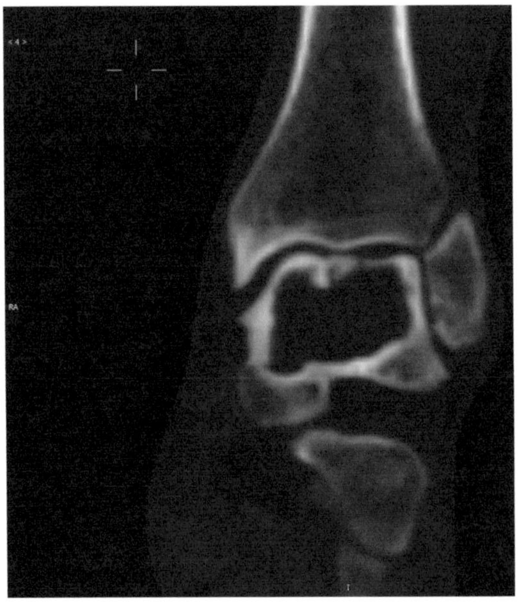

Fig. 31.6 Coronal CT image of the left ankle in bone window

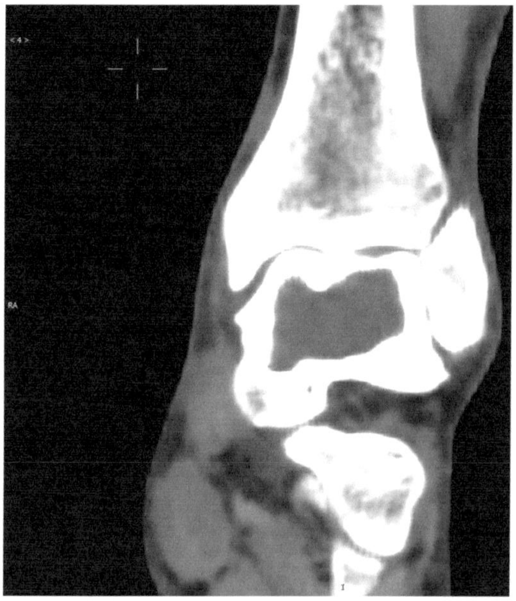

Fig. 31.7 Coronal CT image of the left ankle in soft tissue window

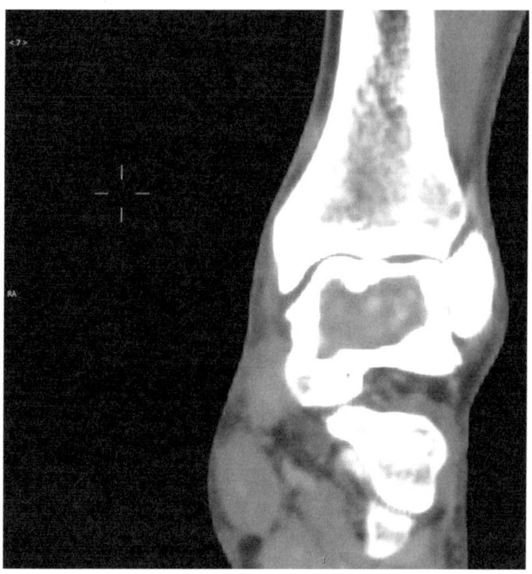

Fig. 31.8 Coronal post-contrast CT image of the left ankle in soft tissue window

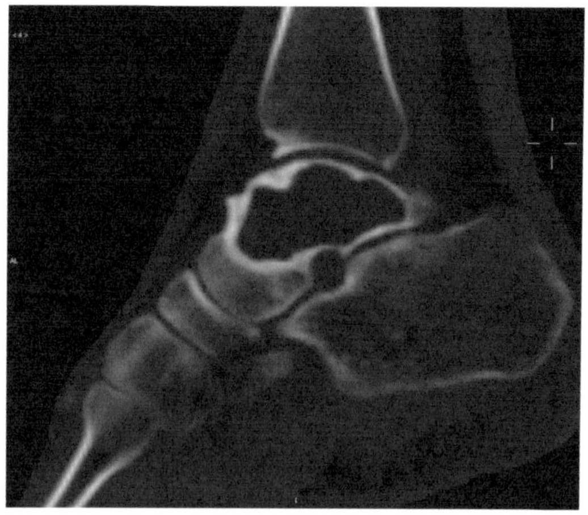

Fig. 31.9 Sagittal CT image of the left ankle in bone window

31.4 Description and Discussion from Residents

Radiographs show lytic lesion of the left talus with clear margin and suspected focal cortical disruption. The CT images demonstrated soft tissue density within the lesion with peripheral residual bone crest and nodular avid enhancement. Given patient's age, location of the lesion, and enhancement pattern, our top consideration is giant cell tumor of bone with chondroid lesion in the differential diagnosis.

31.5 Analysis and Comments from Professor Cheng Xiao-Guang

Patient is a young male. The lesion is at the left talus with lytic bone destruction and homogeneous internal density and clear peripheral sclerosis with nodular enhancement, favoring benign bone tumor. The enhancement pattern is consistent with giant cell tumor of bone; but the *lack of expansion* of the lesion, peripheral sclerosis is not consistent with typical giant cell tumor of bone. Chondroblastoma, vascular tumor are in the differential diagnoses, however the degree of enhancement associated with these two entities is usually less than giant cell tumor of bone.

31.6 Diagnosis

Giant cell tumor of bone.

Suggested Reading

Jeon JY, Chung HW, Kwon JW, et al. Imaging findings of various talus bone tumors-clinico-radiologic features of talus bone tumors. Clin Imaging. 2016;40(4):666–77.

Galvan D, Mullins C, Dudrey E, et al. Giant cell tumor of the talus: A case report. Radiol Case Rep. 2020;15(7):825–831.

Giant Cell Tumor of Bone: Case 7

32

32.1 Medical History

Patient is a 30-year-old male. He sprained his left foot about 2 years ago with swelling and no significant pain and no fever. The swelling worsened about 6 months ago, and he was seen at a local hospital and radiographs showed lesion at the left cuboid.

32.2 Physical Examination

Mild swelling around the lateral aspect of the left foot with focal palpable hard mass with indistinct border and positive point tenderness.

32.3 Imaging Findings

32.3.1 Radiograph

Radiographs of the left foot demonstrated lytic bone destruction of the left cuboid with internal heterogeneous density and patchy high density and clear margin with peripheral sclerosis (Figs. 32.1 and 32.2).

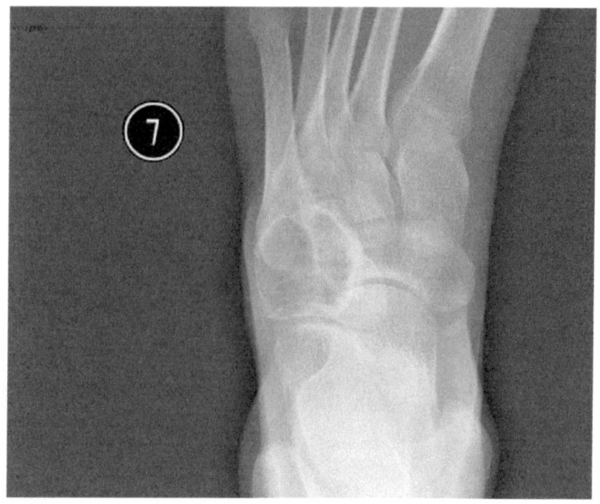

Fig. 32.1 Frontal view of the left foot

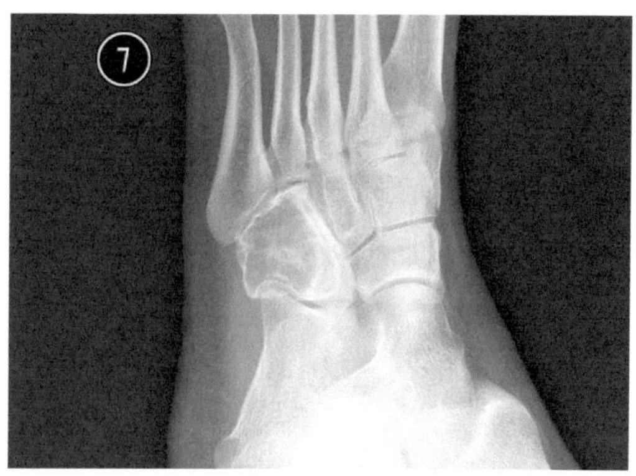

Fig. 32.2 Oblique view of the left foot

32.3.2 CT Imaging

CT images of the left foot demonstrated bone destruction of the cuboid with mild expansion, internal slight heterogeneous density with multiple septations and some septations are calcified and some peripheral sclerosis. No periosteal

X. Cheng et al., *Imaging of Bone Tumors in Wrist, Hand, Ankle and Foot*,
https://doi.org/10.1007/978-981-99-6407-9_32

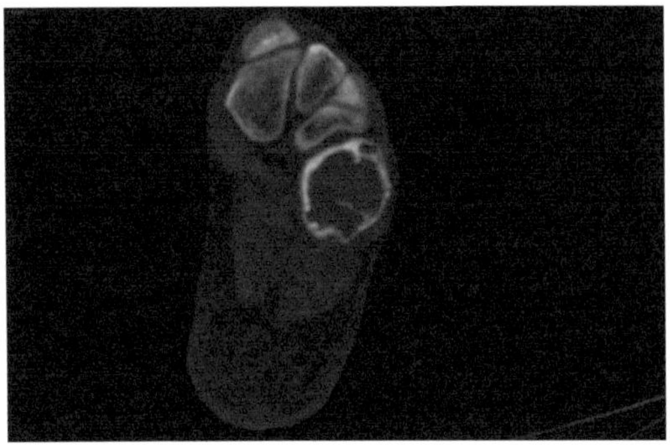

Fig. 32.3 Axial CT image of the left foot in bone window

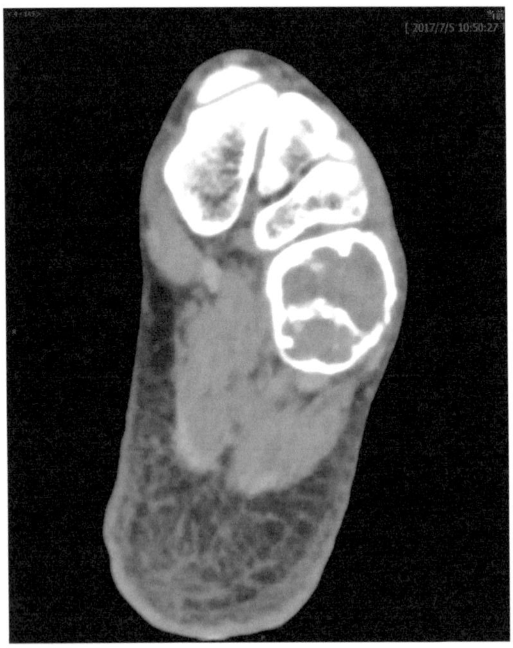

Fig. 32.4 Axial CT image of the left foot in soft tissue window

reaction or associated soft tissue mass is noted. Enhancements are noted around the septations (Figs. 32.3, 32.4, 32.5, 32.6, 32.7, and 32.8).

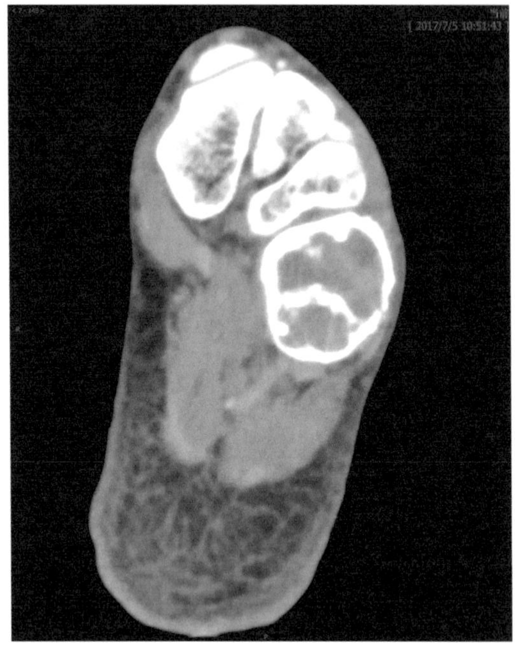

Fig. 32.5 Axial post-contrast CT image of the left foot in soft tissue window

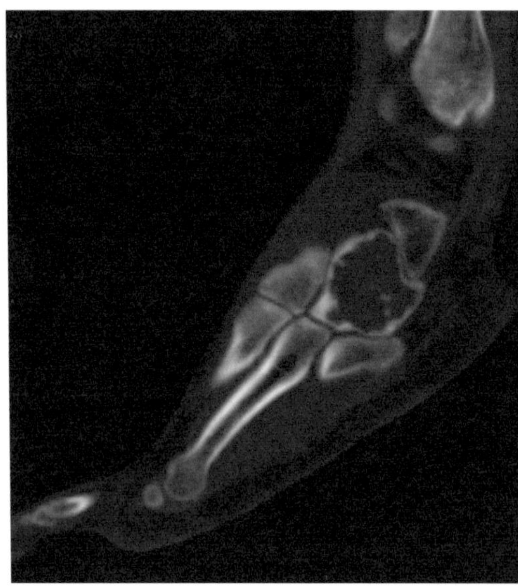

Fig. 32.6 Sagittal CT image of the left foot in bone window

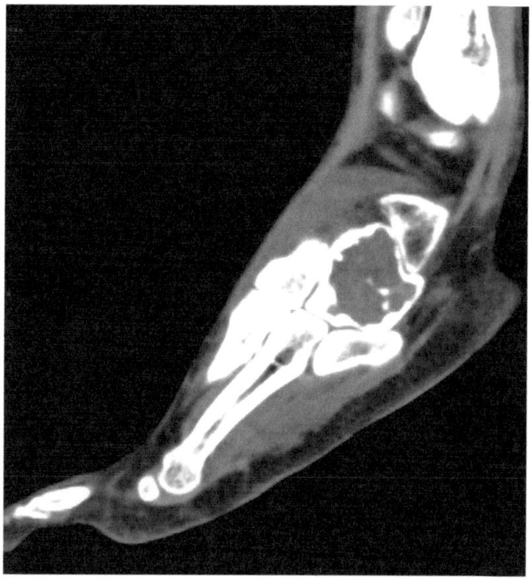

Fig. 32.7 Sagittal CT image of the left foot in soft tissue window

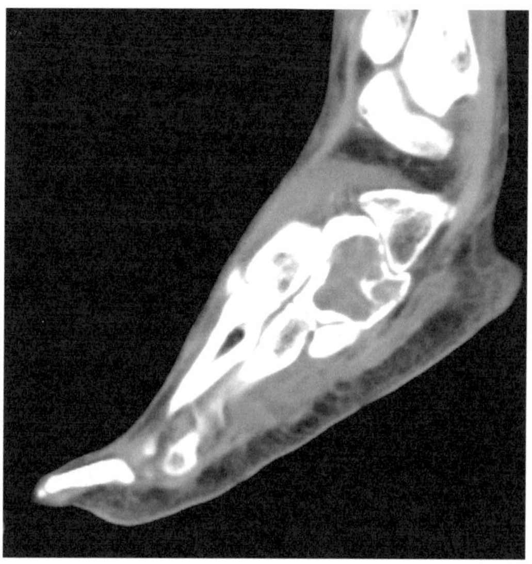

Fig. 32.8 Sagittal post-contrast CT image of the left foot in soft tissue window

32.4 Description and Discussion from Residents

Radiographs showed lytic lesion of the left cuboid with internal residual patchy bone crest and peripheral sclerosis. There were thinning of the cortex without disruption with clear margin and smooth articular surface. CT images showed internal heterogeneous densities with multiple areas of cystic low densities and scattered patchy high densities (could be residual bone or calcification) and mild enhancement. Given the above findings, this is likely a benign bone neoplasm or neoplasm-like lesion. Our top consideration is aneurysmal bone cyst and giant cell tumor of bone, chondroblastoma, and other non-aggressive bone neoplasm in the differential diagnoses.

32.5 Analysis and Comments from Professor Cheng Xiao-Guang

Patient is a young male. Radiographs demonstrated expansile lytic bone destruction of the cuboid with peripheral sclerosis and clear margin with preserved articular surface, favoring benign (non-aggressive) bone neoplasm, or neoplasm-like lesion. CT images show internal heterogeneous density with residual bone crest and scattered calcification and mild enhancement, suggesting chondroid lesion with giant cell tumor of bone and aneurysmal bone cyst in the differential diagnoses. Typically, there is avid enhancement with classic giant cell tumor of bone, not seen in the current case.

32.6 Diagnosis

Giant cell tumor of bone.

Suggested Reading

Nishibori H, Kato H, Kawaguchi M, et al. T2*-weighted MR imaging findings of giant cell tumors of bone: radiological-pathological correlation. Jpn J Radiol. 2019;37(6):473–480.

Paul AJ, Shreemal BB, Titus VTK. Foot and ankle giant cell tumors are not so aggressive after all: A retrospective study. J Foot Ankle Surg. 2021;60(1):176–181.

33 Intraosseous Lipoma: Case 8

33.1 Medical History

Patient is a 50-year-old female. She had discomfort around the left heel with swelling for more than 4 months and worsened for 2 months.

33.2 Physical Examination

Apparent point tenderness around the anterior inferior aspect of the left lateral ankle.

33.3 Imaging Findings

33.3.1 Radiograph

Radiographs demonstrated focal lucency at the left calcaneus with clear margin, peripheral sclerosis with intact cortex and no related periosteal reaction (Figs. 33.1 and 33.2).

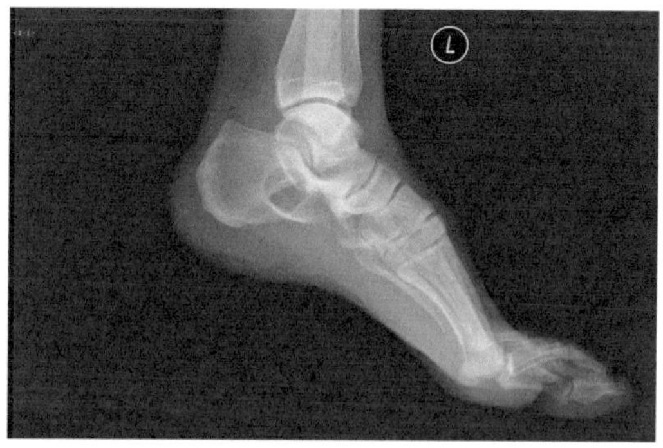

Fig. 33.1 Lateral view of the left foot

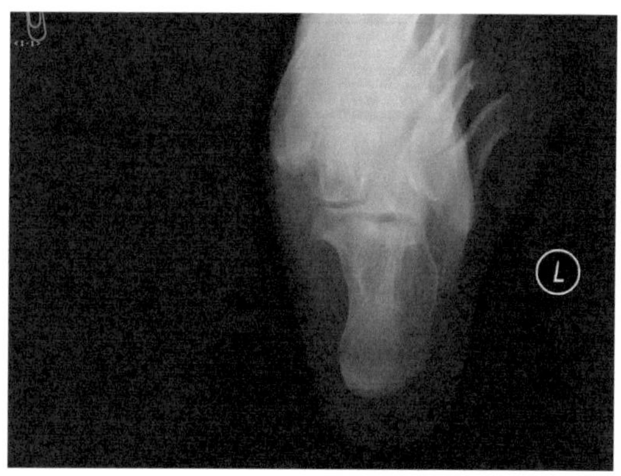

Fig. 33.2 Axial view of the left calcaneus

X. Cheng et al., *Imaging of Bone Tumors in Wrist, Hand, Ankle and Foot*,
https://doi.org/10.1007/978-981-99-6407-9_33

33.3.2 CT Imaging

CT images of the left foot demonstrated focal lucent lesion at the calcaneus with internal low density and focal mature fat density with clear margin and peripheral sclerosis. No enhancement was seen (Figs. 33.3, 33.4, and 33.5).

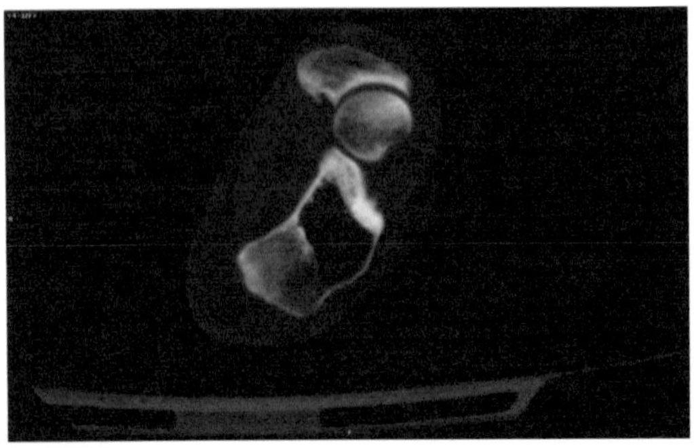

Fig. 33.3 Axial CT image of the left calcaneus in bone window

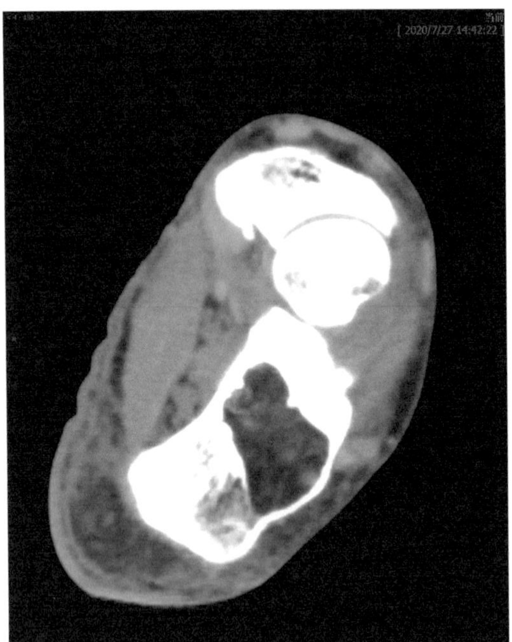

Fig. 33.4 Axial CT image of the left calcaneus in soft tissue window

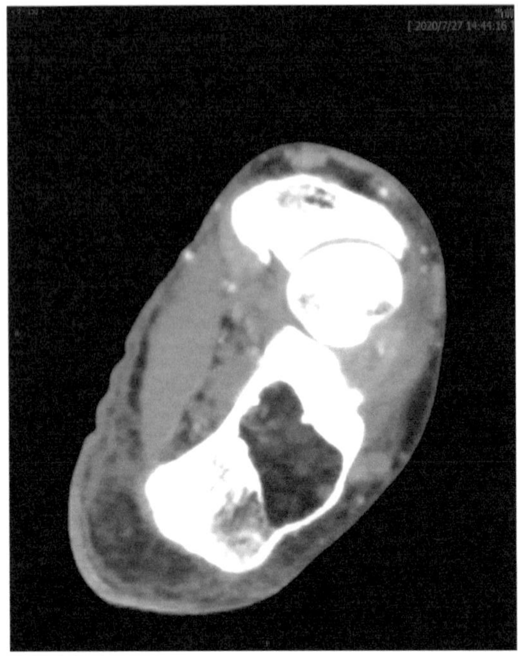

Fig. 33.5 Axial post-contrast CT image of the left calcaneus in soft tissue window

33.4 Description and Discussion from Residents

Radiographs show focal lucent lesion of the lateral left calcaneus with clear margin and peripheral sclerosis, consistent with a benign lesion. CT images demonstrated intact cortex without soft tissue swelling and predominant fat density within the lesion and no enhancement, consistent with intraosseous lipoma. Physiological decreased bone density in the calcaneus is in the differential diagnose. However, there was clear bone destruction with no trabeculae internally and thus, physiological decreased bone density in the calcaneus can be excluded.

33.5 Analysis and Comments from Professor Cheng Xiao-Guang

Radiographs show an asymmetrical focal lucency in the left calcaneus with clear margin, consistent with a benign lesion. There was internal mixed fat and fibrous tissue densities with no enhancement on CT images. Intraosseous lipoma is most common, however with internal complex densities, this could be angiolipoma. When evaluating lateral view of the radiograph, we need to remember to differentiate this with pseudocyst of the calcaneus. Similar to Ward's triangle of proximal femur, this is a region between major trabecular groups of the calcaneus and with aging and osteopenia, there will be increasing fat in the region, forming focal lucency. However, usually there is no clear border with calcaneal pseudocyst on CT images.

33.6 Diagnosis

Intraosseous lipoma.

Suggested Reading

Weinfeld GD, Yu GV, Good JJ. Intraosseous lipoma of the calcaneus: a review and report of four cases. J Foot Ankle Surg. 2002;41(6):398–411.

Azzopardi C, Patel A, James S, et al. A radiological diagnostic approach to tumours and tumour-like lesions of the calcaneus. Br J Radiol. 2021;94(1127):20210330.

34 Intraosseous Hemangioma: Case 9

34.1 Medical History

Patient is a 48-year-old female. She twisted her right foot about 1 month ago with pain and swelling without restricted range of motion. She was treated with local topical medication without relief.

34.2 Physical Examination

Point tenderness around the tip of the lateral right ankle and anterior ankle.

34.3 Imaging Findings

34.3.1 Radiograph

Radiographs demonstrated focal decreased bone density of the right calcaneus with clear margin and mild peripheral sclerosis (Figs. 34.1 and 34.2).

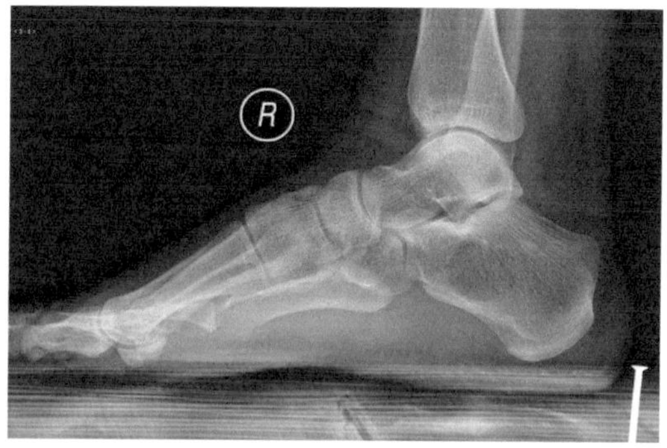

Fig. 34.1 Lateral view of the right foot

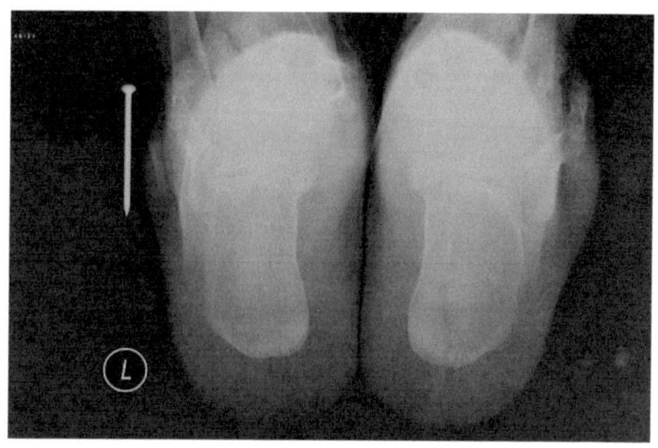

Fig. 34.2 Axial view of both calcaneus

X. Cheng et al., *Imaging of Bone Tumors in Wrist, Hand, Ankle and Foot*,
https://doi.org/10.1007/978-981-99-6407-9_34

34.3.2 CT Imaging

CT images of the right foot demonstrated low density bone destruction at the calcaneus with clear margin and focal mild sclerosis with internal heterogeneous density with predominant fat density and multiple patchy linear densities. No enhancement was seen (Figs. 34.3, 34.4, 34.5, 34.6, 34.7, and 34.8).

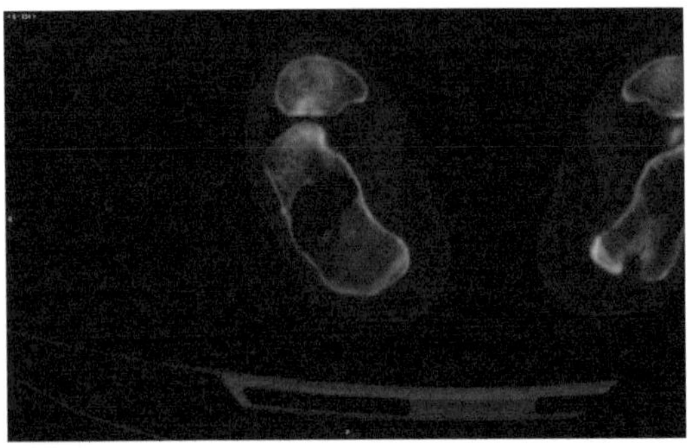

Fig. 34.3 Axial CT image of the right foot in bone window

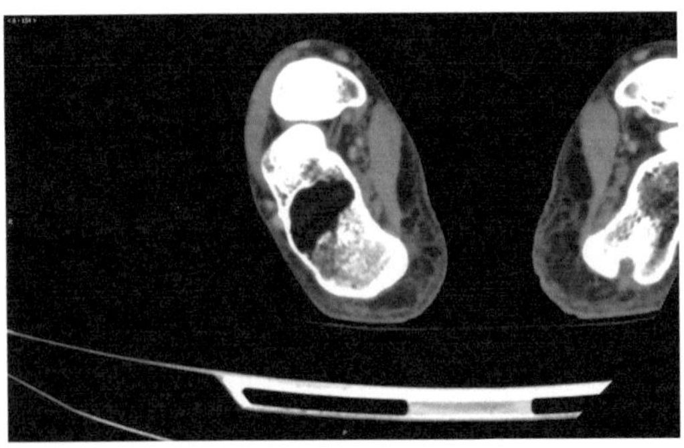

Fig. 34.4 Axial CT image of the right foot in soft tissue window

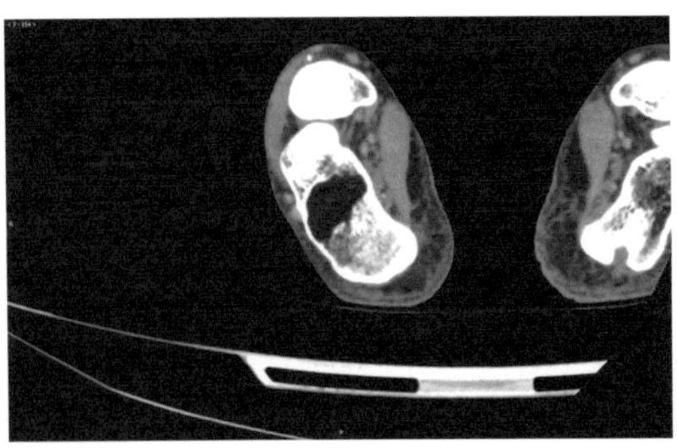

Fig. 34.5 Axial post-contrast CT image of the right foot in soft tissue window

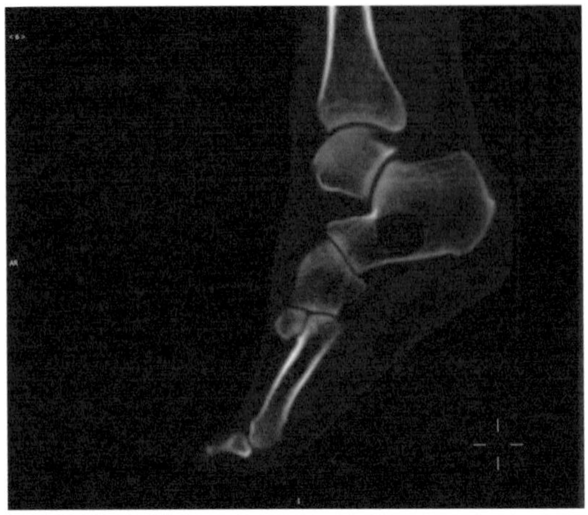

Fig. 34.6 Sagittal CT image of the right foot in bone window

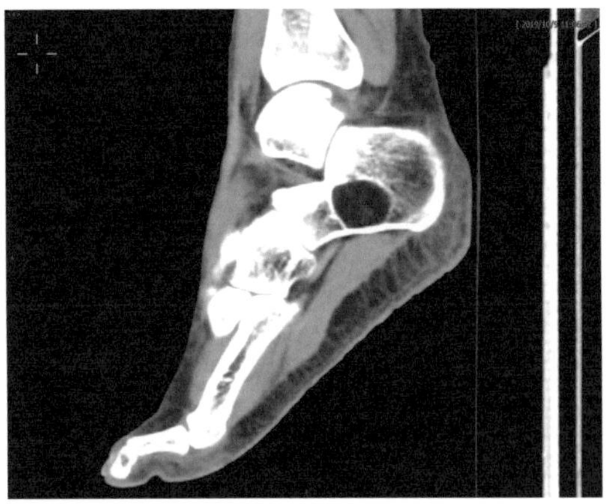

Fig. 34.7 Sagittal CT image of the right foot in soft tissue window

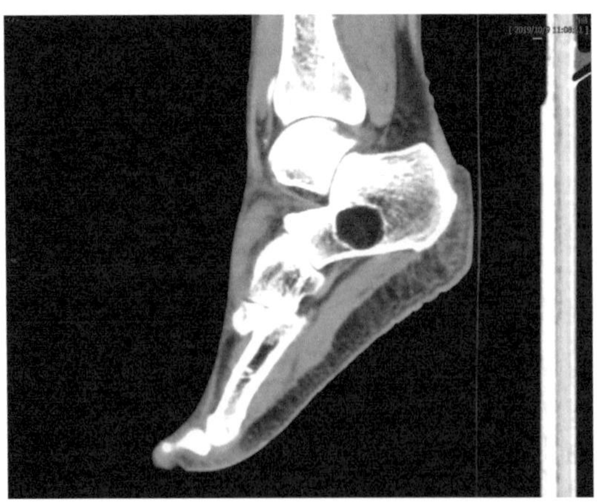

Fig. 34.8 Sagittal post-contrast CT image of the right foot in soft tissue window

34.4 Description and Discussion from Residents

Radiographs show focal lucent bone destruction with clear, sharp margin, and subtle peripheral sclerosis. Internal predominant fat density with some fibrous densities was noted on CT images, and no enhancement was seen. Our top consideration is intraosseous lipoma with liposclerosing myxofibrous tumor and vascular lesion in the differential diagnoses.

34.5 Analysis and Comments from Professor Cheng Xiao-Guang

Radiographs show low density bone destruction in the right calcaneus with clear margin and can be seen in simple bone cyst, intraosseous lipoma, intraosseous hemangioma, calcaneal pseudocyst. Internal predominant fat was noted on the CT scan without enhancement, consistent with benign lesion. My top consideration is intraosseous lipoma; however, the final diagnoses will be based on pathology.

34.6 Diagnosis

Intraosseous hemangioma.

Suggested Reading

Hod N, Ashkenazi I, Cohen I, et al. Interesting appearance of osseous hemangioma of the calcaneus on bone scintigraphy: correlative imaging with radiography CT and MRI. Clin Nucl Med. 2006;31(7):420–2.

Azzopardi C, Patel A, James S, et al. A radiological diagnostic approach to tumours and tumour-like lesions of the calcaneus. Br J Radiol. 2021;94(1127):20210330.

35 Osteosarcoma: Case 10

35.1 Medical History

Patient is a 55-year-old male. He was seen at the outpatient clinic for right calcaneal destruction with pain for half a year.

35.2 Physical Examination

Not done.

35.3 Imaging Findings

35.3.1 Radiograph

Radiographs demonstrated mixed sclerotic and lytic bone destruction at the posterior inferior right calcaneus. There was internal heterogeneous density with focal globular sclerosis (Figs. 35.1 and 35.2).

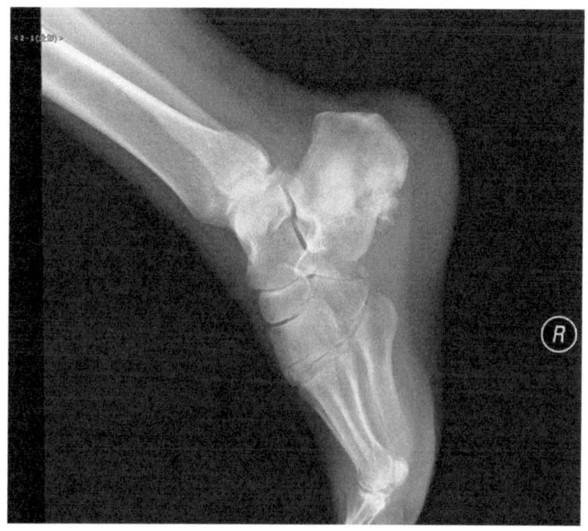

Fig. 35.1 Lateral view of the right foot

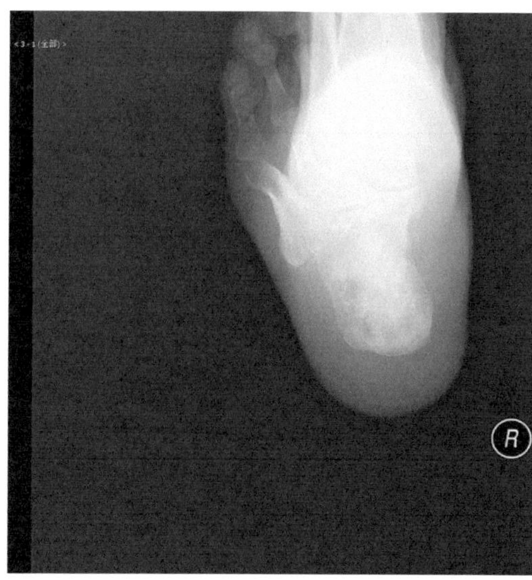

Fig. 35.2 Axial view of the right calcaneus

X. Cheng et al., *Imaging of Bone Tumors in Wrist, Hand, Ankle and Foot*,
https://doi.org/10.1007/978-981-99-6407-9_35

35.3.2 CT Imaging

CT images of the right foot demonstrated bone forming destruction at the calcaneus with irregular periosteal reaction and soft tissue mass. Heterogeneous enhancement was noted at the soft tissue mass with avid enhancement peripherally (Figs. 35.3, 35.4, 35.5, 35.6, 35.7, 35.8, and 35.9).

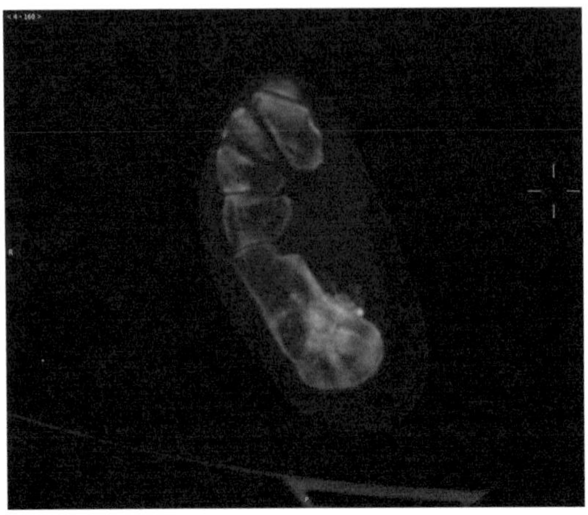

Fig. 35.3 Axial CT image of the right calcaneus in bone window

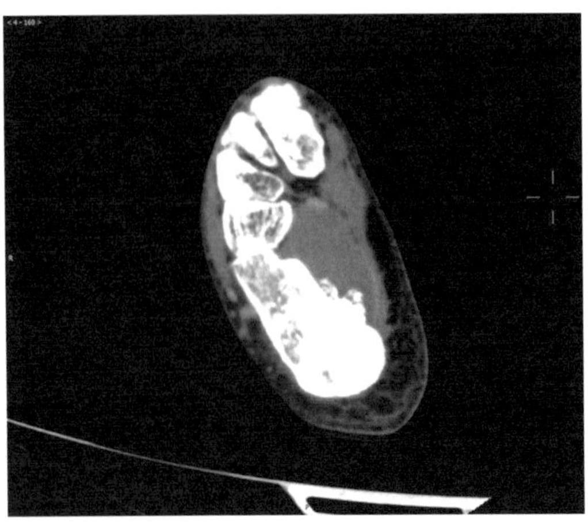

Fig. 35.4 Axial CT image of the right calcaneus in soft tissue window

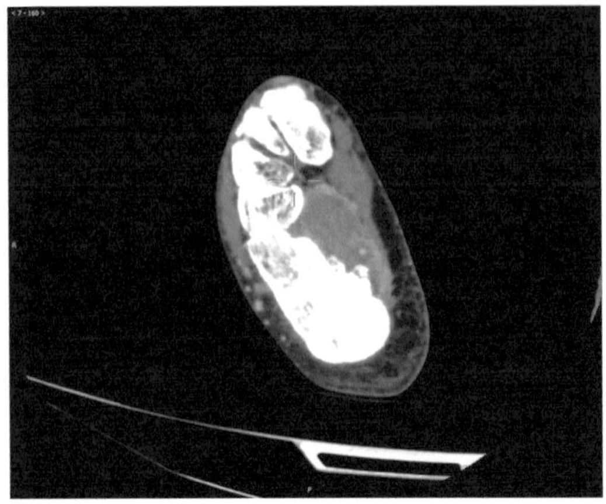

Fig. 35.5 Axial post-contrast CT image of the right calcaneus in soft tissue window

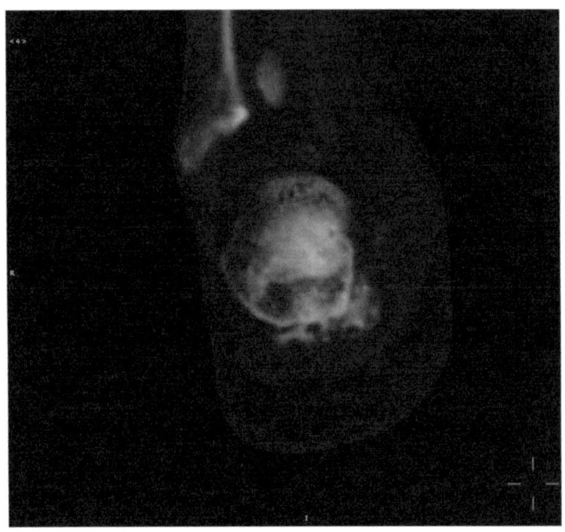

Fig. 35.6 Coronal CT image of the right calcaneus in bone window

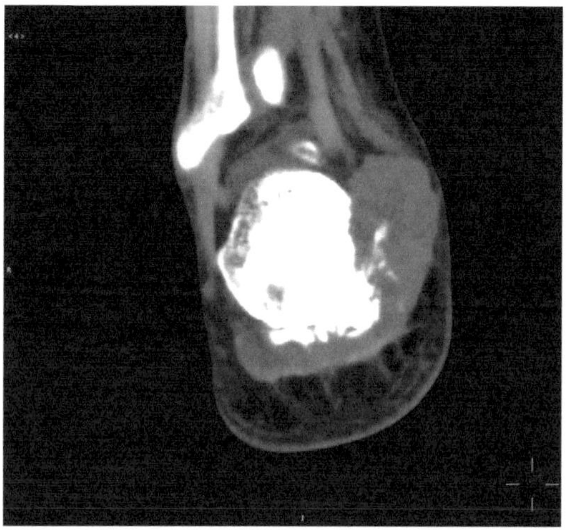

Fig. 35.7 Coronal CT image of the right calcaneus in soft tissue window

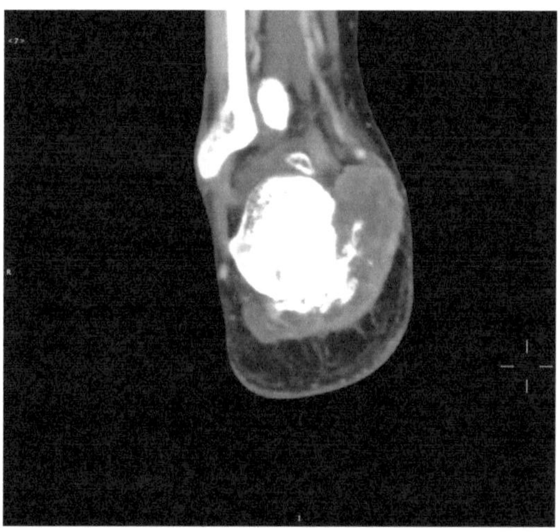

Fig. 35.8 Coronal post-contrast CT image of the right calcaneus in soft tissue window

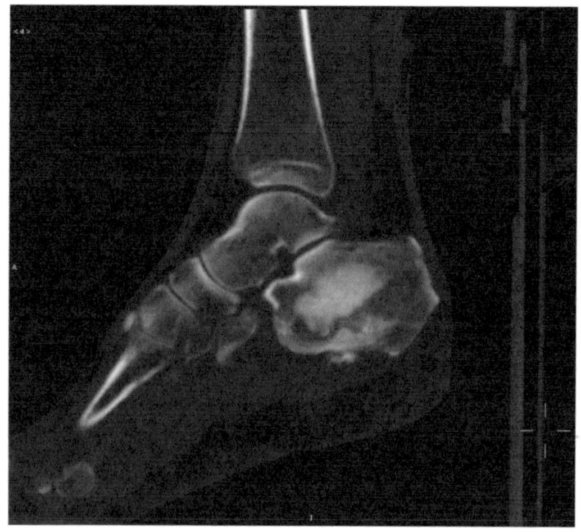

Fig. 35.9 Sagittal CT image of the right calcaneus in bone window

35.4 Description and Discussion from Residents

Radiographs show mixed bone destruction at the calcaneus with predominant bone formation and discontinuous cortex inferiorly. Soft tissue mass was noted medial to the calcaneus on CT images with mild enhancement. Given patient's age, osteosarcoma is our top consideration and osteoblastic metastatic lesion in the differential diagnose. Osteoblastic metastatic lesion is rare in the calcaneus.

35.5 Analysis and Comments from Professor Cheng Xiao-Guang

Patient is an older male. There was mixed bone destruction at the right calcaneus with soft tissue mass. Osteoid matrix production by tumor was noted (need to be differentiated from chondroid matrix) with mild enhancement of the soft tissue mass. The lesion demonstrated aggressiveness, and my top consideration is osteosarcoma with chondrosarcoma and metastatic disease in the differential diagnose.

35.6 Diagnosis

Osteosarcoma.

Suggested Reading

Choong PF, Qureshi AA, Sim FH, et al. Osteosarcoma of the foot: a review of 52 patients at the Mayo Clinic. Acta Orthop Scand. 1999;70(4):361–4.

Singer AD, Datir A, Tresley J, et al. Benign and malignant tumors of the foot and ankle. Skeletal Radiol. 2016;45(3):287–305.

36 Metastatic Disease: Case 11

36.1 Medical History

Patient is a 59-year-old female. She presented with right heel pain with history of status post-surgery from left renal cell cancer.

36.2 Physical Examination

Not done.

36.3 Imaging Findings

36.3.1 Radiograph

Radiographs demonstrated large area of decreased bone density at the right calcaneus with internal septations and inferior cortical irregularity (Figs. 36.1 and 36.2).

36.3.2 CT Imaging

CT images of the right foot demonstrated large area of lytic bone destruction at the right calcaneus with internal some linear high densities and corti-

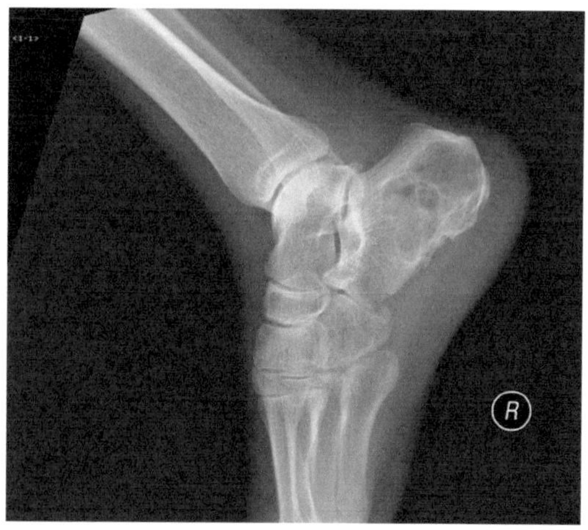

Fig. 36.1 Lateral view of the right foot

X. Cheng et al., *Imaging of Bone Tumors in Wrist, Hand, Ankle and Foot*,
https://doi.org/10.1007/978-981-99-6407-9_36

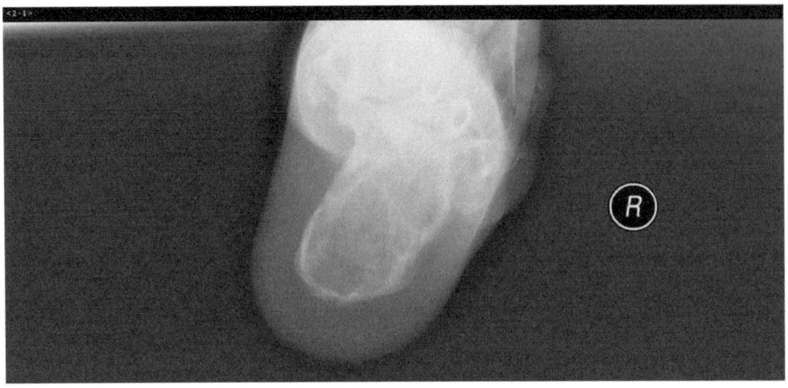

Fig. 36.2 Axial view of the right calcaneus

cal destruction with thickening of the adjacent soft tissue. Small area of avid enhancement was noted (Figs. 36.3, 36.4, 36.5, 36.6, 36.7, and 36.8).

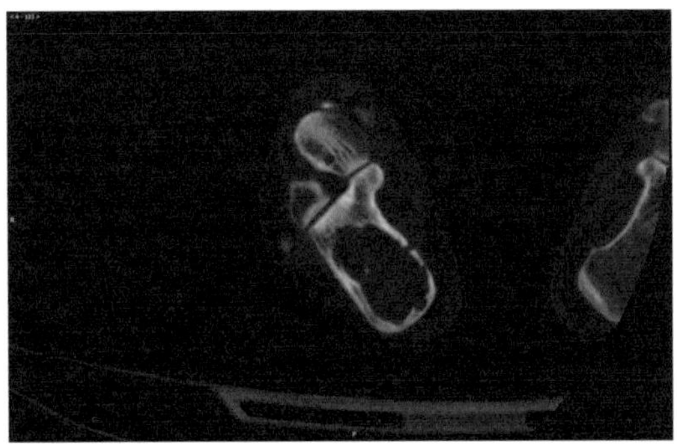

Fig. 36.3 Axial CT image of the right calcaneus in bone window

36.4 Description and Discussion from Residents

Radiographs showed lytic destruction of the right calcaneus with heterogeneous densities with indistinct margin. The lesion showed relative clear margin with peripheral sclerosis on CT images with residual bone crest and internal soft tissue densities. Majority of the lesion showed no enhancement, and no soft tissue mass was noted. The lesion did not show aggressiveness on imaging, however, with patient's age and renal cancer history, metastatic lesion cannot be excluded and giant cell tumor of bone and chondrosarcoma are in the differential diagnose.

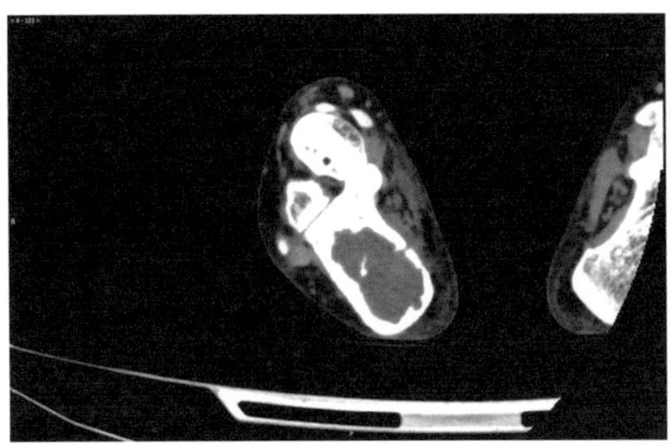

Fig. 36.4 Axial CT image of the right calcaneus in soft tissue window

36.5 Analysis and Comments from Professor Cheng Xiao-Guang

Patient is an older female. Radiographs showed indistinct margin of the lesion at the right calcaneus without clear peripheral sclerosis. Lytic

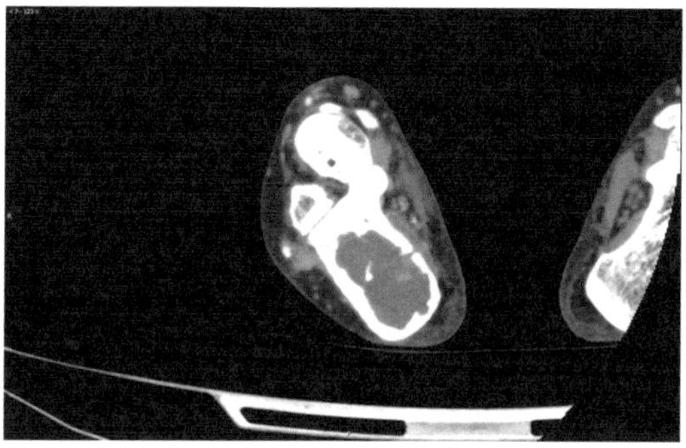

Fig. 36.5 Axial post-contrast CT image of the right calcaneus in soft tissue window

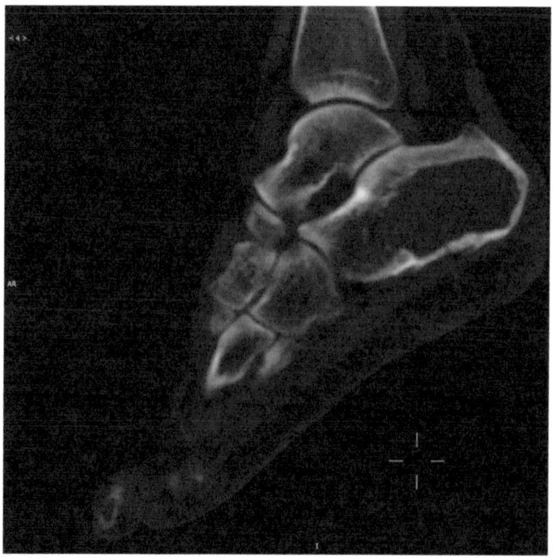

Fig. 36.6 Sagittal CT image of the right calcaneus in bone window

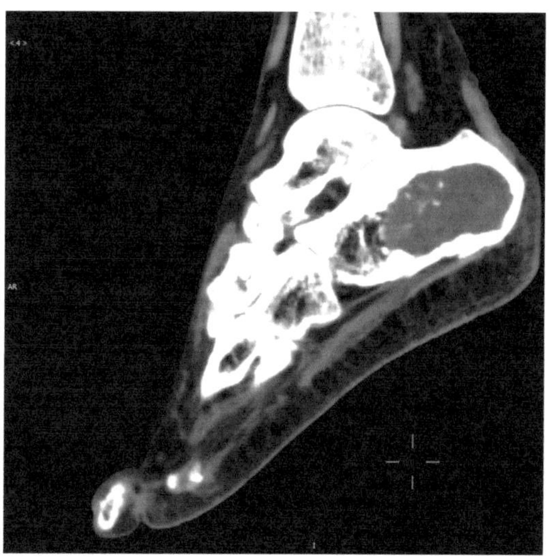

Fig. 36.7 Sagittal CT image of the right calcaneus in soft tissue window

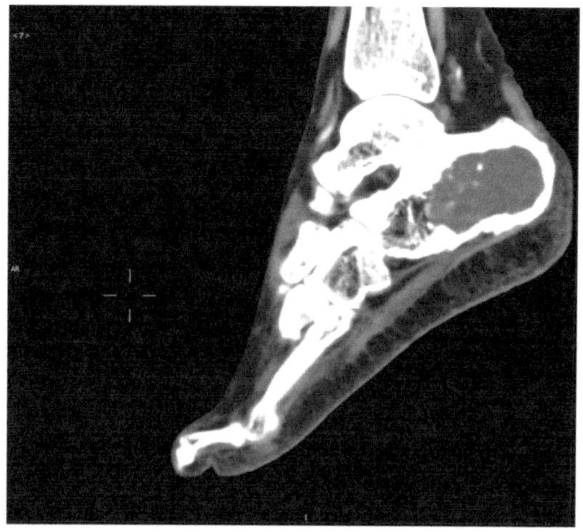

Fig. 36.8 Sagittal post-contrast CT image of the right calcaneus in soft tissue window

bone destruction was seen on CT images with internal heterogeneous densities with linear high densities and small focal enhancement. My top consideration is low grade tumor, given patient's history, metastatic disease from renal cell cancer is a possibility and chondrosarcoma is in the differential diagnose.

36.6 Diagnosis

Metastatic disease.

Suggested Reading

Decoene J, Ameye F, Lerut E, et al. Renal cell carcinoma with synchronous metastasis to the calcaneus and metachronous metastases to the ovary and gallbladder. Case Rep Med. 2011;2011:671645.

Bahrabadi M, Otoukesh B, Moghtadaei M, et al. Foot metastasis: review of 38 cases. Arch Bone Jt Surg. 2021;9(1):122–125.

Diffuse Large B Cell Lymphoma: Case 12

37

37.1 Medical History

Patient is a 51-year-old male. He had noticed left foot mass with episodic pain about 2 years ago without inciting event. He had night sweat, and the symptoms affected him walking then and he was seen at a local hospital and radiographs revealed no abnormalities. The pain at left foot worsened about 1 year ago, and it was diagnosed as gout at the local hospital and he was treated with anti-inflammatory and pain medication with mild relieved symptoms. He had an MRI at the local hospital about 1 month ago and found bone destruction around the left calcaneus with soft tissue mass.

37.2 Physical Examination

Not done.

37.3 Imaging Findings

37.3.1 Radiograph

Radiograph demonstrated diffuse decrease bone density of the left foot. There was mixed bone destruction at the anterior calcaneus with indistinct margin (Fig. 37.1).

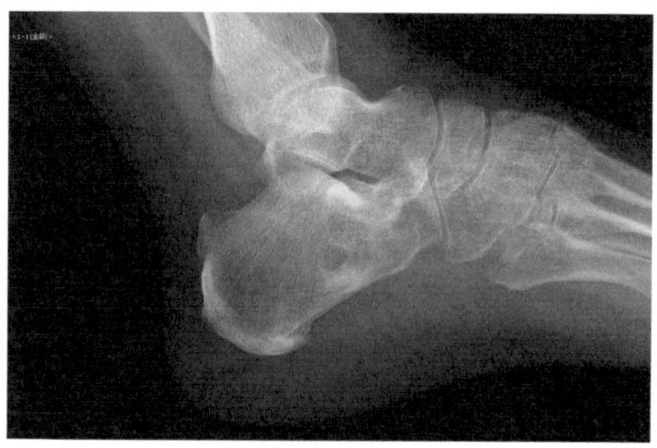

Fig. 37.1 Lateral view of the left foot

X. Cheng et al., *Imaging of Bone Tumors in Wrist, Hand, Ankle and Foot*,
https://doi.org/10.1007/978-981-99-6407-9_37

37.3.2 CT Imaging

CT images of the left foot demonstrated mixed bone destruction of the calcaneus with indistinct margin. There was permeative destruction of the cortex with soft tissue mass and mild enhancement (Figs. 37.2, 37.3, 37.4, 37.5, 37.6, 37.7, 37.8, 37.9, and 37.10).

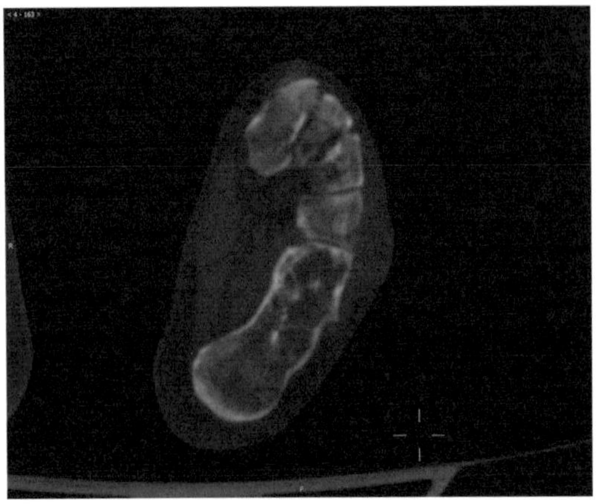

Fig. 37.2 Axial CT image of the left foot in bone window

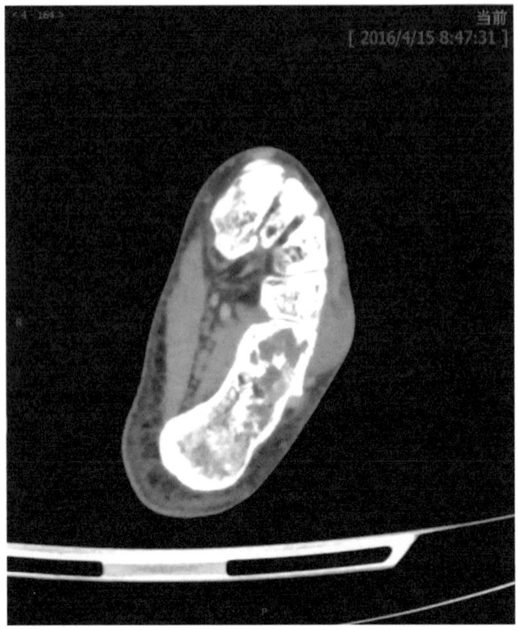

Fig. 37.3 Axial CT image of the left foot in soft tissue window

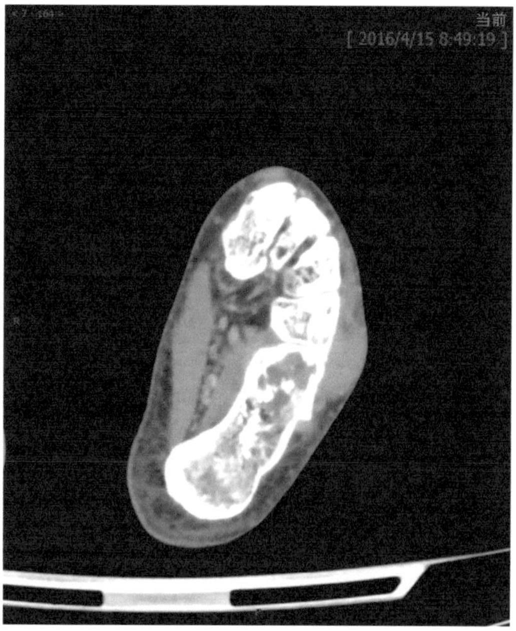

Fig. 37.4 Axial post-contrast CT image of the left foot in soft tissue window

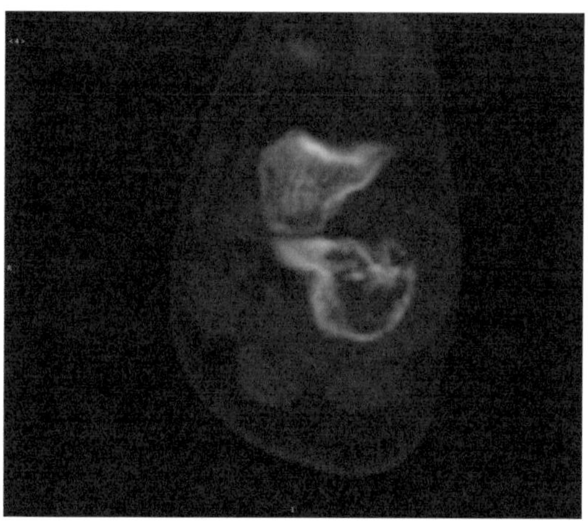

Fig. 37.5 Coronal CT image of the left foot in bone window

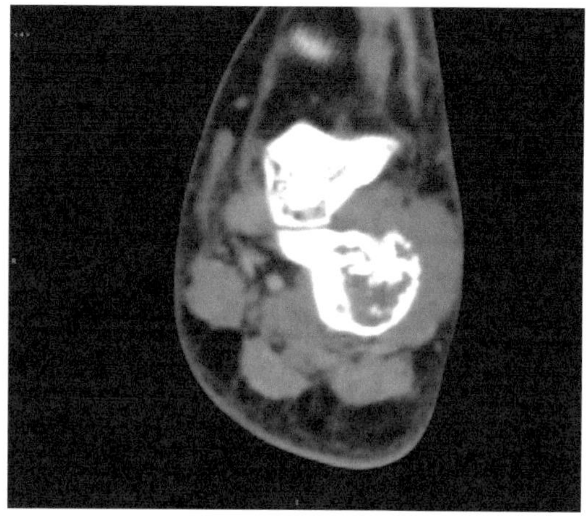

Fig. 37.6 Coronal CT image of the left foot in soft tissue window

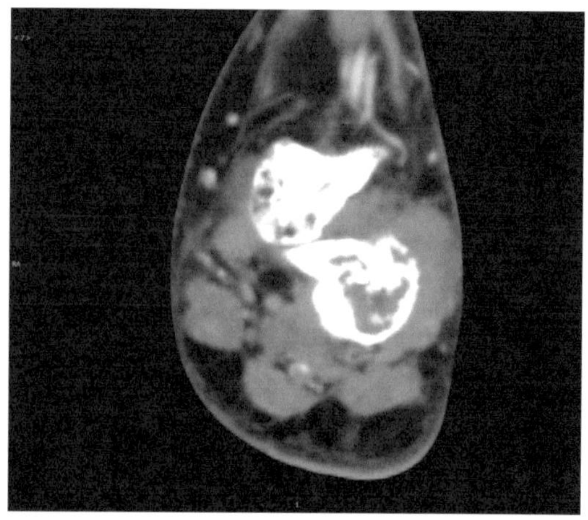

Fig. 37.7 Coronal post-contrast CT image of the left foot in soft tissue window

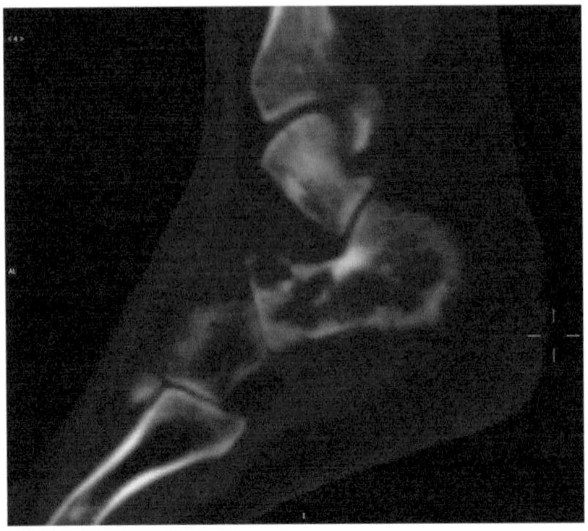

Fig. 37.8 Sagittal CT image of the left foot in bone window

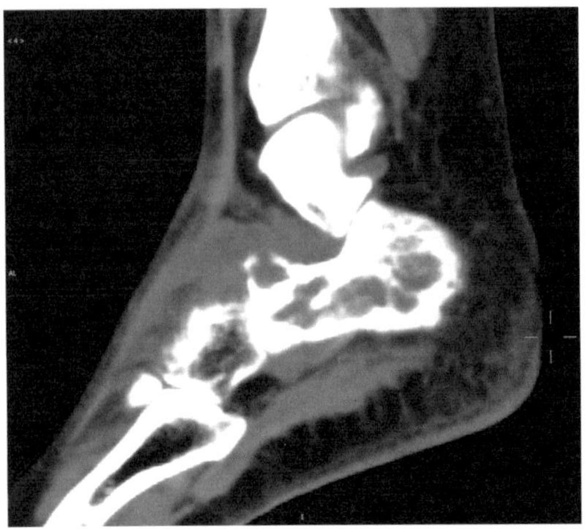

Fig. 37.9 Sagittal CT image of the left foot in soft tissue window

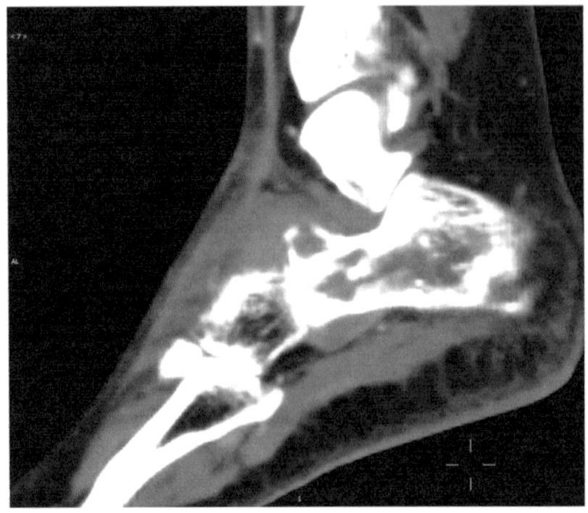

Fig. 37.10 Sagittal post-contrast CT image of the left foot in soft tissue window

37.4 Description and Discussion from Residents

Radiograph showed heterogeneous bone density at anterior left calcaneus with focal lytic bone destruction of indistinct border, favoring aggressive lesion. Multiple foci of lytic bone destruction were noted on the CT images with indistinct border. There was a soft tissue mass without apparent cortical destruction and moderate enhancement. Our top consideration is intramedullary small blue cell malignant neoplasm such as lymphoma with Ewing sarcoma in the differential diagnose. Given there was ivory like osteoblastic density, osteosarcoma is also included in the differential diagnoses.

37.5 Analysis and Comments from Professor Cheng Xiao-Guang

Patient is an older male. Multiple foci of bone destruction noted in the left calcaneus with mixed density and indistinct border and adjacent soft tissue mass with moderate enhancement and no enhancement in the region of lytic bone destruction. Given clinical history, this is consistent with a malignant tumor. Differential diagnoses include metastatic disease, osteosarcoma, and undifferentiated pleomorphic sarcoma.

37.6 Diagnosis

Diffuse large B cell lymphoma.

Suggested Reading

Krishnan A, Shirkhoda A, Tehranzadeh J, et al. Primary bone lymphoma: radiographic-MR imaging correlation. Radiographics. 2003;23(6):1371–83.

Blume P, Charlot-Hicks F, Mohammed S. Case report and review of primary bone diffuse large B-cell lymphoma involving the calcaneus. J Foot Ankle Surg. 2013;52(5):666–72.

38 Ewing Sarcoma: Case 13

38.1 Medical History

Patient is a 30-year-old female. She experienced severe left foot pain 3 years ago without clearly inciting event. The pain is not activity related and can happen at night during rest time. There was swelling at the dorsal aspect of the foot and ankle without fever or numbness. She was seen at local hospital and was treated with oral pain killer and IV fluid. The symptoms recurred. She had CT and MRI exams of the foot about 1 year ago and was notified of bone necrosis and biopsy revealed inflammation. The pain increased in severity in the past 4 months with apparent soft tissue mass with tenderness. She could not bear weight and walking. She received an open bone biopsy about 1 month ago.

38.2 Physical Examination

There was protrusion at the dorsal and plantar aspects of the left foot with palpable masses. The dorsal mass measured about 10 cm × 10 cm × 6 cm. The plantar mass measured 8 cm × 6 cm × 4 cm. There was no clear border of the masses, nonmobile, rubbery, with tenderness and local increased skin temperature.

38.3 Imaging Findings

38.3.1 Radiograph

Radiographs of the left foot demonstrated diffuse decreased bone densities. There was general thinning of the cortex. There was irregular shape of multiple tarsal bones with clear adjacent soft tissue swelling (Figs. 38.1 and 38.2).

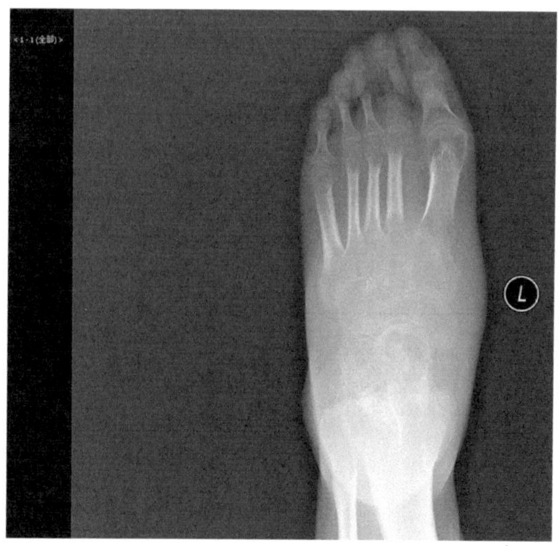

Fig. 38.1 Frontal view of the left foot

X. Cheng et al., *Imaging of Bone Tumors in Wrist, Hand, Ankle and Foot*,
https://doi.org/10.1007/978-981-99-6407-9_38

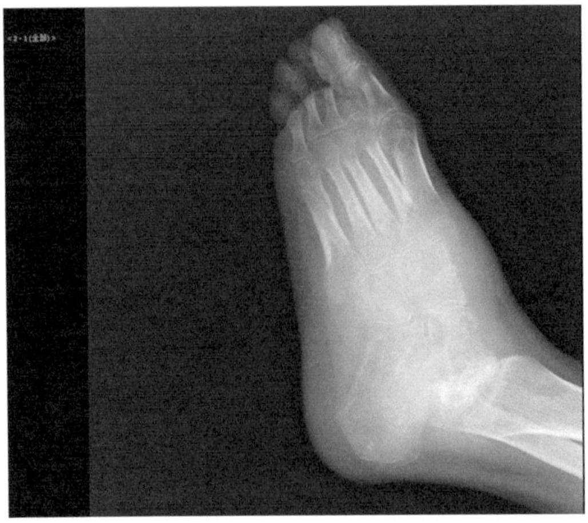

Fig. 38.2 Oblique view of the left foot

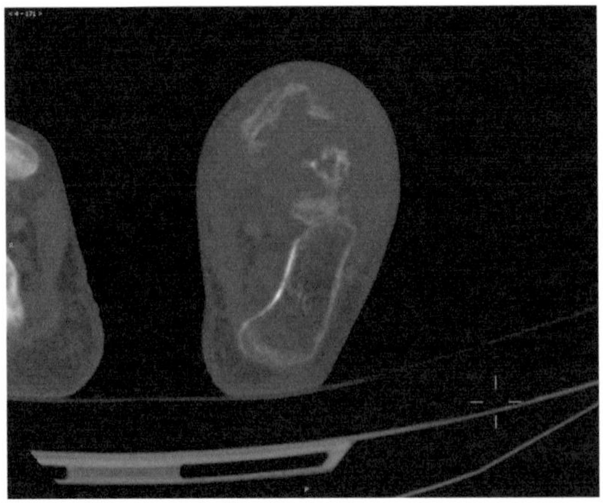

Fig. 38.3 Axial CT image of the left foot in bone window

38.3.2 CT Imaging

CT images of the left foot demonstrated lytic bone destruction of multiple bones in the mid and hindfoot with cortical thinning and focal cortical disruption with soft tissue mass. The articular surfaces were preserved. Overall, there was irregular margin and heterogenous enhancement (Figs. 38.3, 38.4, 38.5, 38.6, 38.7, 38.8, 38.9, 38.10, 38.11).

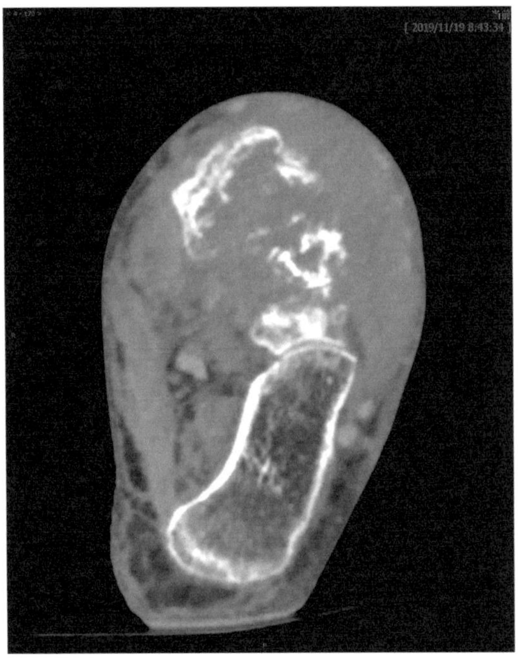

Fig. 38.4 Axial CT image of the left foot in soft tissue window

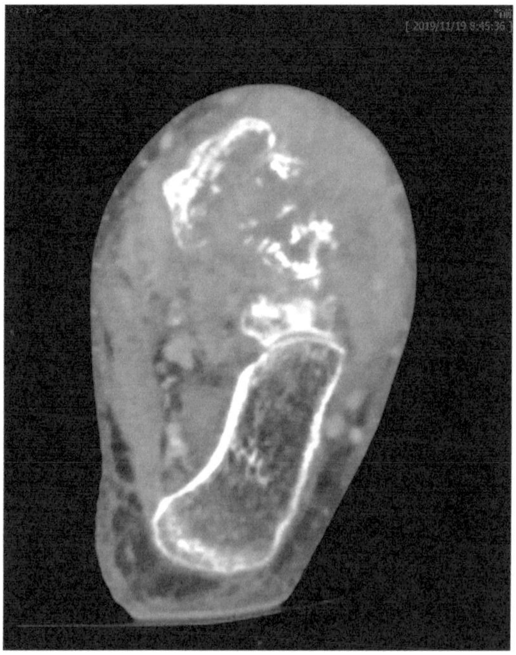

Fig. 38.5 Axial post-contrast CT image of the left foot in soft tissue window

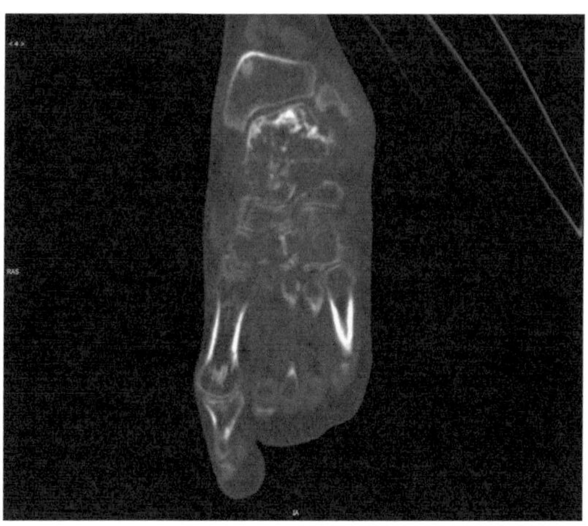

Fig. 38.6 Long axis CT image of the left foot in bone window

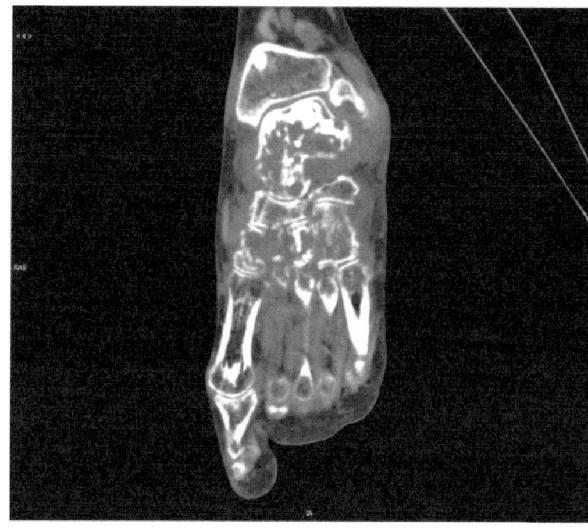

Fig. 38.7 Long axis CT image of the left foot in soft tissue window

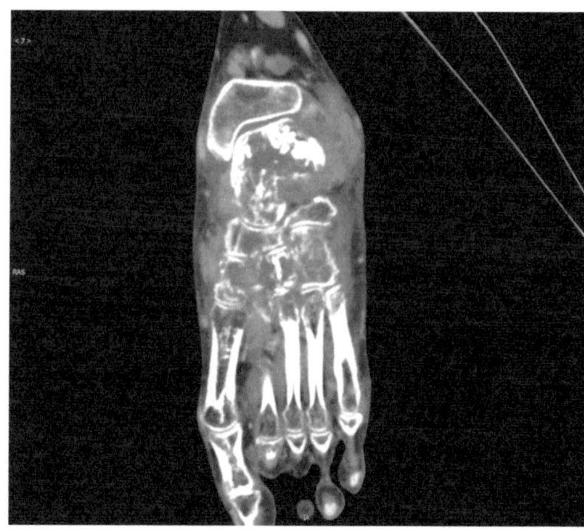

Fig. 38.8 Long axis post-contrast CT image of the left foot in soft tissue window

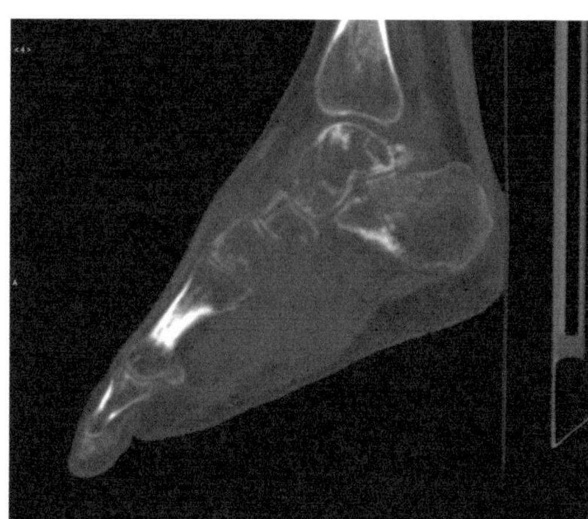

Fig. 38.9 Sagittal CT image of the left foot in bone window

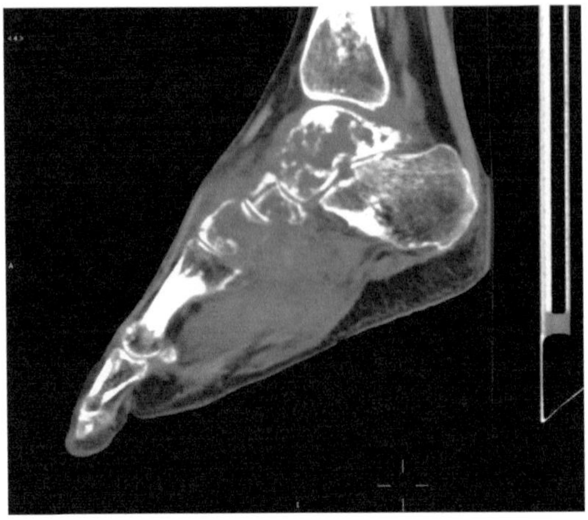

Fig. 38.10 Sagittal CT image of the left foot in soft tissue window

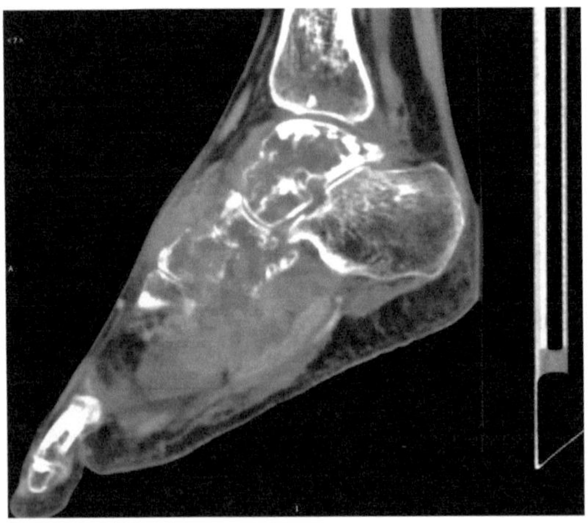

Fig. 38.11 Sagittal post-contrast CT image of the left foot in soft tissue window

38.4 Description and Discussion from Residents

Radiographs demonstrate osteopenia of the left foot, centered around mid-foot with bone destruction and soft tissue swelling. CT images demonstrate multiple bone destruction, cortical thinning, and large soft tissue mass around the tarsal bones. Overall, the lesion demonstrates heterogenous densities with heterogenous enhancement, and internal necrosis. The combination of findings is most suggestive of aggressive lesion, with inflammation in the differential diagnosis.

38.5 Analysis and Comments from Professor Cheng Xiao-Guang

The patient is a young female. Radiographs show severe osteopenia of the left foot with multiple bone destruction and apparent soft tissue swelling but preserved joint space, thus inflammatory arthropathy can be excluded. Diffuse lytic bone destruction of multiple tarsal bones on CT images with soft tissue mass and heterogenous enhancement are most suggestive of aggressive tumor. The lesion involves multiple bones, suggesting lymphoma or similar aggressive tumor. Synovial sarcoma and metastatic lesion are included in the differential diagnoses.

38.6 Diagnosis

Ewing sarcoma.

Suggested Reading

Baraga JJ, Amrami KK, Swee RG, et al. Radiographic features of Ewing's sarcoma of the bones of the hands and feet. Skeletal Radiol. 2001;30(3):121–6.

Kubo T, Furuta T, Johan MP, et al. Percent slope analysis of dynamic magnetic resonance imaging for assessment of chemotherapy response of osteosarcoma or Ewing sarcoma: systematic review and meta-analysis. Skeletal Radiol. 2016;45(9):1235–42.

39 Ewing Sarcoma: Case 14

39.1 Medical History

Patient is an 11-year-old boy. He presented with a right foot dorsal mass about 5 months ago without clearly inciting event.

39.2 Physical Examination

There was focal protuberance between the right first and second metatarsals. Prior biopsy scar was noted in the region. There was a focal palpable mass, soft, without clear margin and nontender. Normal motion preserved of the joints.

39.3 Imaging Findings

39.3.1 Radiograph

Radiographs of the right foot demonstrated cortical thickening of the second metatarsal with narrowing of the intramedullary cavity and adjacent soft tissue swelling (Figs. 39.1 and 39.2).

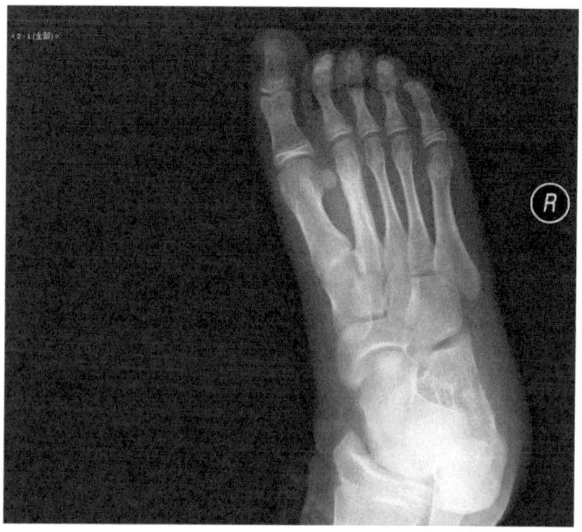

Fig. 39.1 Frontal view of the right foot

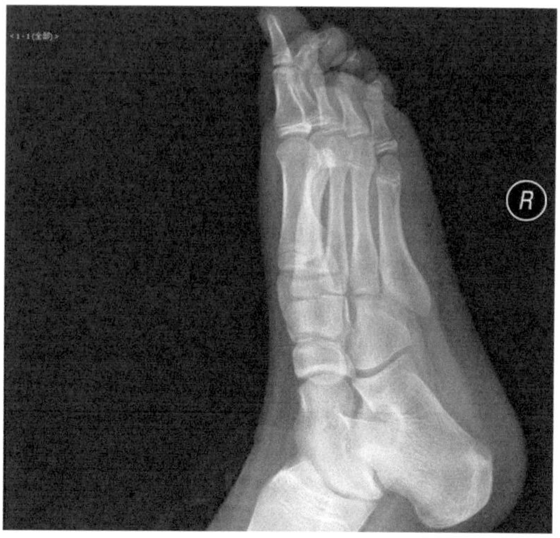

Fig. 39.2 Oblique view of the right foot

X. Cheng et al., *Imaging of Bone Tumors in Wrist, Hand, Ankle and Foot*,
https://doi.org/10.1007/978-981-99-6407-9_39

39.3.2 CT Imaging

CT images of the right foot demonstrated increased densities of the cortex and medullary cavity of the second metatarsal with surrounding soft tissue mass and peripheral mild enhancement (Figs. 39.3, 39.4, 39.5, 39.6, 39.7, 39.8, 39.9, and 39.10).

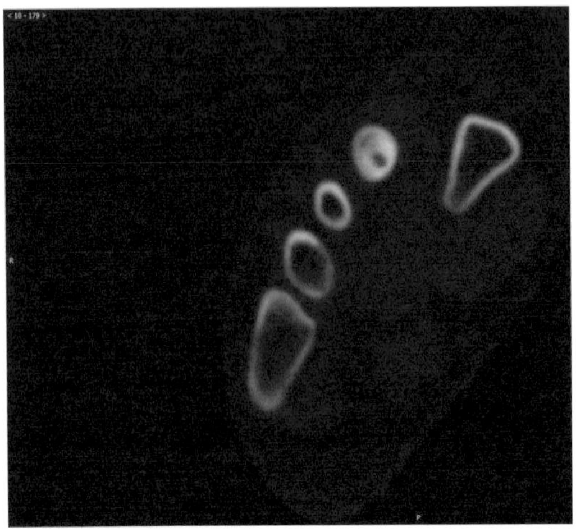

Fig. 39.3 Short axis CT image of the right foot in bone window

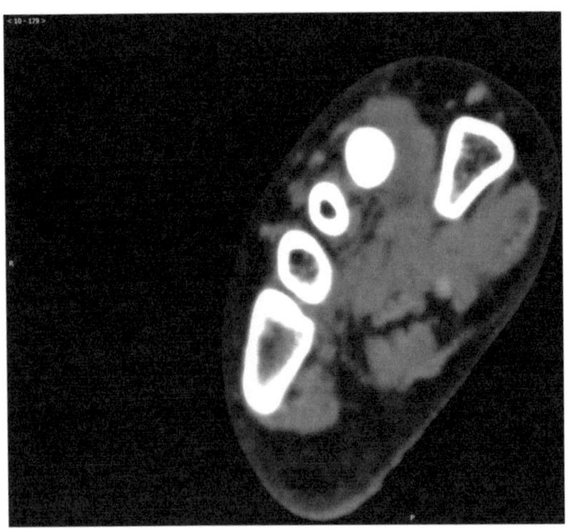

Fig. 39.4 Short axis CT image of the right foot in soft tissue window

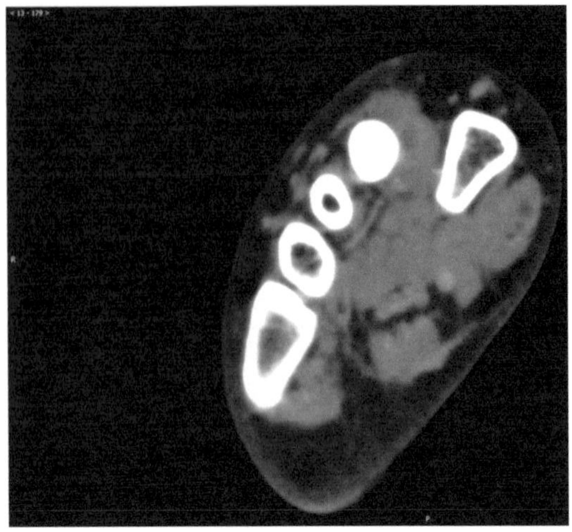

Fig. 39.5 Short axis post-contrast CT image of the right foot in soft tissue window

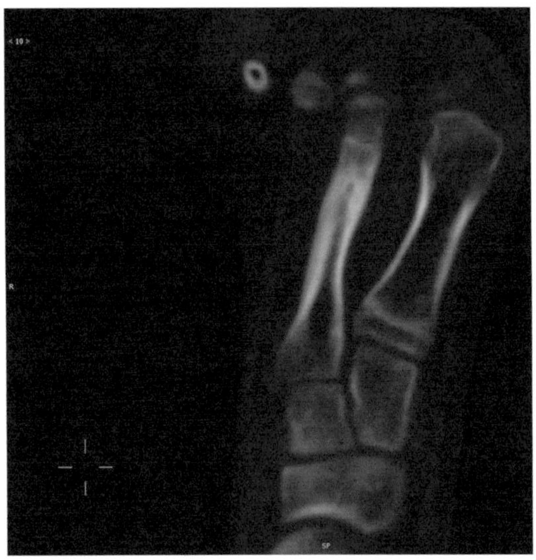

Fig. 39.6 Long axis CT image of the right foot in bone window

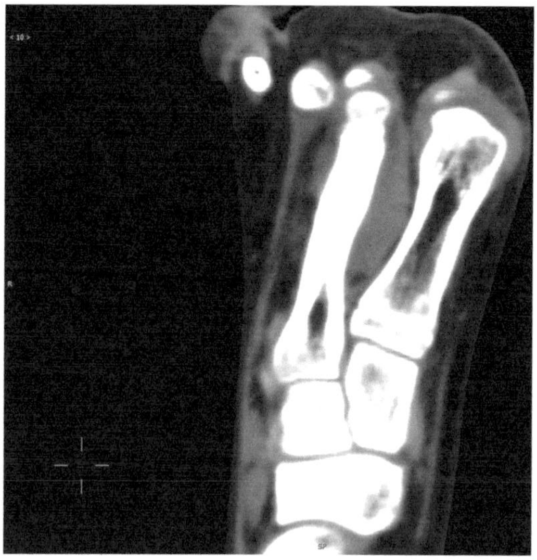

Fig. 39.7 Long axis CT image of the right foot in soft tissue window

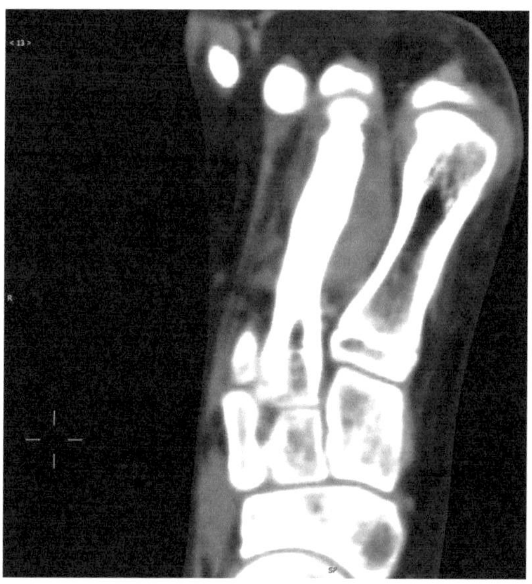

Fig. 39.8 Long axis post-contrast CT image of the right foot in soft tissue window

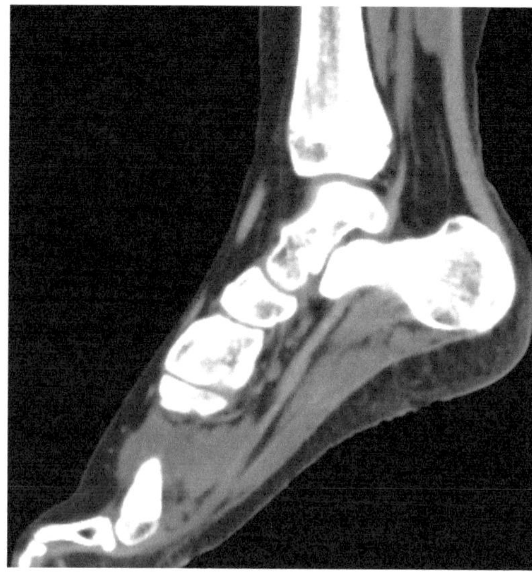

Fig. 39.9 Sagittal CT image of the right foot in soft tissue window

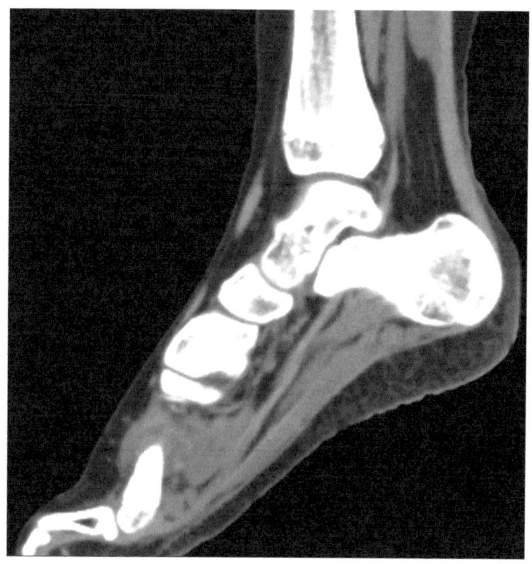

Fig. 39.10 Sagittal post-contrast CT image of the right foot in soft tissue window

39.4 Description and Discussion from Residents

The radiographs demonstrated thickening of the second metatarsal shaft with cortical thickening and narrowing of the medullary canal. There was circular cortical thickening on CT images. The soft tissue mass appeared more in the medial aspect. There was mild enhancement.

39.5 Analysis and Comments from Professor Cheng Xiao-Guang

The patient is a young boy. There was increased density of the second metatarsal of the right foot with surrounding soft tissue mass and mild enhancement on CT images. Given the patient's age and location of the lesion, Ewing sarcoma is the top consideration. Differential diagnosis includes infection and desmoid fibromatosis of soft tissue, and further evaluation with MRI would be helpful.

39.6 Diagnosis

Ewing sarcoma.

Suggested Reading

Baraga JJ, Amrami KK, Swee RG, et al. Radiographic features of Ewing's sarcoma of the bones of the hands and feet. Skeletal Radiol. 2001;30(3):121–6.

Mogavero M, Khlopas H, Fallat LM. A Rare presentation of Ewing's sarcoma presenting in the third metatarsal. J Foot Ankle Surg. 2022;61(2):421–425.

40 Myoepithelial Carcinoma of Bone: Case 15

40.1 Medical History

Patient is a 23-year-old male. He accidentally noticed a mass at the dorsum of his left foot about 3 years ago. Later, he developed pain after walking and activities with relief after rest. He sought no medical advice. The pain increased in the last 2 months, alleviated by rest.

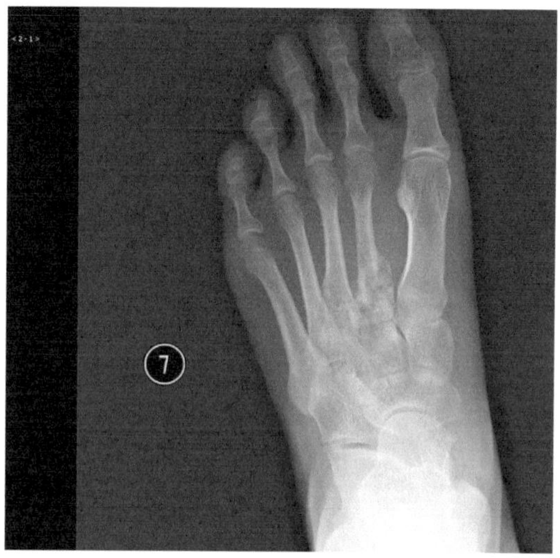

Fig. 40.1 Frontal view of the left foot

40.2 Physical Examination

There was mild swelling at the dorsum of the left foot with a deep palpable mass, measuring about 3 cm × 2 cm × 2 cm. The mass had no clear margin, hard, firm, and with tenderness.

40.3 Imaging Findings

40.3.1 Radiograph

Radiographs of the left foot demonstrated expansile bone destruction at the base and proximal shaft of the second metatarsal. Multiple patchy high densities were noted within the lesion (Figs. 40.1 and 40.2).

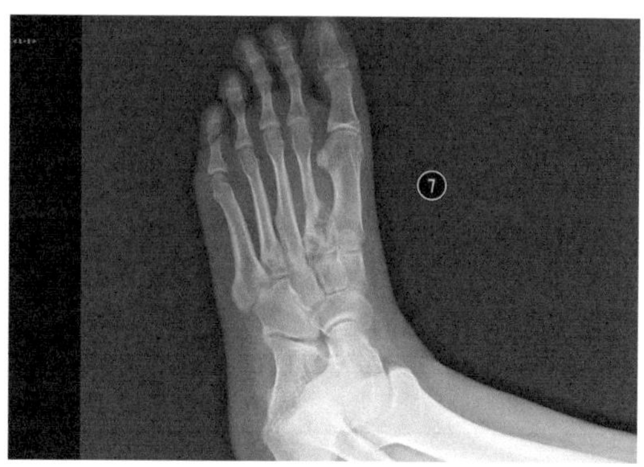

Fig. 40.2 Oblique view of the left foot

X. Cheng et al., *Imaging of Bone Tumors in Wrist, Hand, Ankle and Foot*,
https://doi.org/10.1007/978-981-99-6407-9_40

40.3.2 CT Imaging

CT images of the left foot demonstrated expansile bone destruction at base and proximal shaft of the second metatarsal with internal multiple calcifications and destruction of the cortex. There was a dorsal and lateral soft tissue mass with avid enhancement (Figs. 40.3, 40.4, 40.5, 40.6, 40.7, 40.8, and 40.9).

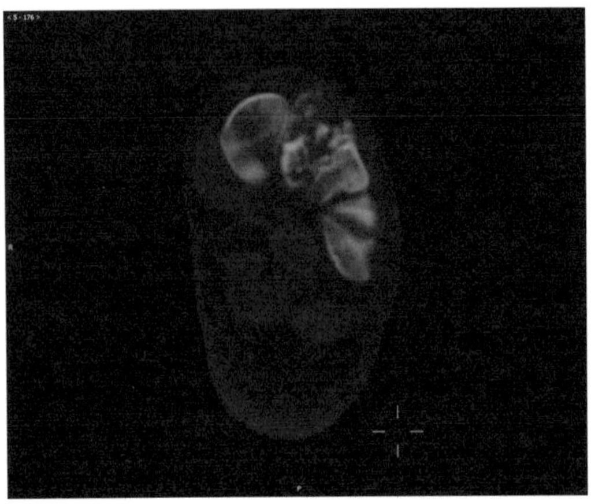

Fig. 40.3 Short axis CT image of the left foot in bone window

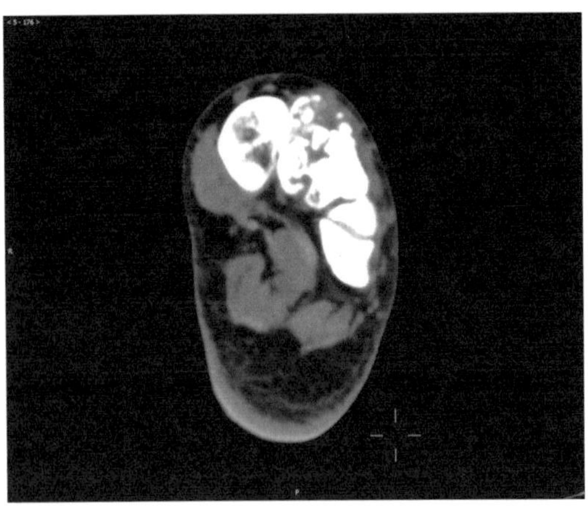

Fig. 40.4 Short axis CT image of the left foot in soft tissue window

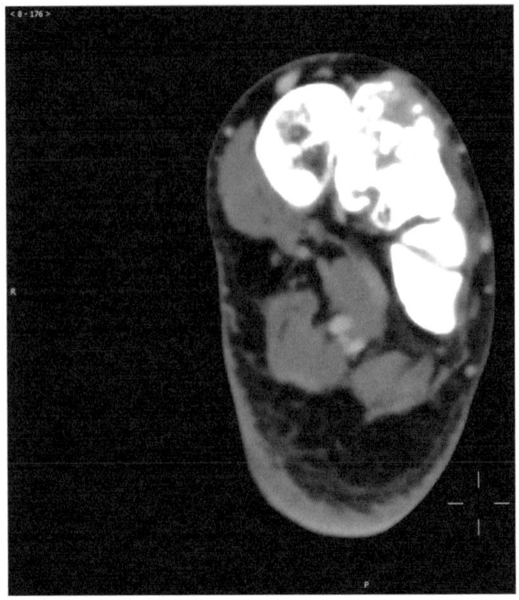

Fig. 40.5 Short axis post-contrast CT image of the left foot in soft tissue window

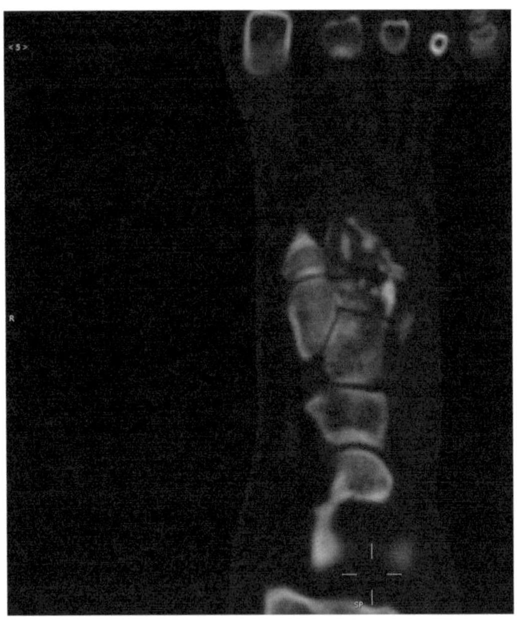

Fig. 40.6 Long axis CT image of the left foot in bone window

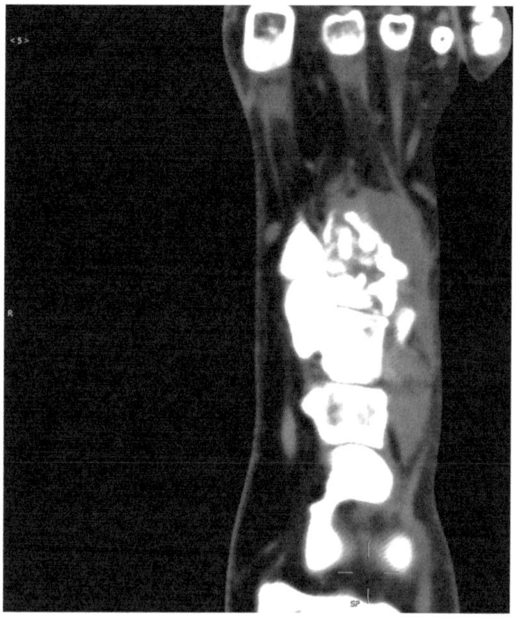

Fig. 40.7 Long axis CT image of the left foot in soft tissue window

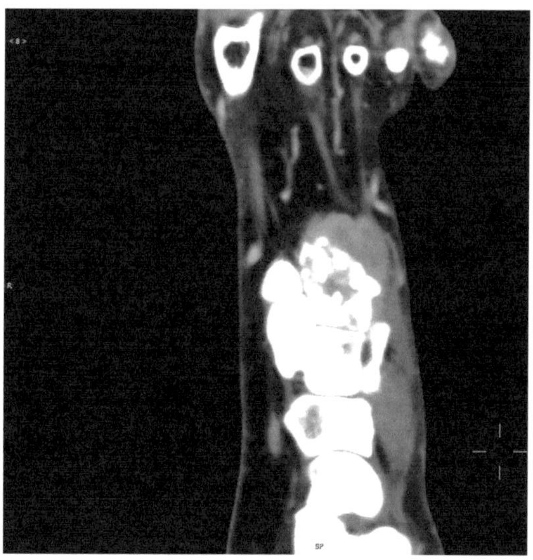

Fig. 40.8 Long axis post-contrast CT image of the left foot in soft tissue window

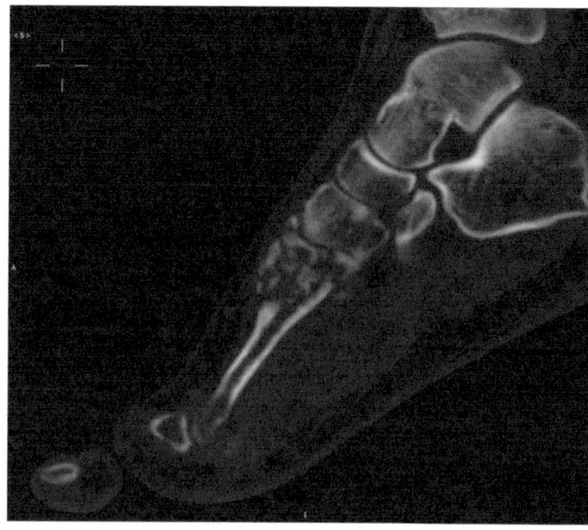

Fig. 40.9 Sagittal CT image of the left foot in bone window

40.4 Description and Discussion from Residents

The radiographs demonstrated expansile bone destruction of the second metatarsal base and proximal shaft with heterogenous densities, irregular margin, and irregular cortex, favoring benign lesion. One of the considerations is chondroid lesion. However, the irregular morphology of the multiple high densities within the lesion on CT images is different from chondroid matrix. There were cortical break and soft tissue mass with avid enhancement. Given the patient's long course of the lesion, the possibility of aggressive lesion is less, it could be infection or granulomatous lesion, with chondrosarcoma in the differential diagnosis.

40.5 Analysis and Comments from Professor Cheng Xiao-Guang

The patient is a young male with long history with the lesion. Radiographs showed bone destruction of the proximal second metatarsal with irregular margin. Multiple patchy high densities are noted on CT images with adjacent soft tissue mass and avid enhancement. The imaging findings are most suggestive of aggressive tumor such as osteosarcoma with chondrosarcoma in the differential diagnosis. However, the patient's age and the morphology of the calcification are not typical of the above entities. With long history of the lesion, non-aggressive lesion with combined pathological fracture can't be excluded. Given the patient's age and the location of the lesion, our consideration of benign lesions includes enchondroma, osteoblastoma, and chondroblastoma. With the above nonspecific imaging findings, the final diagnosis would be combined with pathology and clinical findings.

40.6 Diagnosis

Myoepithelial carcinoma of the bone.

Suggested Reading

Rekhi B, Joshi S, Panchwagh Y, et al. Clinicopathological features of five unusual cases of intraosseous myoepithelial carcinomas, mimicking conventional primary bone tumours, including EWSR1 rearrangement in one case. APMIS. 2016;124(4):278–90.

Song W, Flucke U, Suurmeijer AJH. Myoepithelial Tumors of Bone. Surg Pathol Clin. 2017;10(3):657–674.

41 Bizarre Parosteal Osteochondromatous Proliferation: Case 16

41.1 Medical History

Patient is a 33-year-old male. He started to experience discomfort at the bottom of the left foot after activities about 6 months ago. About 3 months ago, he noticed a small mass at the bottom of the mid left foot in the size of a peanut without pain at rest but became painful after activities or long-distance walking.

41.2 Physical Examination

There is a deep, palpable mass at the bottom of the left foot, measuring about 3 cm × 2 cm × 2 cm with clear margin, rubbery, non-mobile with mild point tenderness.

41.3 Imaging Findings

41.3.1 Radiograph

Radiographs demonstrated circular high densities around the third and fourth metatarsals and with adjacent cortical thickening (Figs. 41.1, 41.2, and 41.3).

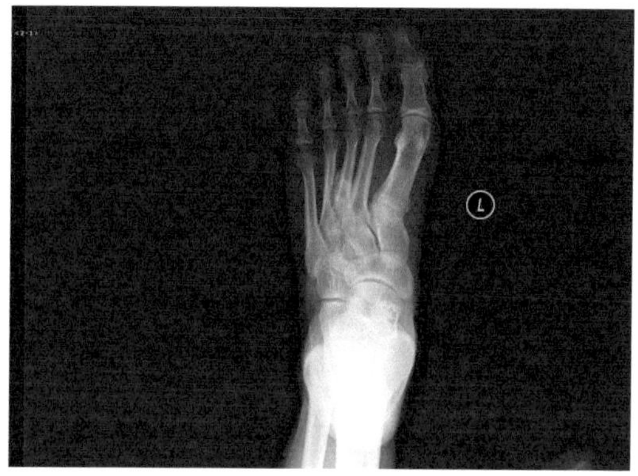

Fig. 41.1 Frontal view of the left foot

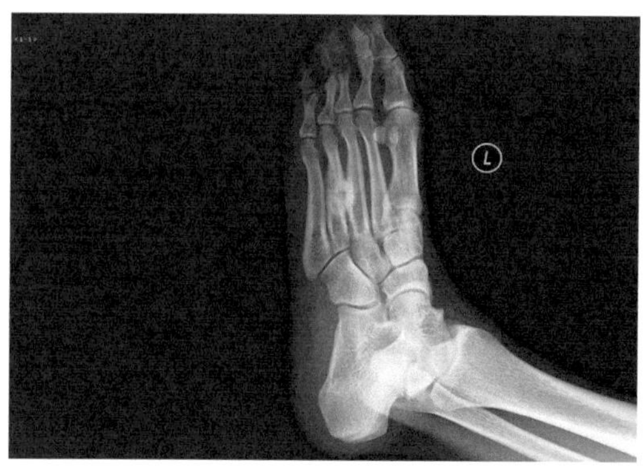

Fig. 41.2 Oblique view of the left foot

X. Cheng et al., *Imaging of Bone Tumors in Wrist, Hand, Ankle and Foot*,
https://doi.org/10.1007/978-981-99-6407-9_41

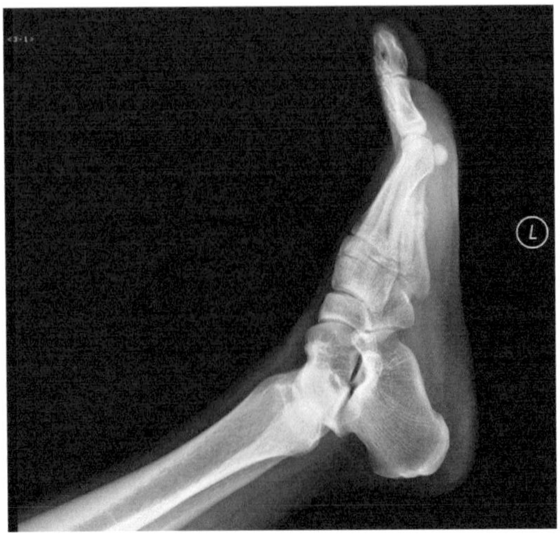

Fig. 41.3 Lateral view of the left foot

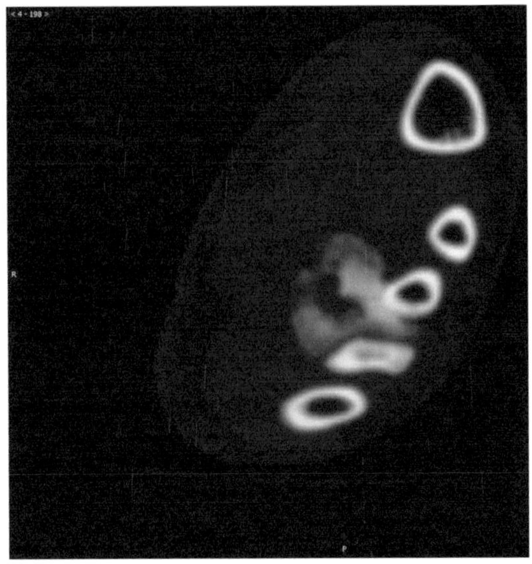

Fig. 41.4 Short axis CT image of the left foot in bone window

41.3.2 CT Imaging

CT images of the left foot demonstrated patchy bone densities around the region between third and fourth metatarsals. It appears to be connected to the third metatarsal cortex and fourth metatarsal demonstrated compression changes. There was an internal low density with irregular margin and adjacent soft tissue swelling and no clear enhancement (Figs. 41.4, 41.5, 41.6, 41.7, and 41.8).

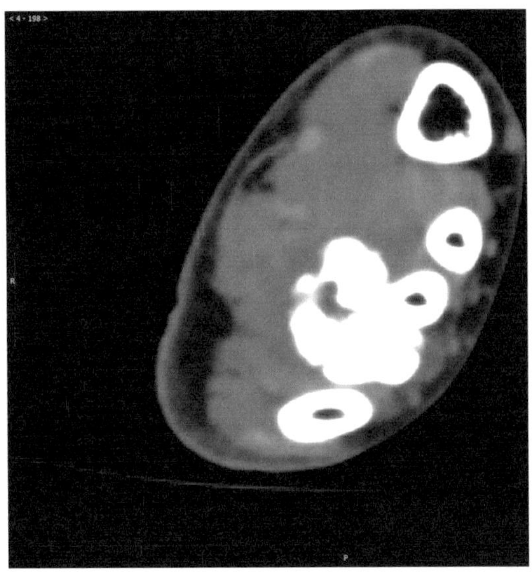

Fig. 41.5 Short axis CT image of the left foot in soft tissue window

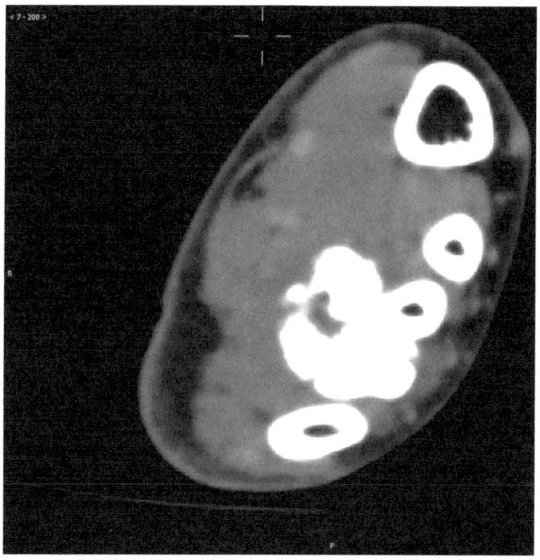

Fig. 41.6 Short axis post-contrast CT image of the left foot in soft tissue window

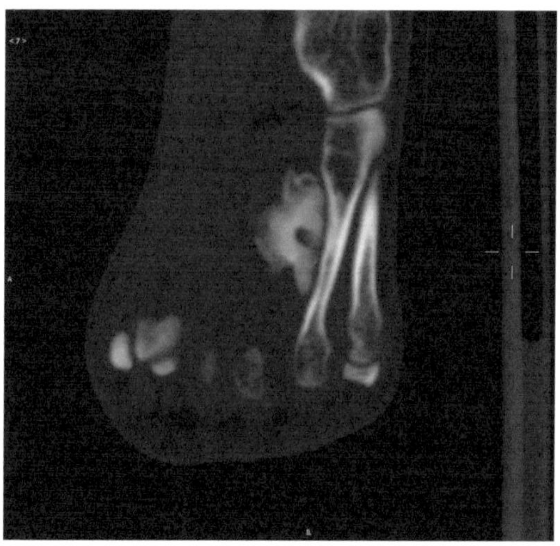

Fig. 41.7 Long axis CT image of the left foot in bone window

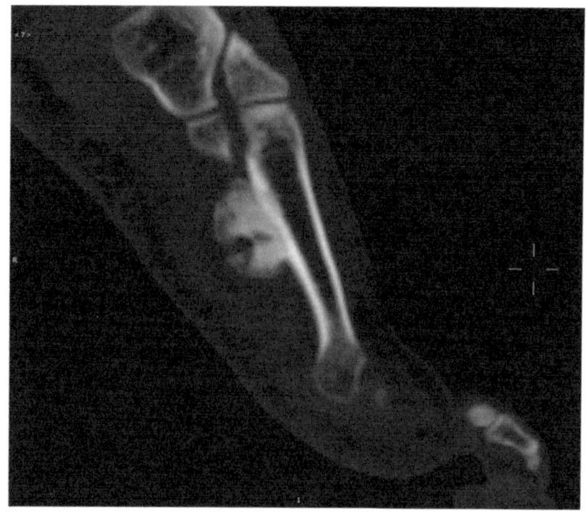

Fig. 41.8 Sagittal CT image of the left foot in bone window

41.3.3 MR Imaging

MR images of the left foot demonstrated cortical thickening of the third metatarsal with patchy lesion with internal heterogenous signals containing fat. In the center and most peripheral of the lesion, there was high T2 signal with enhancement. There was marrow edema of the third and fourth metatarsals with adjacent soft tissue swelling (Figs. 41.9, 41.10, 41.11, 41.12, 41.13, and 41.14).

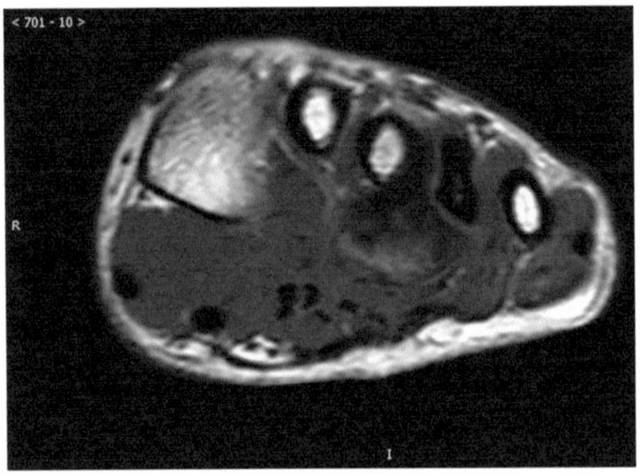

Fig. 41.9 Short axis T1-weighted image of the left foot

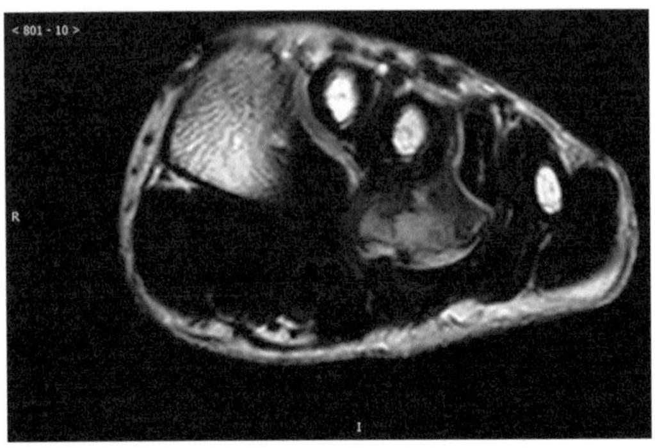

Fig. 41.10 Short axis T2-weighted image of the left foot

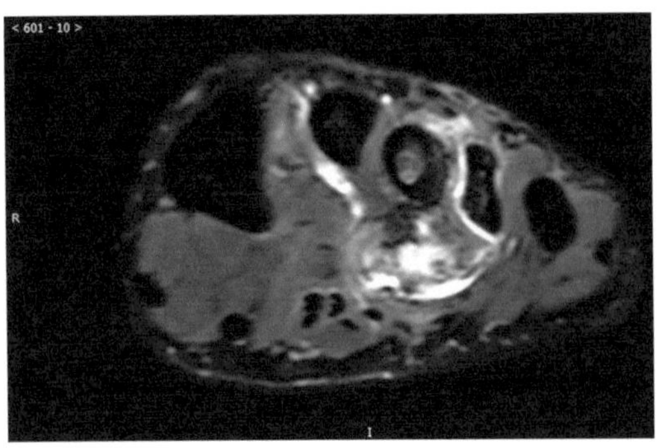

Fig. 41.11 Short axis fat-suppressed T2-weighted image of the left foot

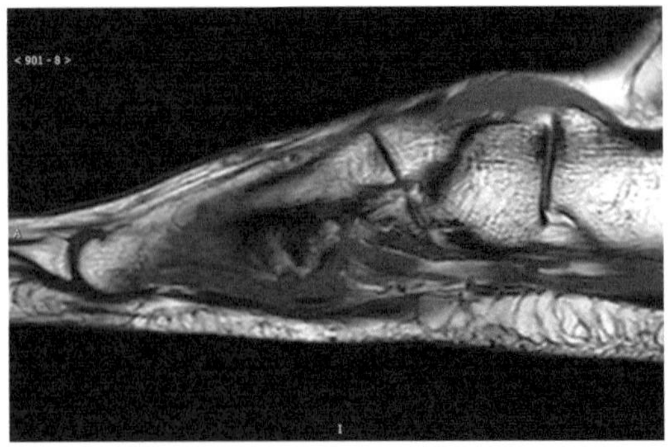

Fig. 41.12 Sagittal T1-weighted image of the left foot

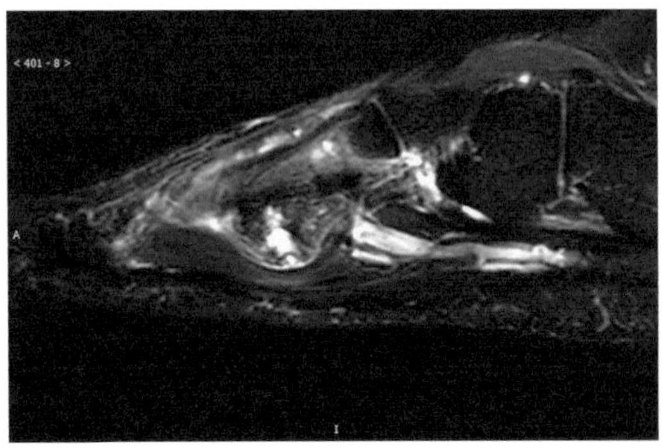

Fig. 41.13 Sagittal fat-suppressed T2-weighted image of the left foot

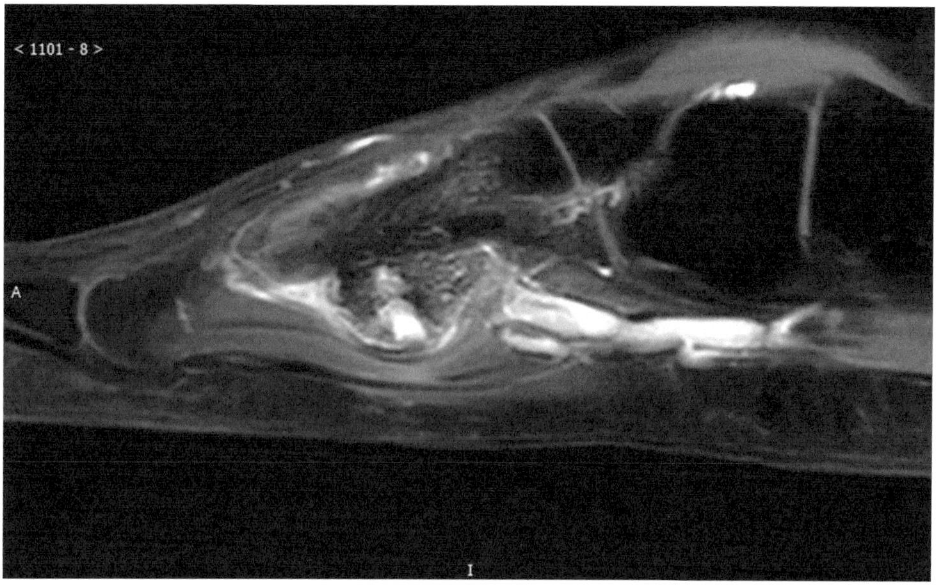

Fig. 41.14 Sagittal post-contrast fat-suppressed T1-weighted image of the left foot

41.4 Description and Discussion from Residents

Radiographs show bone densities around third and fourth metatarsals with cortical thickening. There was a large area of irregular bone densities on CT images with close relationship with the cortex of the third metatarsal and no enhancement. On MR images, the lesion shows clear margin with adjacent soft tissue swelling, most suggestive of benign lesion, such as osteochondroma with myositis ossificans in the differential diagnosis.

41.5 Analysis and Comments from Professor Cheng Xiao-Guang

Patchy bone densities around the third and fourth metatarsals of the left foot are in close relationship with the third metatarsal. Internal densities were inhomogeneous on CT images and fat component demonstrated on MR images. The first consideration is bizarre parosteal osteochondromatous proliferation (Nora's disease). The disease usually involves small tubular bones of the hands and feet. The typical presentation is para-osteal mass with internal large amounts of calcification/ossification and continuous at the base with cortex but no intra-medullary communication. Myositis ossificans is in the differential diagnosis, which in most circumstances shows no intimate relationship with the cortex.

41.6 Diagnosis

Bizarre parosteal osteochondromatous proliferation (Nora's disease).

Suggested Reading

Torreggiani WC, Munk PL, Al-Ismail K, et al. MR imaging features of bizarre parosteal osteochondromatous proliferation of bone (Nora's lesion). Eur J Radiol. 2001;40(3):224–31.

Başdelioğlu K, Yıldırım ANT, Reddy K, et al. Bizarre parosteal osteochondromatous proliferation (Nora's lesion) of the foot: a case report and literature review of Nora's lesion of the foot. Cureus. 2022;14(4):e24197.

42 Aneurysmal Bone Cyst: Case 17

42.1 Medical History

Patient is a 10-year-old boy. His family noticed a left foot dorsal mass when he was about one and half years old and was seen at our hospital. Radiographs were taken at the time and the patient was told to do regular follow ups. He was seen at the local hospital once the following year. He developed left foot swelling with pain after skiing when he was 5 years old and pain was relieved by rest. He was seen again at our hospital and left fourth metatarsal bone biopsy was done. This was followed by steroid infusion, curettage with filling of artificial bone material. He was seen 2 months post operative at the local hospital and recurrence was thought at the time. He did not receive any treatment then. He suffered from pain with limited activities in the past 1 year.

42.2 Physical Examination

The left fourth and fifth toes are slightly shorter when compared to the contralateral side. There was a 3 cm × 3 cm deep, hard and palpable mass dorsal to the fourth and fifth metatarsals.

42.3 Imaging Findings

42.3.1 Radiograph

Radiographs demonstrated apparent expansion and deformity of the fourth metatarsal with internal lytic bone destruction and multiple areas of high densities in the shape of septations. There is marked thinning of the cortex and no periosteal reaction or soft tissue mass. The lesion demonstrated a clear margin. There appears to be communication with the fifth metatarsal. There is similar lytic expansile changes of the fifth metatarsal (Figs. 42.1, 42.2, and 42.3).

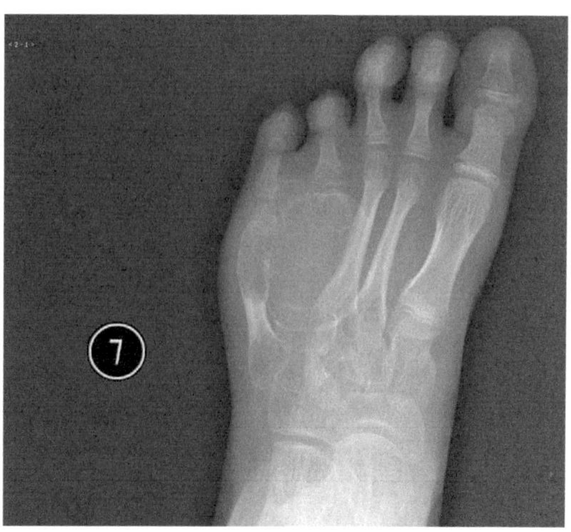

Fig. 42.1 Frontal view of the left foot

X. Cheng et al., *Imaging of Bone Tumors in Wrist, Hand, Ankle and Foot*,
https://doi.org/10.1007/978-981-99-6407-9_42

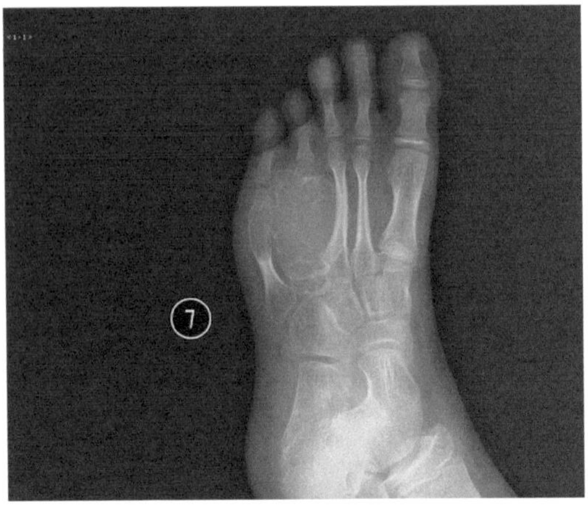

Fig. 42.2 Oblique view of the left foot

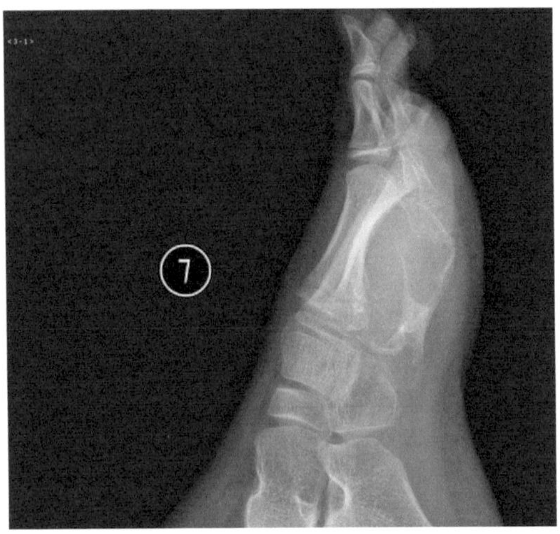

Fig. 42.3 Lateral view of the left foot

42.3.2 CT Imaging

CT images of the left foot demonstrated apparent lytic expansile lesion of the fourth metatarsal and also similar changes of the distal fifth metatarsal. There were internal inhomogeneous densities with focal fluid-like low densities. There is marked thinning of the overlying cortex without periosteal reaction or associated soft tissue mass (Figs. 42.4, 42.5, 42.6, 42.7, 42.8, and 42.9).

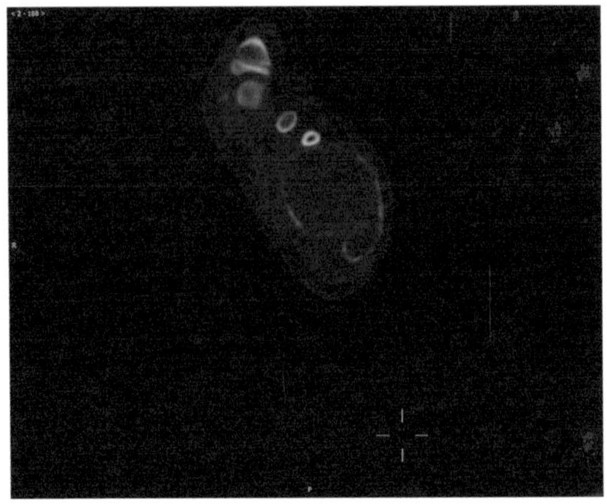

Fig. 42.4 Short axis CT image of the left foot in bone window

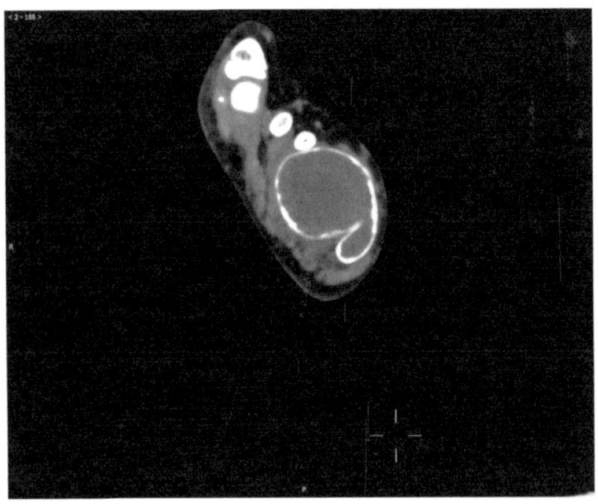

Fig. 42.5 Short axis CT image of the left foot in soft tissue window

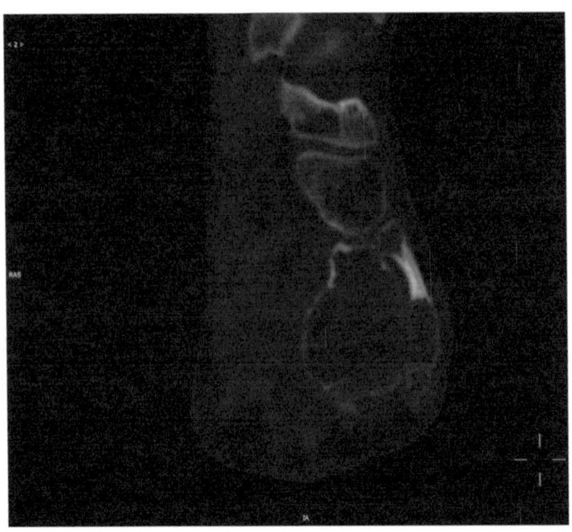

Fig. 42.6 Long axis CT image of the left foot in bone window

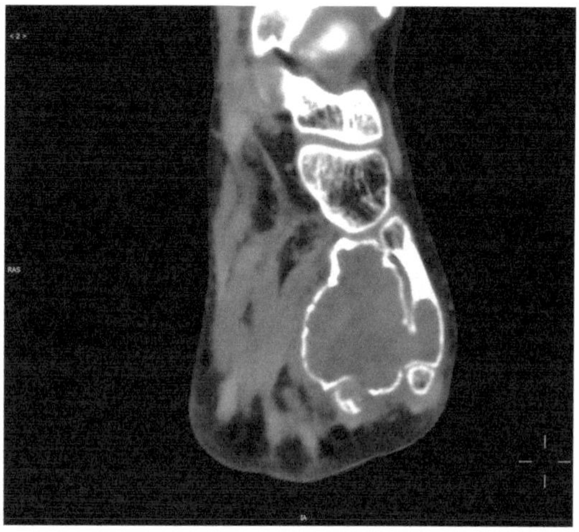

Fig. 42.7 Long axis CT image of the left foot in soft window

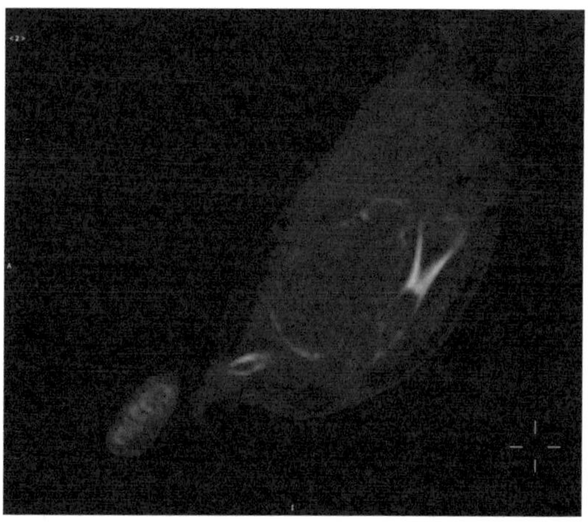

Fig. 42.8 Sagittal CT image of the left foot in bone window

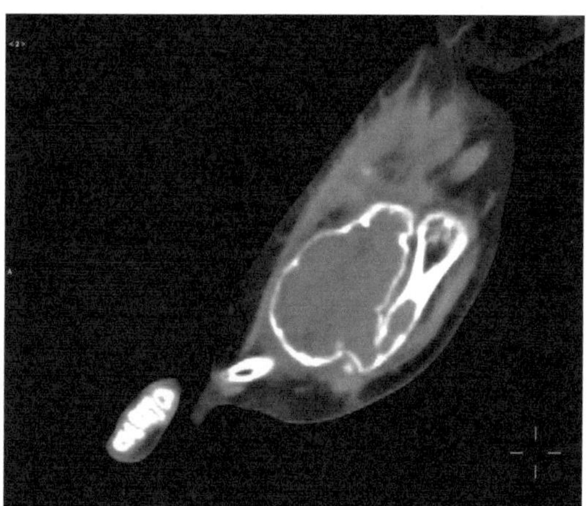

Fig. 42.9 Sagittal CT image of the left foot in soft tissue window

42.3.3 MR Imaging

MR images of the left foot demonstrated expansile lytic process of the fourth metatarsal and fifth metatarsal. Fluid signal noted in majority of the lesion with internal multiple septations and peripheral and septation enhancement (Figs. 42.10, 42.11, 42.12, and 42.13).

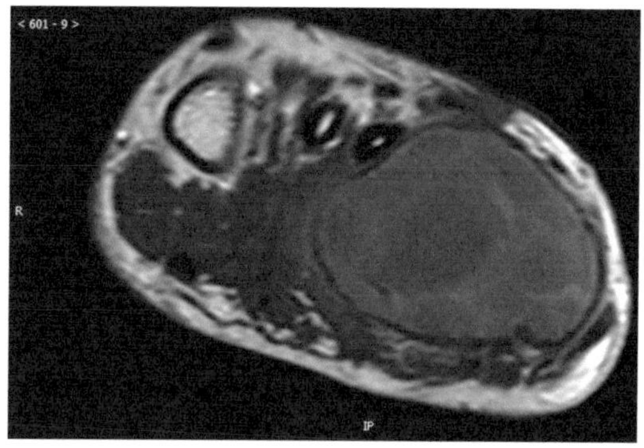

Fig. 42.10 Short axis T1-weighted image of the left foot

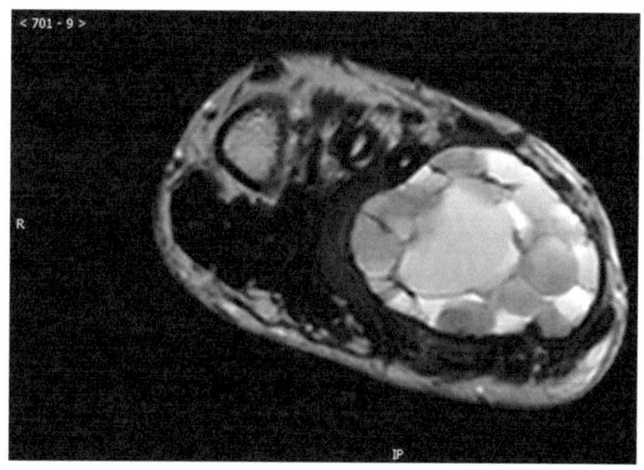

Fig. 42.11 Short axis T2-weighted image of the left foot

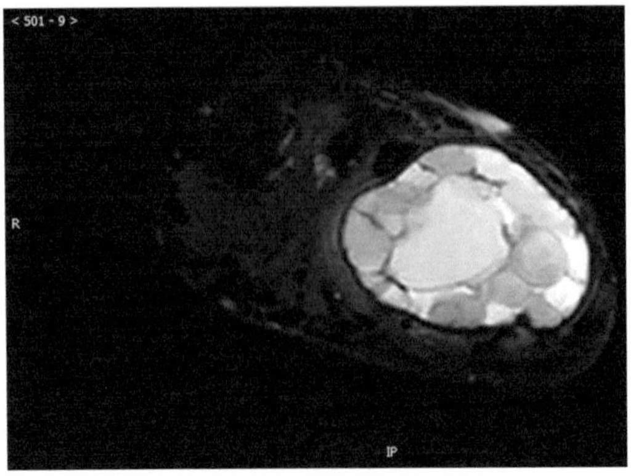

Fig. 42.12 Short axis fat-suppressed T2-weighted image of the left foot

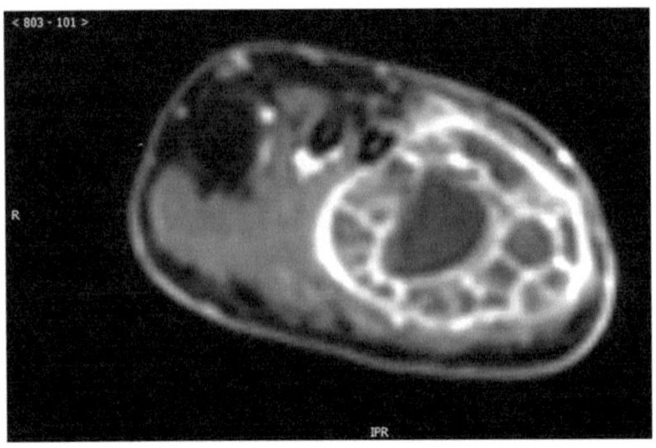

Fig. 42.13 Short axis post-contrast fat-suppressed T1-weighted image of the left foot

42.4 Description and Discussion from Residents

Radiographs show expansile lytic process of the fourth and fifth metatarsals with thinning of the cortex and communication between the two bones. There was a clear margin and adjacent pressive changes. Internal inhomogeneous densities with continuous overlying cortex and no associated soft tissue mass were noted on CT images. Cystic septations noted on MR images with internal fluid-fluid levels and avid enhancement along the septations. Our top consideration is aneurysmal bone cyst. However, given the multiple area of solid components and the location of the foot, other considerations include giant cell reparative granuloma (solid aneurysmal bone cyst) and telangiectatic osteosarcoma.

42.5 Analysis and Comments from Professor Cheng Xiao-Guang

Patient is a boy. Radiographs showed an expansile lytic process of the fourth metatarsal with involvement of the fifth metatarsal. There was a clear margin with compressive changes of the adjacent osseous structures. CT images showed internal inhomogeneous densities but no calcification or bone fragments with continuous overlying cortex. Multiple cystic septations were noted on MR images with avid enhancement along the septations. Overall, the findings are consistent with aneurysmal bone cyst, with telangiectatic osteosarcoma and giant cell tumor of bone in the differential diagnoses. Given the imaging features, the lesion did not appear aggressive, and we favor benign process. Giant cell tumor of tbone usually affects adult patients at the end of long bones with internal more solid components, not consistent with current case.

42.6 Diagnosis

Aneurysmal bone cyst.

Suggested Reading

Reda B. Cystic bone tumors of the foot and ankle. J Surg Oncol. 2018;117(8):1786–1798.

Deventer N, Toporowski G, Gosheger G, et al. Aneurysmal bone cyst of the foot: A series of 10 cases. Foot Ankle Surg. 2022;28(2):276–280.

43 Osteoid Osteoma: Case 18

43.1 Medical History

Patient is a 22-year-old male. He started to experience pain around latera left fifth toe without inciting event about 11 months ago. The pain increases at night and worsened about 4 months ago. He was seen multiple times at the local hospital and revealed nothing significant. Process related to the fifth metatarsal was noted about 1 month ago.

43.2 Physical Examination

Swelling of the distal left foot laterally with a palpable mass, which is hard, with irregular border, non-mobile and with point tenderness.

43.3 Imaging Findings

43.3.1 Radiograph

Radiographs demonstrated focal high densities along the mid and distal left fifth metatarsal with cortical thickening and adjacent soft tissue swelling (Figs. 43.1 and 43.2).

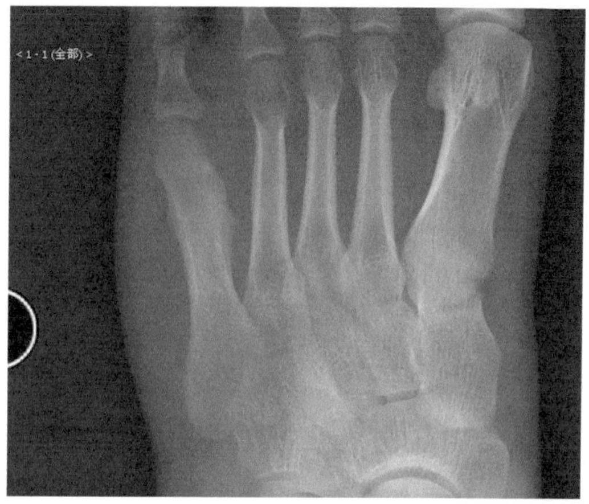

Fig. 43.1 Frontal view of the left foot

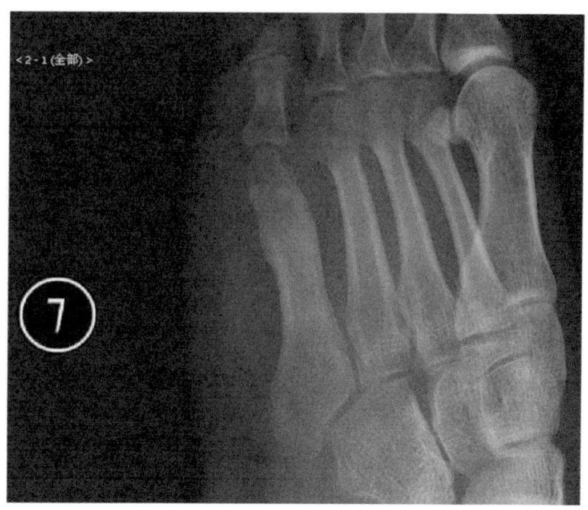

Fig. 43.2 Oblique view of the left foot

X. Cheng et al., *Imaging of Bone Tumors in Wrist, Hand, Ankle and Foot*,
https://doi.org/10.1007/978-981-99-6407-9_43

43.3.2 CT Imaging

CT images of the left foot demonstrated pointed high densities of the distal fifth metatarsal with surrounding lower densities and osseous sclerosis of the medullary cavity with dense periosteal reaction and soft tissue swelling. Peripheral avid enhancement was noted (Figs. 43.3, 43.4, and 43.5).

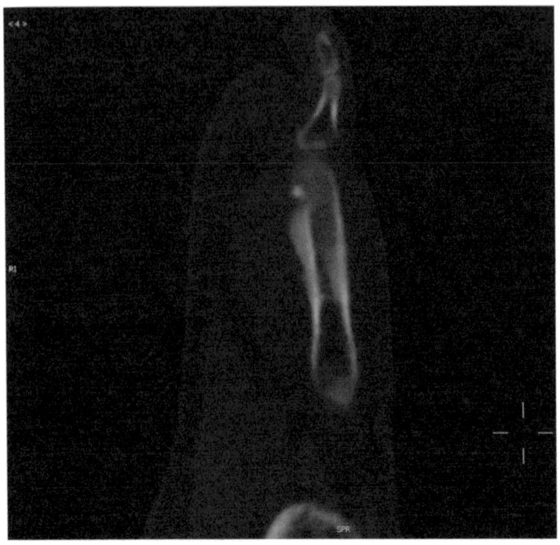

Fig. 43.3 Sagittal CT image of the left foot in bone window

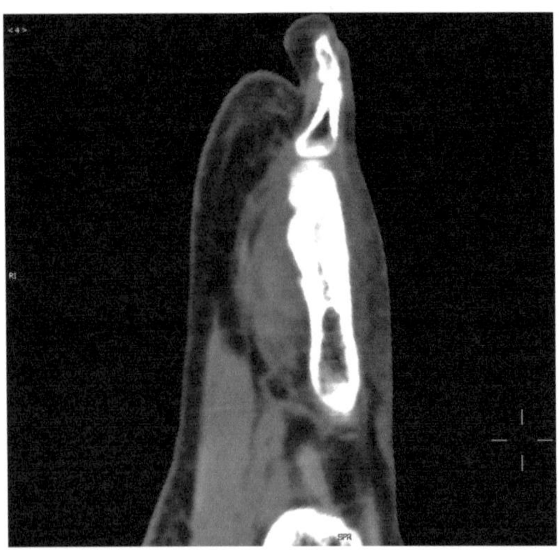

Fig. 43.4 Sagittal CT image of the left foot in soft tissue window

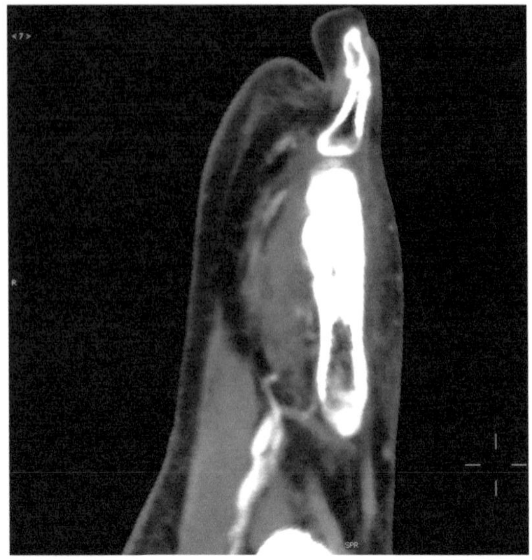

Fig. 43.5 Sagittal post-contrast CT image of the left foot in soft tissue window

43.4 Description and Discussion from Residents

Radiographs show periosteal reaction along the fifth metatarsal without narrowing of the medullar cavity. There were punctate high densities distally with adjacent soft tissue swelling. Apparent thickening of the cortex with soft tissue swelling was seen on CT images with mild enhancement. The punctate high densities could represent calcification in osteoid osteoma. However, the punctate densities located at the distal portion of the periosteal reaction and are not in the center, not typical of osteoid osteoma. Further evaluation with MRI is recommended. Differential diagnosis includes chronic sclerosing osteomyelitis, stress fracture, and hemangioma.

43.5 Analysis and Comments from Professor Cheng Xiao-Guang

Patient is a young male. There was cortical thickening of the fifth metatarsal with apparent periosteal reaction and increased density of the medullary cavity with adjacent soft tissue swelling and mild enhancement. The above findings favor chronic inflammatory changes, such as osteoid osteoma. Hemangioma is in the differential diagnosis. MRI exam would be helpful for narrow down the diagnosis.

43.6 Diagnosis

Osteoid osteoma.

Suggested Reading

Shukla S, Clarke AW, Saifuddin A. Imaging features of foot osteoid osteoma. Skeletal Radiol. 2010;39(7):683–9.

Payo-Ollero J, Moreno-Figaredo V, Llombart-Blanco R, et al. Osteoid osteoma in the ankle and foot. An overview of 50 years of experience. Foot Ankle Surg. 2021;27(2):143–149.

44 Tuberculosis: Case 19

44.1 Medical History

Patient is a 65-year-old female. She experienced left knee and left foot pain without clear inciting event about 11 months ago and the pain was activity related, more apparent when squatting with focal mild protuberance. She was seen at local hospital and radiographs done which revealed no abnormality. She received a steroid injection without much relief. The dorsal swelling of the left foot worsened, and she was treated with pain killer without much relief. The pain and swelling worsened about 1 month ago.

44.2 Physical Examination

Focal protuberance of the left foot and left knee.

44.3 Imaging Findings

44.3.1 Radiograph

Radiographs demonstrated lytic bone destruction at the base of the third metatarsal and anterior left proximal tibia medially. There was an indistinct margin of the lesions and without periosteal reaction. Peripheral sclerosis was noted around the tibial lesion but not seen around the lesion of the third metatarsal (Figs. 44.1, 44.2, 44.3, and 44.4).

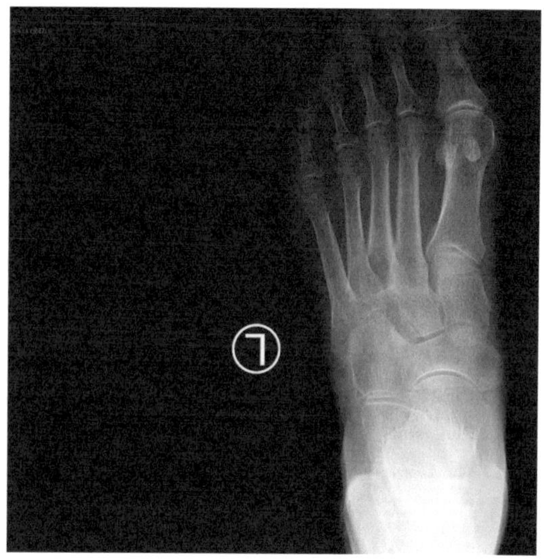

Fig. 44.1 Frontal view of the left foot

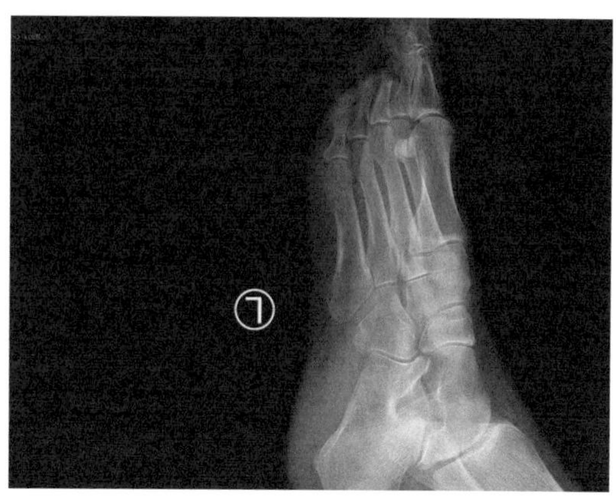

Fig. 44.2 Oblique view of the left foot

X. Cheng et al., *Imaging of Bone Tumors in Wrist, Hand, Ankle and Foot*,
https://doi.org/10.1007/978-981-99-6407-9_44

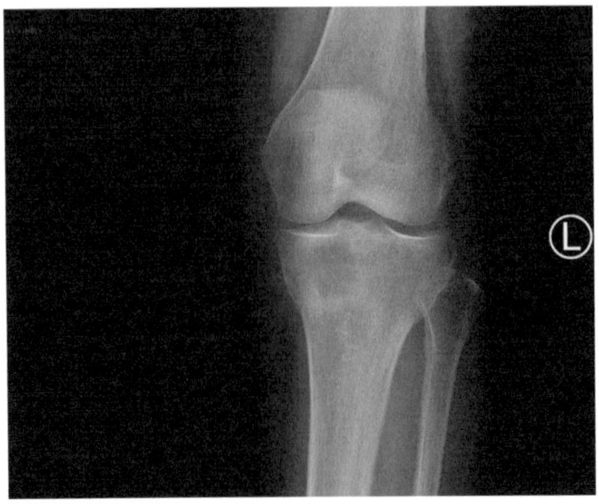

Fig. 44.3 Frontal view of the left knee

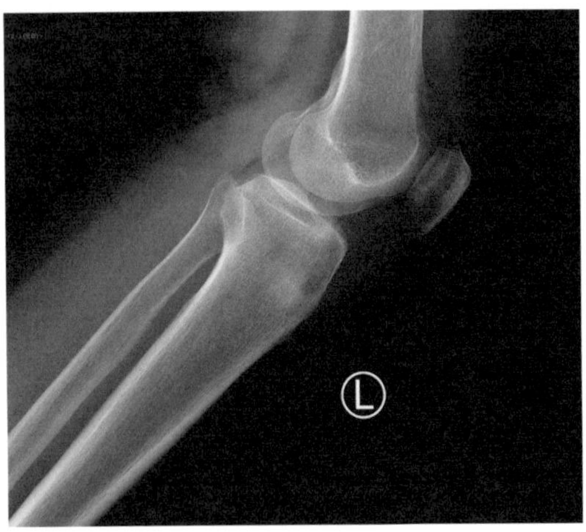

Fig. 44.4 Lateral view of the left knee

44.3.2 CT Imaging

There was lytic bone destruction at the base of the third metatarsal with focal cortical disruption and lesion extending outside the confine of the cortex with peripheral circular enhancement. There was lytic bone destruction of the anterior proximal tibia with focal cortical disruption with peripheral sclerosis and anterior soft tissue swelling with peripheral circular enhancement (Figs. 44.5, 44.6, 44.7, 44.8, 44.9, 44.10, 44.11, 44.12, 44.13, 44.14, 44.15, and 44.16).

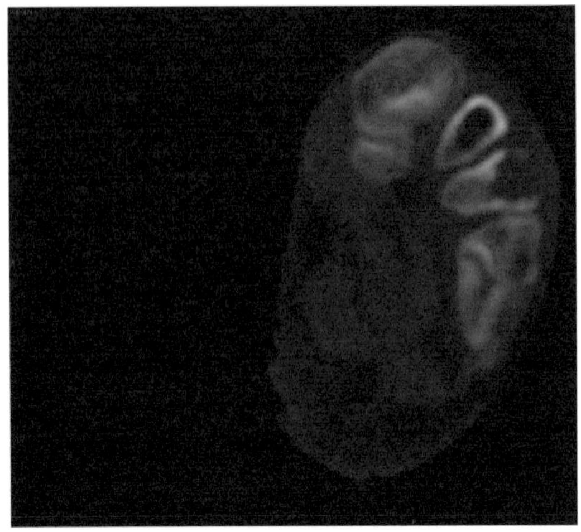

Fig. 44.5 Short axis CT image of the left foot in bone window

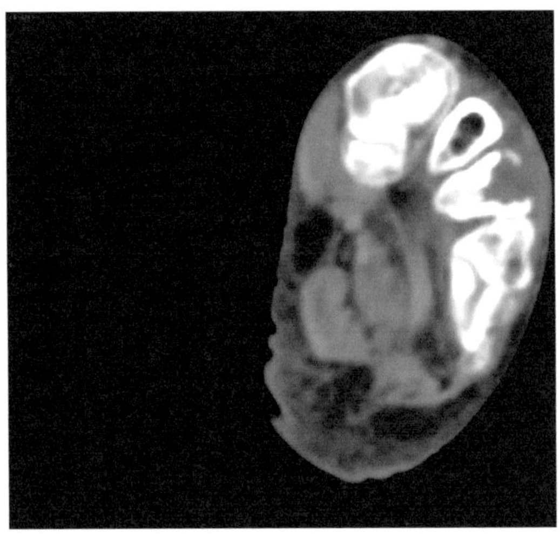

Fig. 44.6 Short axis CT image of the left foot in soft tissue window

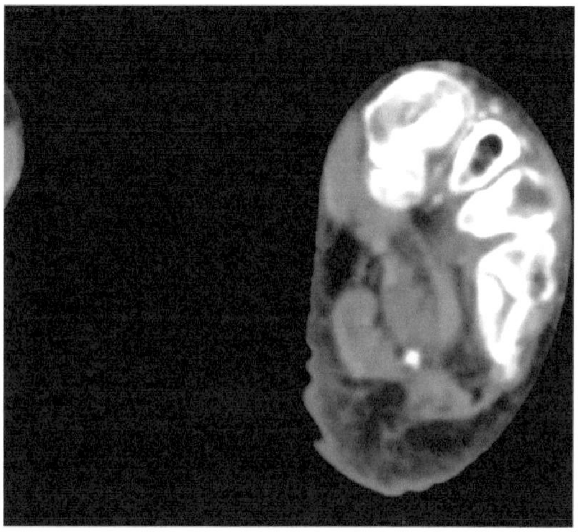

Fig. 44.7 Short axis post-contrast CT image of the left foot in soft tissue window

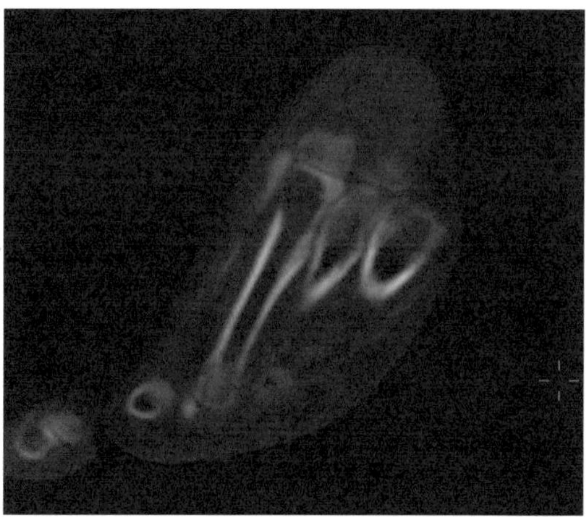

Fig. 44.8 Long axis CT image of the left foot in bone window

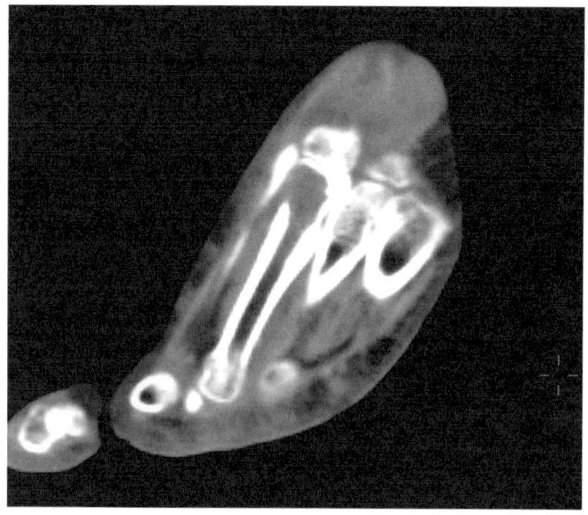

Fig. 44.9 Long axis CT image of the left foot in soft tissue window

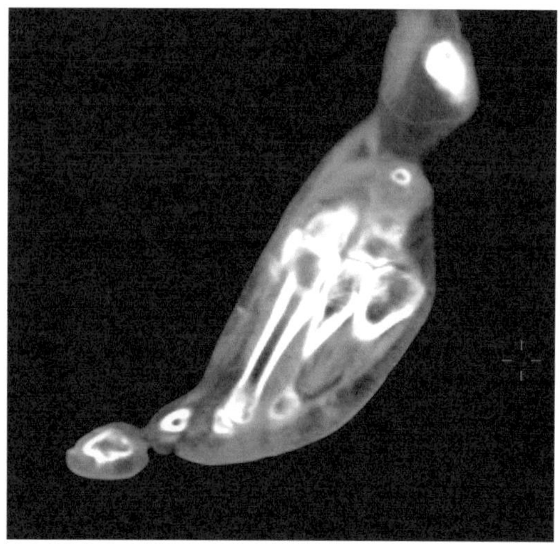

Fig. 44.10 Long axis post-contrast CT image of the left foot in soft tissue window

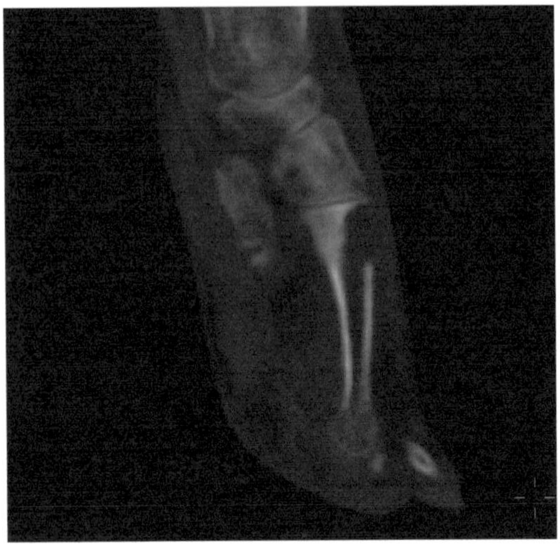

Fig. 44.11 Sagittal CT image of the left foot in bone window

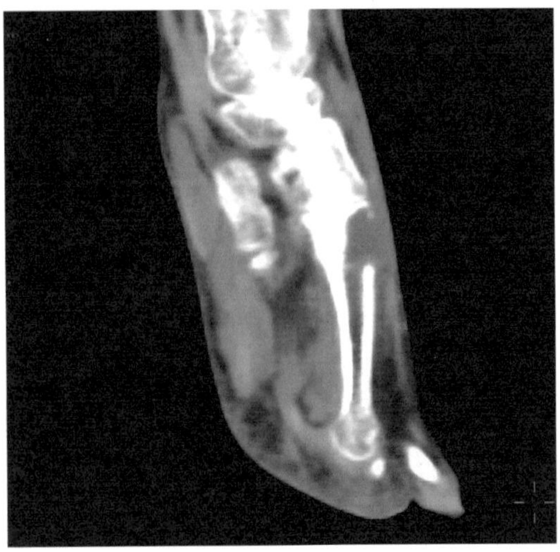

Fig. 44.12 Sagittal CT image of the left foot in soft tissue window

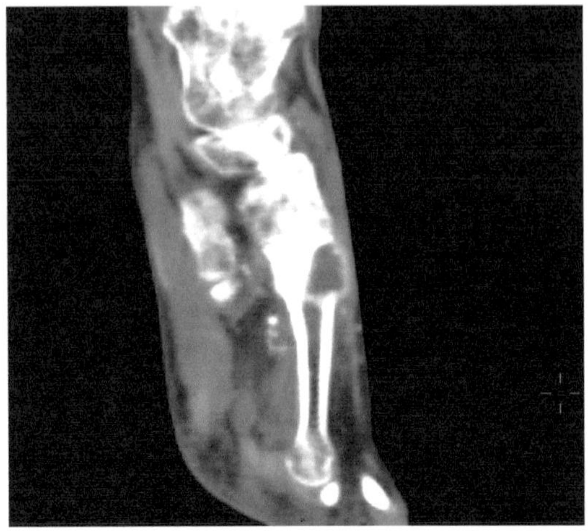

Fig. 44.13 Sagittal post-contrast CT image of the left foot in soft tissue window

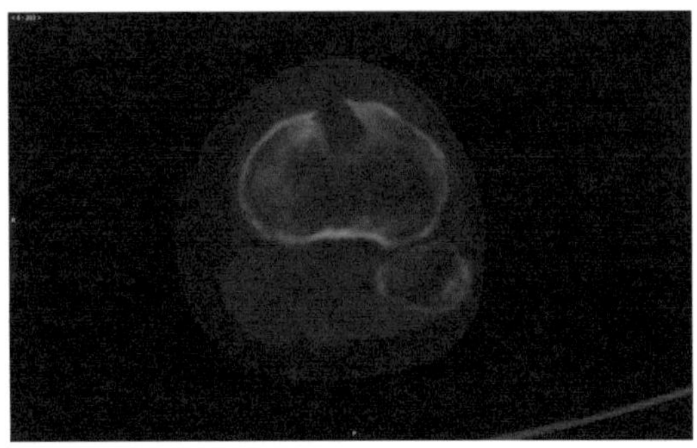

Fig. 44.14 Axial CT image of the left knee in bone window

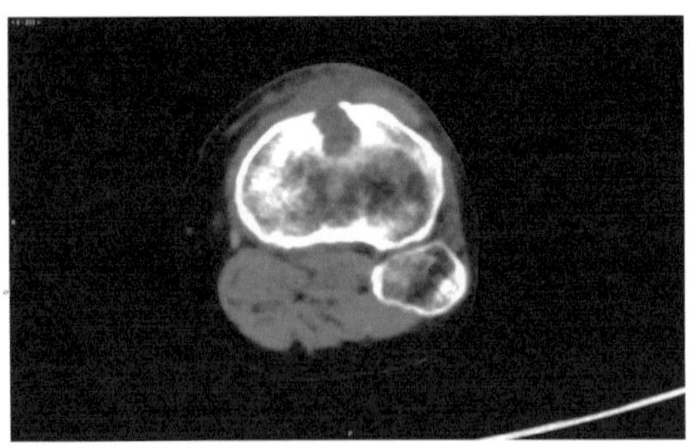

Fig. 44.15 Axial CT image of the left knee in soft tissue window

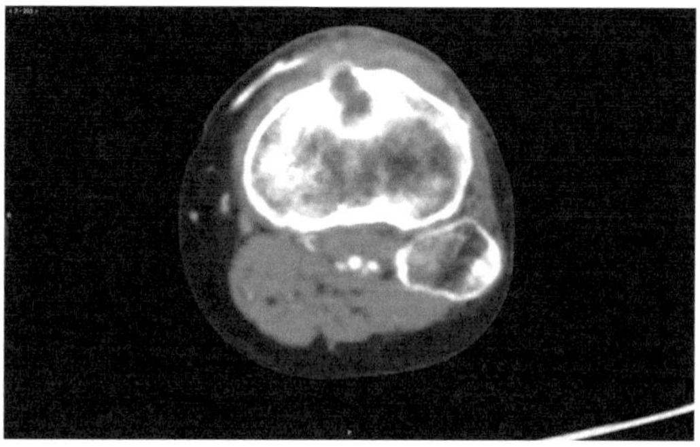

Fig. 44.16 Axial post-contrast CT image of the left knee in soft tissue window

44.4 Description and Discussion from Residents

Radiographs showed eccentric lytic bone destruction of the third metatarsal with irregular margin and no peripheral sclerosis or periosteal reaction. There was focal cortical disruption but the articular surface was maintained. Bone destruction was noted at the proximal tibia anteriorly with peripheral sclerosis with irregular margin. The imaging findings favor low grade neoplasm or metastatic lesion. However, given multiple bone involvements, hyperthyroidism should be considered in the differential diagnosis. Although, without general osteopenia, this could be excluded. There were internal general low densities of the lesions on CT images with focal cortical disruption and reactive edema of surrounding soft tissue and peripheral circular enhancement, all supportive of inflammatory process. Thus, we are considering multifocal infectious process.

44.5 Analysis and Comments from Professor Cheng Xiao-Guang

Patient is an older female with prolonged history. The radiographs showed lesion of the left proximal third metatarsal and proximal left tibia anteriorly with irregular margin. Given the patient's age, first consideration is metastatic disease or other malignant neoplasm, with infection in the differential diagnosis. CT images showed reactive sclerosis and edema changes around the bone destruction with focal cortical disruption and peripheral circular enhancement. Infection is my top consideration, however, given patient's advanced age, differential diagnosis includes metastatic disease and other malignant neoplasm.

44.6 Diagnosis

Necrotizing granulomatous inflammation, first consideration of tuberculosis.

Suggested Reading

Korim M, Patel R, Allen P, et al. Foot and ankle tuberculosis: case series and literature review. Foot (Edinb). 2014;24(4):176–9.

Prakash M, Gupta P, Sen RK, et al. Magnetic resonance imaging evaluation of tubercular arthritis of the ankle and foot. Acta Radiol. 2015;56(10):1236–41.

Faroug R, Psyllakis P, Gulati A, et al. Diagnosis and treatment of tuberculosis of the foot and ankle-A literature review. Foot (Edinb). 2018;37:105–112.

45 Pseudomyogenic Hemangioendothelioma of Bone: Case 20

45.1 Medical History

Patient is a 33-year-old male. He was seen at our out-patient clinic for multiple bone complaints of the left foot.

45.2 Physical Examination

Not done.

45.3 Imaging Findings

45.3.1 Radiograph

Radiographs demonstrated multiple bones of lytic destructions with indistinct border but preserved articular surface (Figs. 45.1 and 45.2).

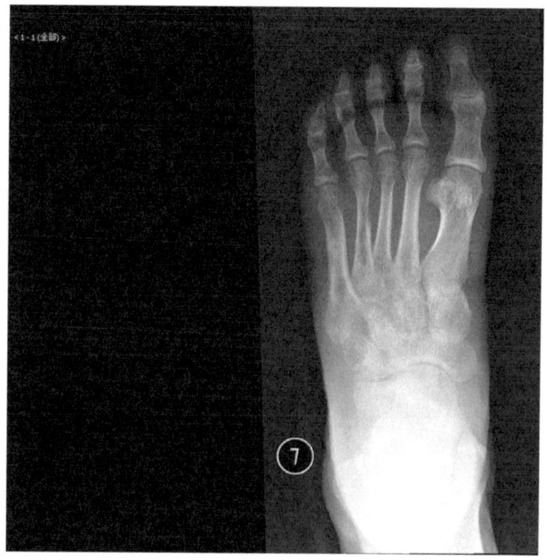

Fig. 45.1 Frontal view of the left foot

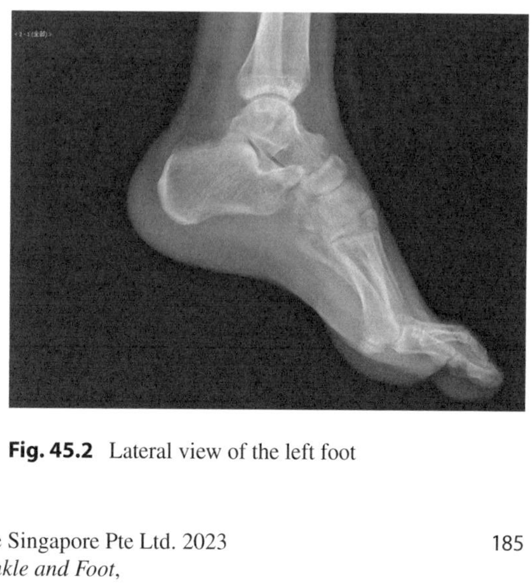

Fig. 45.2 Lateral view of the left foot

X. Cheng et al., *Imaging of Bone Tumors in Wrist, Hand, Ankle and Foot*,
https://doi.org/10.1007/978-981-99-6407-9_45

45.3.2 CT Imaging

There were decreased densities of multiple bones of the left foot with lytic bone destruction of cortex and medullary cavity. There was peripheral mild sclerosis without periosteal reaction or apparent soft tissue mass without enhancement (Figs. 45.3, 45.4, 45.5, 45.6, 45.7, and 45.8).

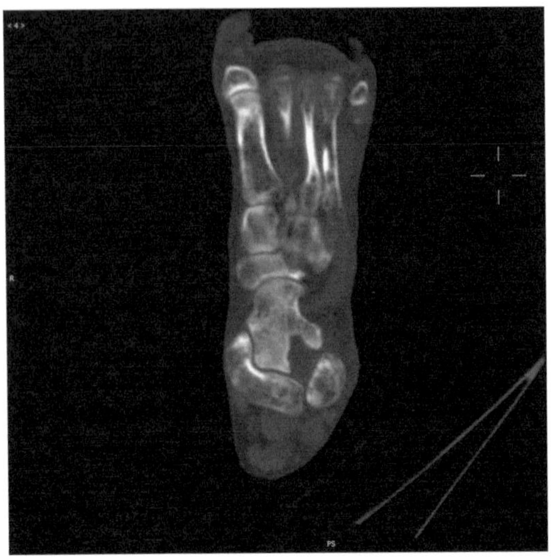

Fig. 45.3 Long axis CT image of the left foot in bone window

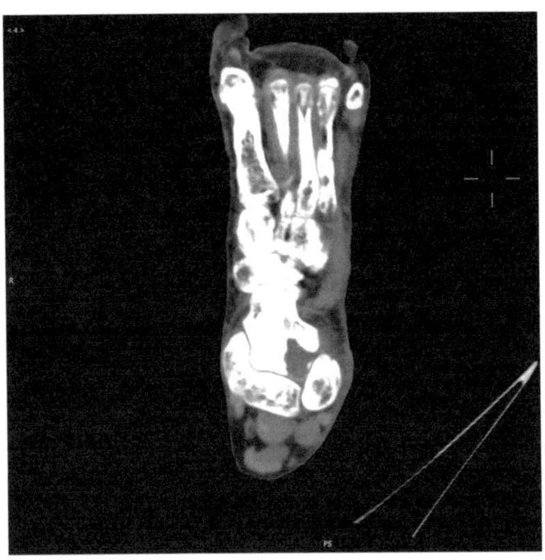

Fig. 45.4 Long axis CT image of the left foot in soft tissue window

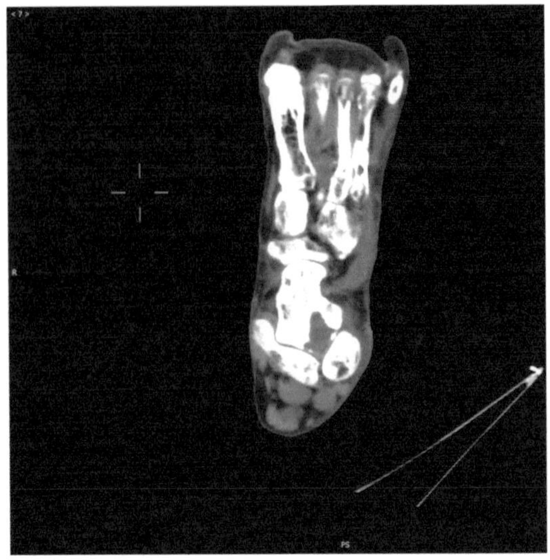

Fig. 45.5 Long axis post-contrast CT image of the left foot in soft tissue window

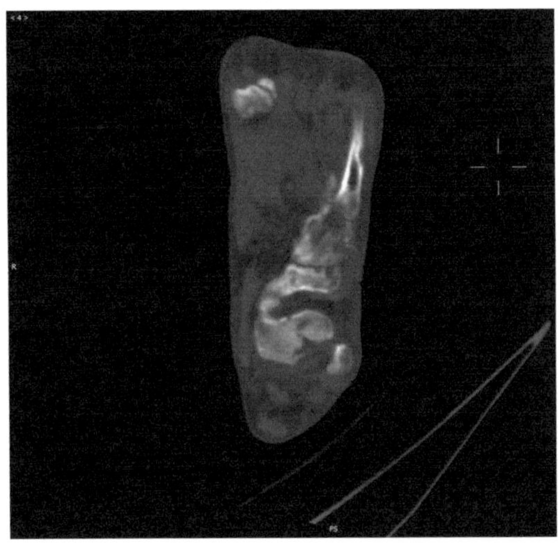

Fig. 45.6 Long axis CT image of the left foot in bone window

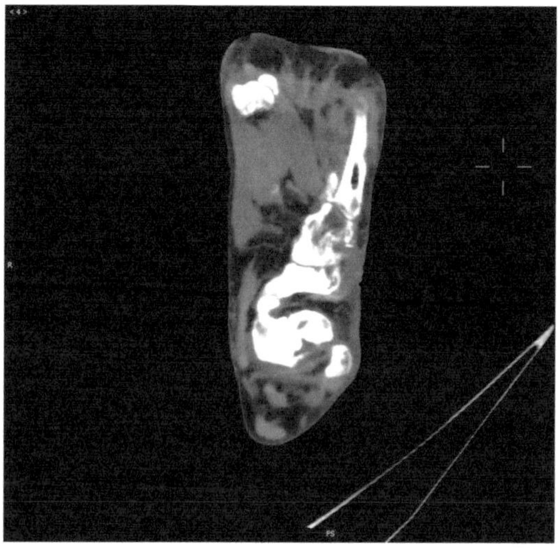

Fig. 45.7 Long axis CT image of the left foot in soft tissue window

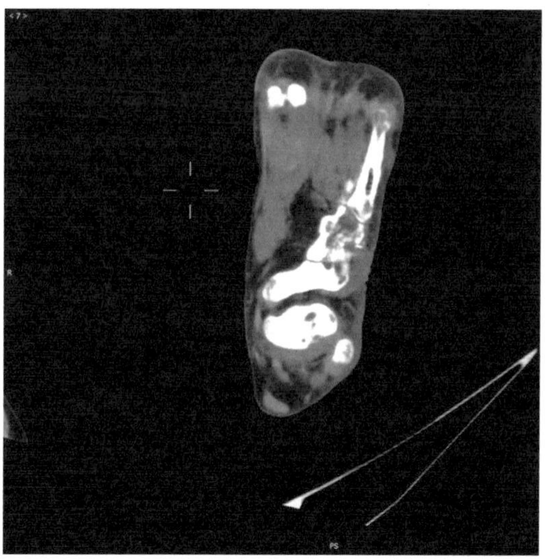

Fig. 45.8 Long axis CT post-contrast image of the left foot in soft tissue window

45.4 Description and Discussion from Residents

Radiographs show multiple bony destructions of the left foot with indistinct margin. CT images show multiple areas of bone destruction along the articular surface with focal beaded morphology. The cortex and the medullary cavity were both affected with peripheral sclerosis and soft tissue mass with mild enhancement. The differential diagnosis includes infection and inflammatory arthropathy. Infectious processes usually show circular peripheral enhancement with central necrosis and sequestrum, not seen in the current case. With inflammatory arthropathy, there were apparent destructions of the articular surfaces and usually with bilateral involvements, not consistent with current case. Other diagnoses included in the differential diagnosis would be vascular lesion, such as hemangioendothelioma.

45.5 Analysis and Comments from Professor Cheng Xiao-Guang

Patient is a young male. There were bone destructions of multiple bones in the left foot with indistinct margin with osteopenia with relative preserved joint space and adjacent soft tissue welling and no avid enhancement. Multiple bone destructions in the foot of a young male, the first consideration would be tuberculosis or gout. However, the imaging findings of the current case are not consistent with gout or tuberculosis. Vascular tumor is a possibility, but with limited clinical information, further evaluation is limited.

45.6 Diagnosis

Pseudomyogenic hemangioendothelioma of bone.

Suggested Reading

Amary MF, O'Donnell P, Berisha F, et al. Pseudomyogenic (epithelioid sarcoma-like) hemangioendothelioma: characterization of five cases. Skeletal Radiol. 2013;42(7):947–57.

Righi A, Gambarotti M, Picci P, et al. Primary pseudomyogenic haemangioendothelioma of bone: report of two cases. Skeletal Radiol. 2015;44(5):727–31.

46 Chondromyxoid Fibroma: Case 21

46.1 Medical History

Patient is a 13-year-old boy. He underwent curettage with bone graft placement of the left first proximal phalanx in local hospital about half a year ago due to more than 1 month of left first toe pain. There was a recurrence of symptoms about 2 months ago.

46.2 Physical Examination

Mild swelling about the left first metatarsophalangeal joint with scar noted medially of 2 cm long and with point tenderness.

46.3 Imaging Findings

46.3.1 Radiograph

Radiographs demonstrated eccentric lytic bone destruction at the base of the first proximal phalanx with clear margin and cortical disruption medially with adjacent soft tissue swelling (Figs. 46.1 and 46.2).

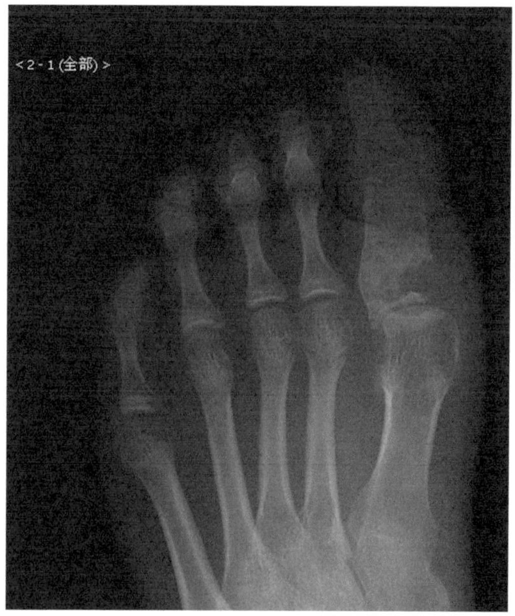

Fig. 46.1 Frontal view of the left foot

X. Cheng et al., *Imaging of Bone Tumors in Wrist, Hand, Ankle and Foot*,
https://doi.org/10.1007/978-981-99-6407-9_46

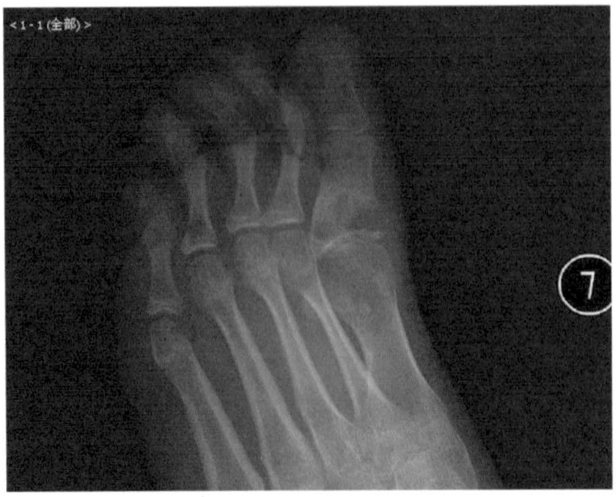

Fig. 46.2 Oblique view of the left foot

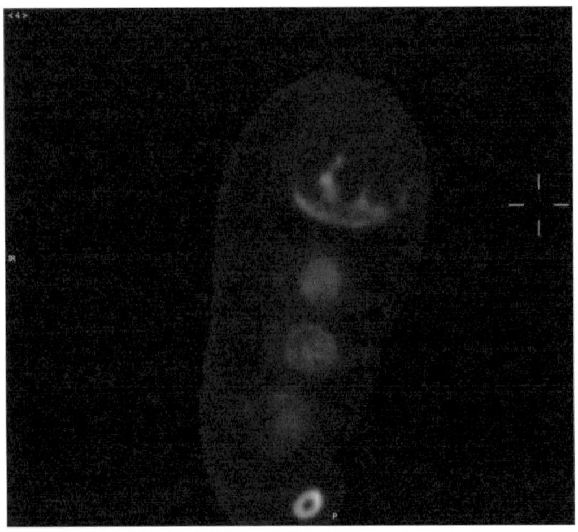

Fig. 46.3 Short axis CT image of the left foot in bone window

46.3.2 CT Imaging

There was eccentric lytic bone destruction of the base of the first proximal phalanx with focal cortical disruption and internal multiple coarse bone crest. There was adjacent soft tissue swelling with mild enhancement (Figs. 46.3, 46.4, 46.5, 46.6, 46.7, and 46.8).

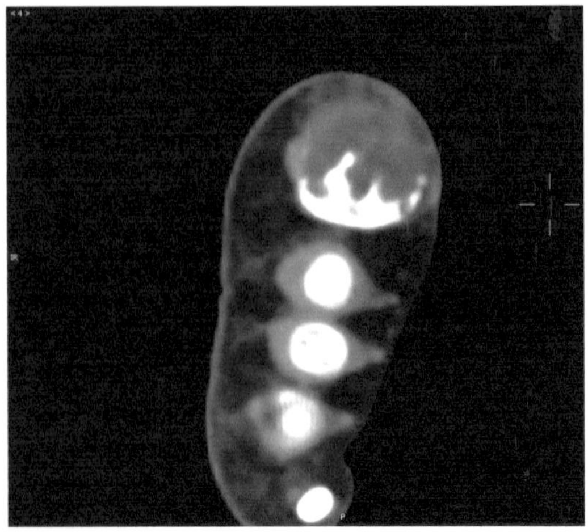

Fig. 46.4 Short axis CT image of the left foot in soft tissue window

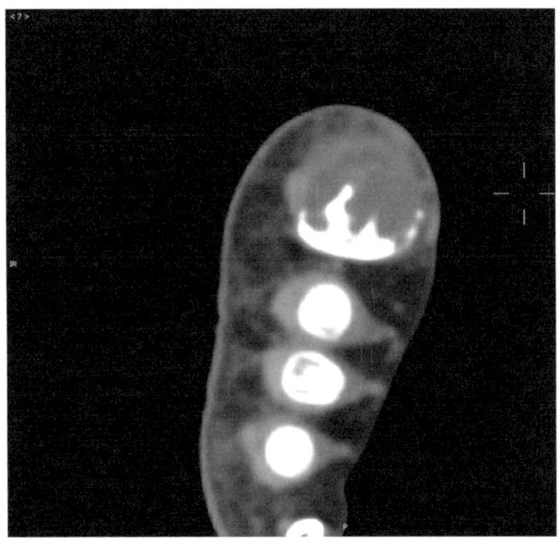

Fig. 46.5 Short axis post-contrast CT image of the left foot in soft tissue window

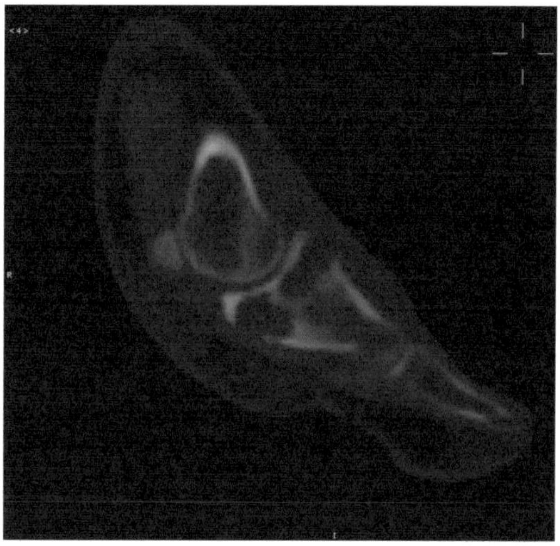

Fig. 46.6 Sagittal CT image of the left foot in bone window

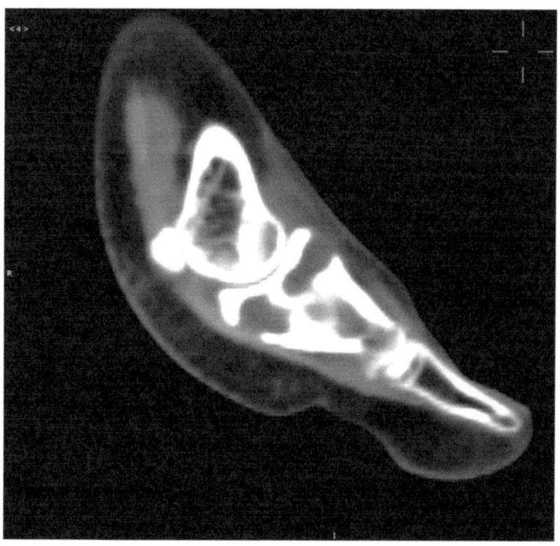

Fig. 46.7 Sagittal CT image of the left foot in soft tissue window

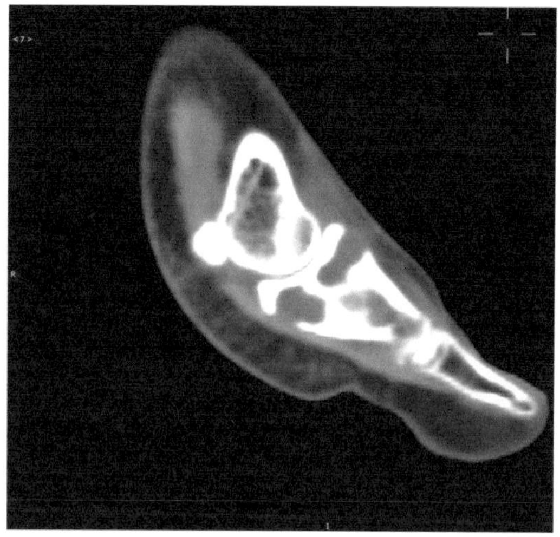

Fig. 46.8 Sagittal post-contrast image of the left foot in soft tissue window

46.4 Description and Discussion from Residents

The patient is a 13-year-old boy with a history of surgery. Radiographs show eccentric and expansile lytic bone destruction at the base of the first proximal phalanx with clear sharp margin and lobular morphology. Internal cortex is discontinuous with adjacent soft tissue swelling and preserved smooth articular surface. The findings support recurrence of a benign process. The lesion appears to be located within the bone on CT images with internal heterogenous densities and focal cystic area of low densities with lobular contour and peripheral sclerosis with clear margin. Moderate enhancement is noted peripherally with no enhancement of the cystic portion. We favor benign osseous process, given patient's age, location, our first consideration would be chondroblastoma, with eosinophilic granuloma and intra-osseous giant cell tumor of the tendon sheath in the differential diagnosis.

46.5 Analysis and Comments from Professor Cheng Xiao-Guang

Patient is a 13-year-old boy. The lesion is located at the base of the first proximal phalanx with a clear margin and no involvement of the articular surface. Focal discontinuous cortex could be post-surgical. The overall imaging findings favor non-aggressive lesion. With non-aggressive neoplasm that tends to occur in the foot in pediatric patients, we first consider chondroblastoma.

46.6 Diagnosis

Chondromyxoid fibroma.

Suggested Reading

O'Connor PJ, Gibbon WW, Hardy G, et al. Chondromyxoid fibroma of the foot. Skeletal Radiol. 1996;25(2):143–8.

Sharma H, Jane MJ, Reid R. Chondromyxoid fibroma of the foot and ankle: 40 years' Scottish bone tumour registry experience. Int Orthop. 2006;30(3):205–9.

Budny AM, Ismail A, Osher L. Chondromyxoid fibroma. J Foot Ankle Surg. 2008;47(2):153–9.

47 Myofibroma: Case 22

47.1 Medical History

Patient is a 33-year-old female. She experienced pain around the right first toe after skiing about 3 years ago. The pain occurs mostly at night and episodic without radiation. About 1 year ago, she had an accident where her cell phone dropped and hit her right foot and swelling about the first toe occurred with worsening pain.

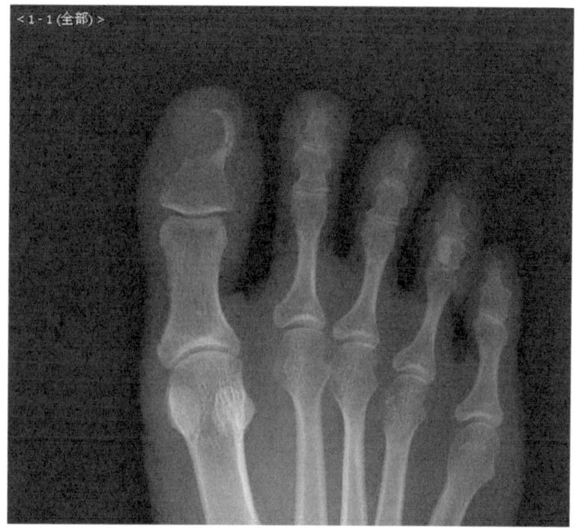

Fig. 47.1 Frontal view of the right foot

47.2 Physical Examination

Swelling at the distal right first toe with increased skin temperature and focal palpable mass, rubbery, firm with indistinct border and point tenderness.

47.3 Imaging Findings

47.3.1 Radiograph

Radiographs demonstrated lytic bone destruction of the right first distal phalanx with destruction of the medial cortex and soft tissue mass with indistinct border (Figs. 47.1 and 47.2).

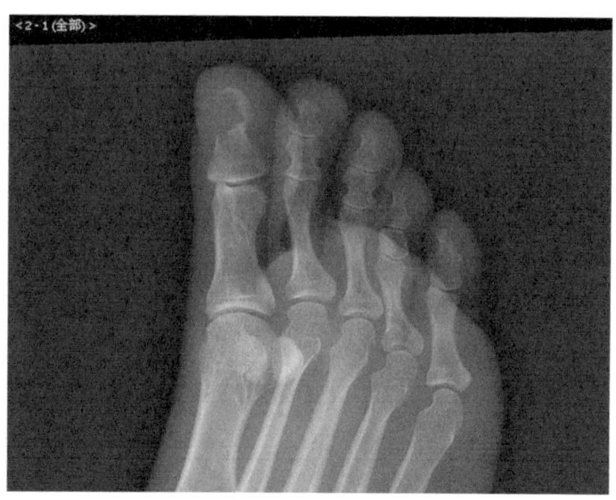

Fig. 47.2 Oblique view of the right foot

X. Cheng et al., *Imaging of Bone Tumors in Wrist, Hand, Ankle and Foot*,
https://doi.org/10.1007/978-981-99-6407-9_47

47.3.2 CT Imaging

There was lytic bone destruction of the first distal phalanx with rather heterogeneous density and medial cortical destruction with soft tissue mass and mild enhancement (Figs. 47.3, 47.4, and 47.5).

47.3.3 MR Imaging

There was bone destruction of the left first distal phalanx with T2 high signal and heterogeneous enhancement, more avid peripheral (Figs. 47.6, 47.7, 47.8, and 47.9).

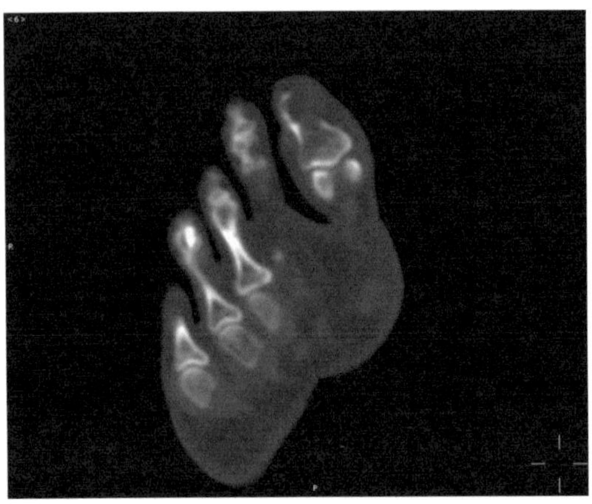

Fig. 47.3 Long axis CT image of the right foot in bone window

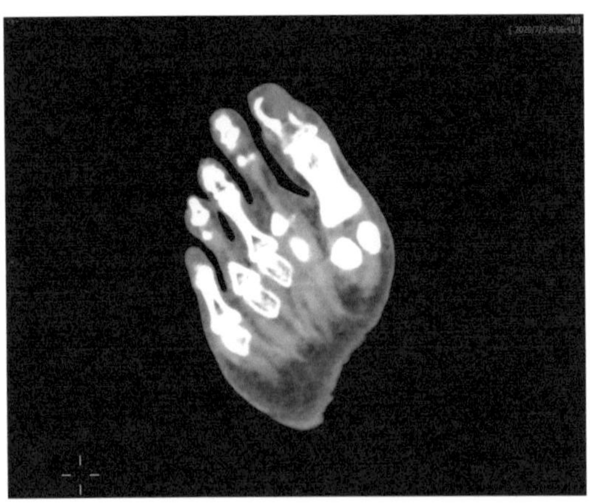

Fig. 47.4 Long axis CT image of the right foot in soft tissue window

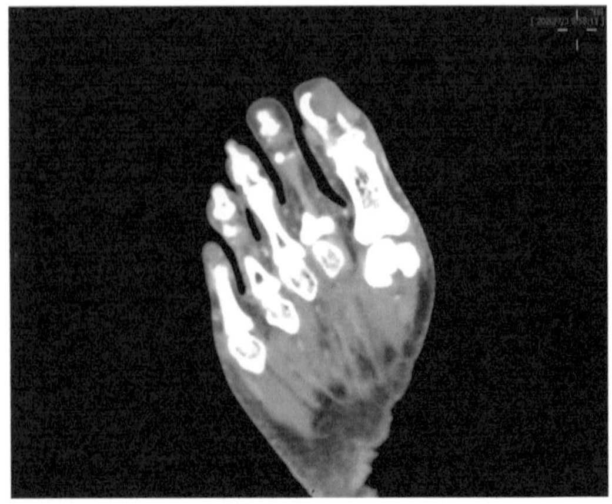

Fig. 47.5 Long axis post-contrast CT image of the right foot in soft tissue window

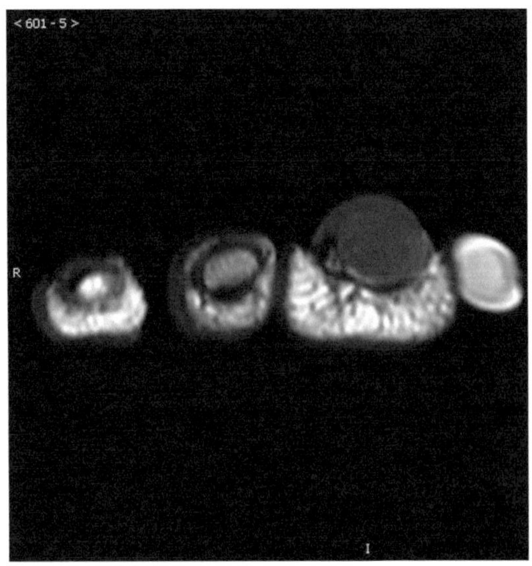

Fig. 47.6 Short axis T1-weighted MR image of the right foot

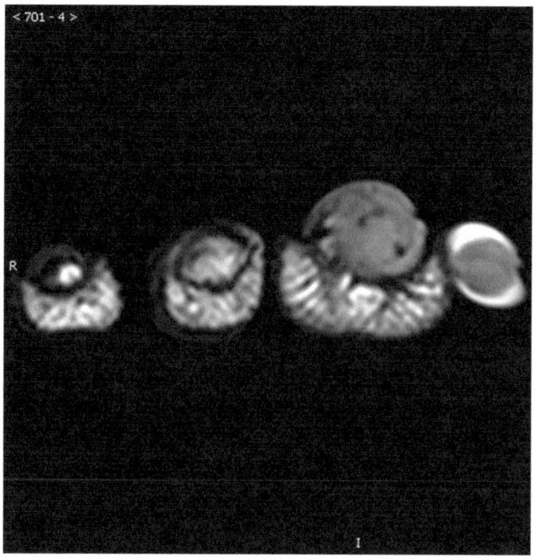

Fig. 47.7 Short axis T2-weighted MR image of the right foot

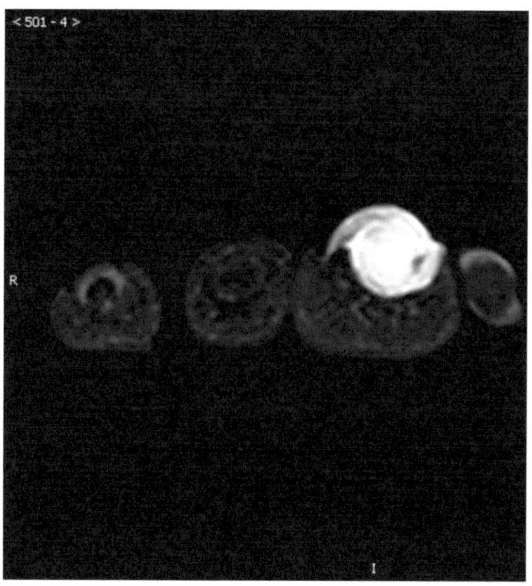

Fig. 47.8 Short axis fat-suppressed T2-weighted MR image of the right foot

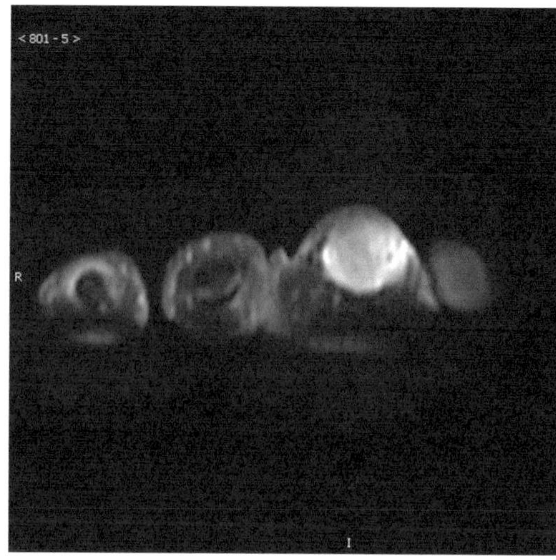

Fig. 47.9 Short axis post-contrast fat-suppressed T1-weighted MR image of the right foot

47.4 Description and Discussion from Residents

Radiographs show eccentric bone destruction of the right first distal phalanx with clear margin and peripheral mild sclerosis. There were rather homogenous densities on the CT images without calcification or fluid-fluid level and mild enhancement. There was internal iso or low T1 and high T2 signal within the lesion with avid enhancement. Overall, we consider neoplasm or neoplasm-like lesion. Given the patient's history of trauma, our first consideration is epidermoid cyst with glomus tumor in the differential diagnosis. Glomus tumors usually occur beneath the nail in the fingers and mostly in the center.

47.5 Analysis and Comments from Professor Cheng Xiao-Guang

Patient is a young female with history of trauma. The lesion is at distal first toe with solid component internally without fat or calcification and mild enhancement. This is suggestive of benign tumor at the distal phalanx, my top consideration is glomus tumor. Given the patient's history of trauma, foreign body granuloma is in the differential diagnosis.

47.6 Diagnosis

Spindle cell tumor (intermediate or locally aggressive), more consistent with perivascular tumor. In perivascular tumors, we favor atypical myofibroma (according to the fifth edition of WHO classification of soft tissue and bone tumors, atypical myofibroma, and glomus tumor all belong to the family of perivascular tumor.

Suggested Reading

Horner CWM, Speller A, McBride T, et al. Rare digital tumours: two case reports and mini review. Hand Surg. 2012;17(2):267–70.

Ma Y, Siegal GP, Wei Sh. Solitary, adult-onset, intraosseous myofibroma of the finger: report of a case and review of literature. Hand (N Y). 2015;10(3):550–4.

48 Hemangioma of Soft Tissue: Case 23

48.1 Medical History

Patient is a 23-year-old male. He started to experience left ankle pain about 15 months ago and worsened after walking, without night pain. Ankle swelling followed and more severe at night and mild in the morning.

48.2 Physical Examination

Mild protuberance of dorsal left ankle with point tenderness.

48.3 Imaging Findings

48.3.1 Radiograph

Radiographs demonstrated soft tissue mass at the anterior aspect of the left ankle with internal multiple high densities and no abnormalities of the adjacent osseous structure (Figs. 48.1 and 48.2).

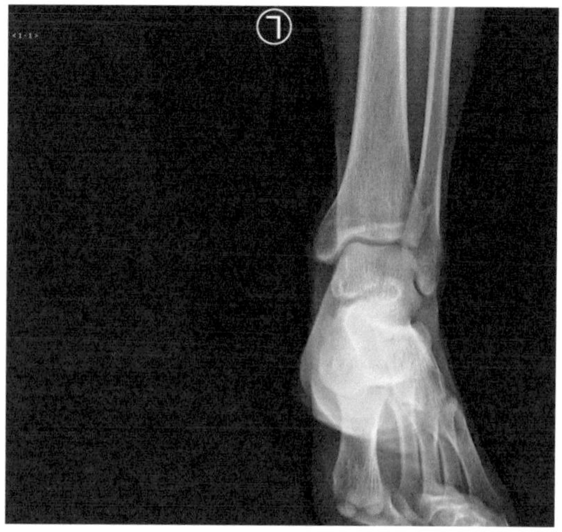

Fig. 48.1 Frontal view of the left ankle

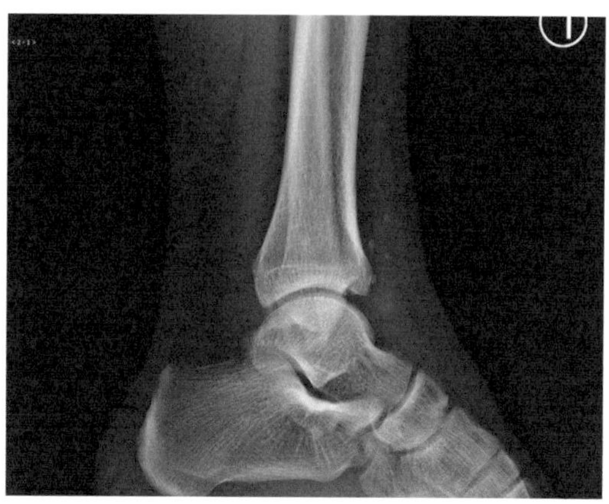

Fig. 48.2 Lateral view of the left ankle

X. Cheng et al., *Imaging of Bone Tumors in Wrist, Hand, Ankle and Foot*,
https://doi.org/10.1007/978-981-99-6407-9_48

48.3.2 CT Imaging

CT images of the left ankle demonstrated an irregular shaped soft tissue mass that was anterior to the distal tibia and talus with internal fat and multiple calcifications. There were compressive changes of the distal tibia. Multiple tubular and circular blood vessel-like enhancements were noted in the lesion (Figs. 48.3, 48.4, 48.5, 48.6, and 48.7).

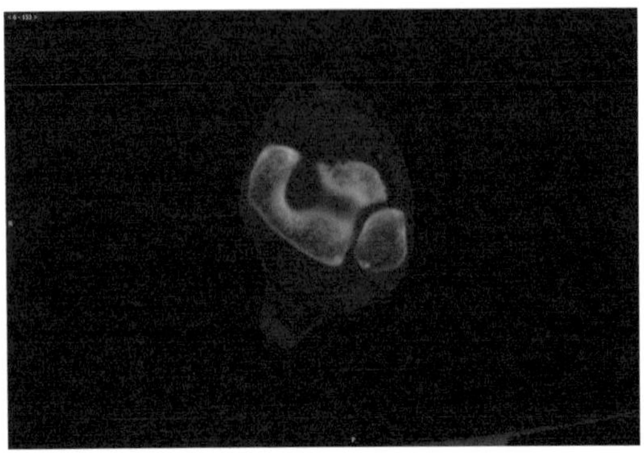

Fig. 48.3 Axial CT image of the left ankle in bone window

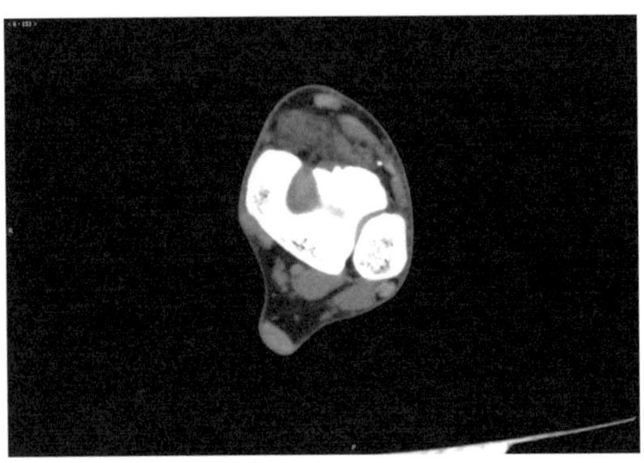

Fig. 48.4 Axial CT image of the left ankle in soft tissue window

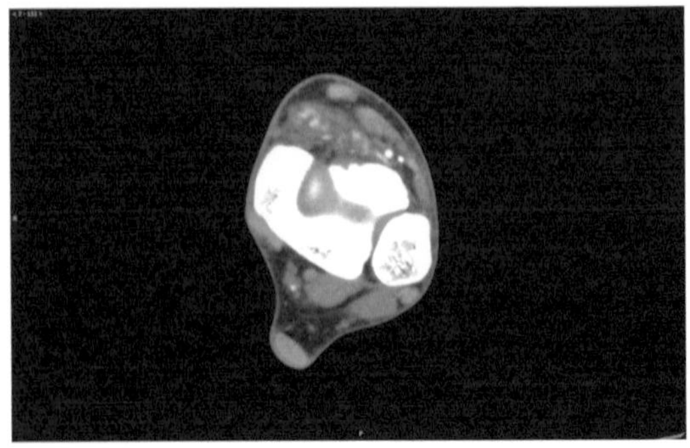

Fig. 48.5 Axial post-contrast CT image of the left ankle in soft tissue window

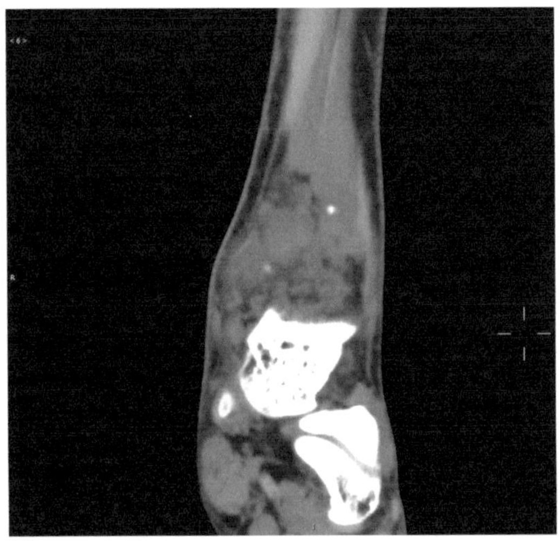

Fig. 48.6 Coronal CT image of the left ankle in soft tissue window

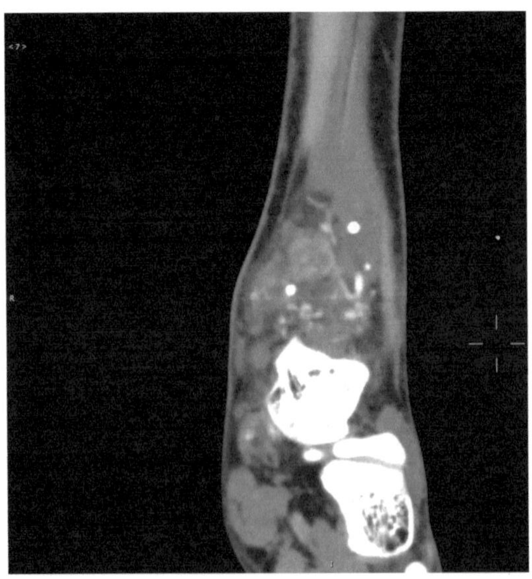

Fig. 48.7 Coronal post-contrast CT image of the left ankle in soft tissue window

48.3.3 MR Imaging

MR images of the left ankle demonstrated a soft tissue mass at anterior left ankle. There was slightly high T2 signal of the lesion with internal multiple circular vessel-like signals and fat signals around the lesion with irregular margin. Multiple tubular and circular vessel-like enhancements were noted (Figs. 48.8, 48.9, 48.10, and 48.11).

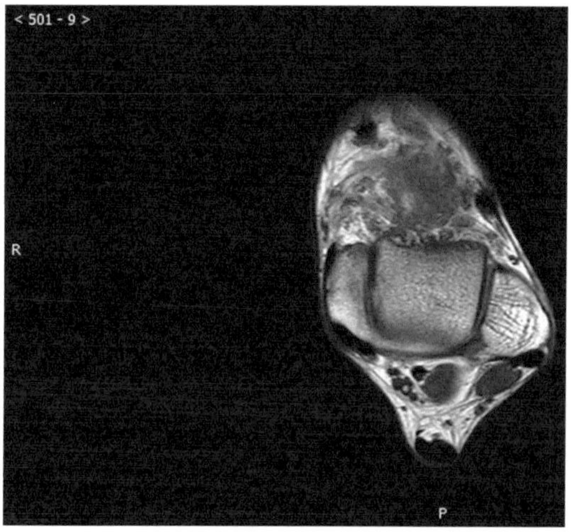

Fig. 48.8 Axial T1-weighted MR images of the left ankle

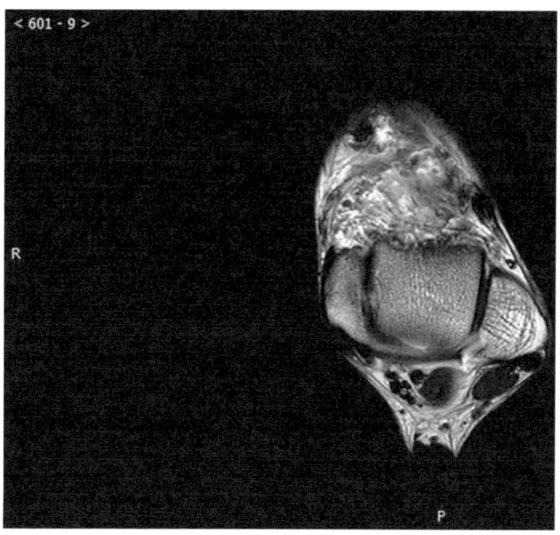

Fig. 48.9 Axial T2-weighted MR images of the left ankle

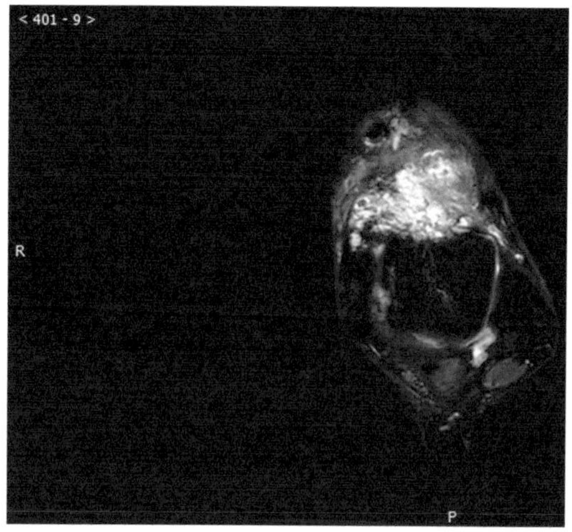

Fig. 48.10 Axial fat-suppressed T2-weighted MR images of the left ankle

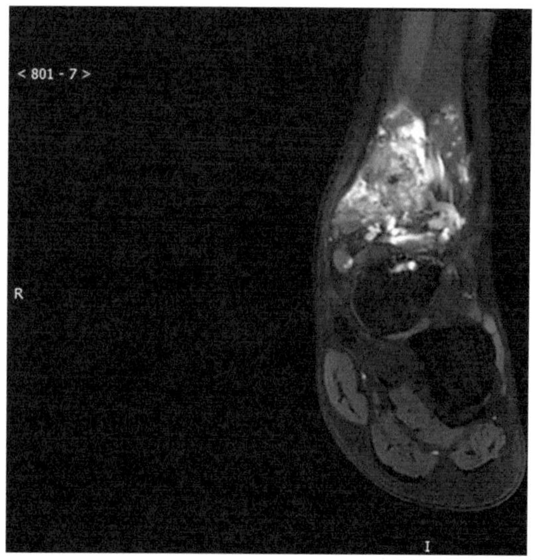

Fig. 48.11 Coronal post-contrast fat-suppressed T1-weighted MR images of the left ankle

48.4 Description and Discussion from Residents

Radiographs demonstrated left ankle anterior soft tissue mass with internal multiple high densities. CT images show that the soft tissue lesion was anterior to the ankle involving deep fascia with compressive changes of the anterior distal tibia. Avid enhancement was noted. MRI images demonstrated the lesion more clearly with irregular isointense T1 and heterogeneous T2 signal and avid enhancement. Our consideration is hemangioma of soft tissue.

48.5 Analysis and Comments from Professor Cheng Xiao-Guang

Patient is a young male. Radiographs demonstrated soft tissue swelling of the anterior left ankle with internal pointed high densities. Based on CT and MRI images, these high densities likely represent phleboliths. Non-contrast CT images show internal heterogeneous densities of the soft tissue mass with internal calcifications and fat densities with circular vessel-like density after enhancement and consistent with hemangioma. MRI images demonstrated the lesion more clearly and further support the diagnosis of hemangioma. Hemangioma is not neoplasm but development anomaly.

48.6 Diagnosis

Hemangioma of soft tissue.

Suggested Reading

Woertler K. Soft tissue masses in the foot and ankle: characteristics on MR Imaging. Semin Musculoskelet Radiol. 2005;9(3):227–42.

Pourbagher A, Pourbagher MA, Karan B, et al. MRI manifestations of soft-tissue haemangiomas and accompanying reactive bone changes. Br J Radiol. 2011;84(1008):1100–8.

Hochman MG, Wu JS. MR imaging of common soft tissue masses in the foot and ankle. Magn Reson Imaging Clin N Am. 2017;25(1):159–181.

49 Tenosynovial Giant Cell Tumor: Case 24

49.1 Medical History

Patient is a 37-year-old male. He experienced right ankle swelling and pain about 8 years ago from ankle sprain. This was followed by multiple ankle sprains. He had another ankle sprain of the right ankle about 1 month ago with ankle swelling and pain.

49.2 Physical Examination

Point tenderness (+) at right medial and lateral malleoli of the right ankle without radiation. Normal range of motion of the subtalar joint. Positive drawer test. Mildly decreased skin pinprick test.

49.3 Imaging Findings

49.3.1 Radiograph

Radiographs demonstrated normal alignment of the right ankle with preserved joint space. Soft tissue mass was noted around the joint. There was lytic osseous destruction of the distal tibia and fibula with clear margin and peripheral sclerosis (Figs. 49.1 and 49.2).

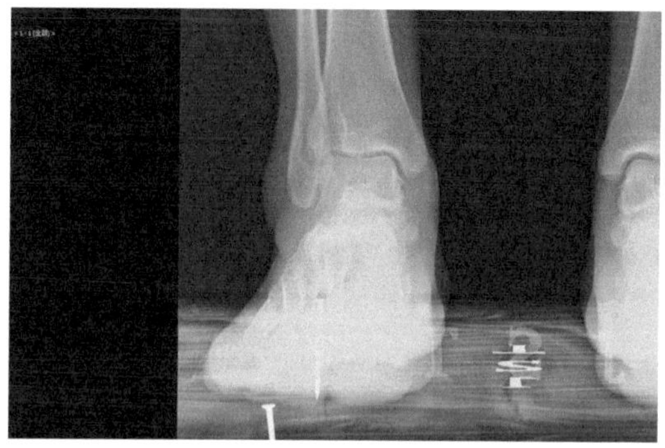

Fig. 49.1 Frontal view of the right ankle

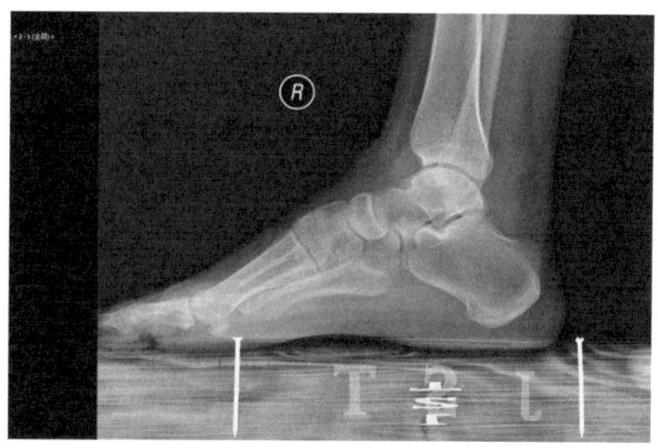

Fig. 49.2 Lateral view of the right ankle

X. Cheng et al., *Imaging of Bone Tumors in Wrist, Hand, Ankle and Foot*,
https://doi.org/10.1007/978-981-99-6407-9_49

49.3.2 CT Imaging

CT images of the right ankle demonstrated thickening of the synovium with multiple nodules and erosions of the distal tibia, fibular, and talus. Heterogeneous enhancement noted, avid more focally (Figs. 49.3, 49.4, 49.5, 49.6, 49.7, and 49.8).

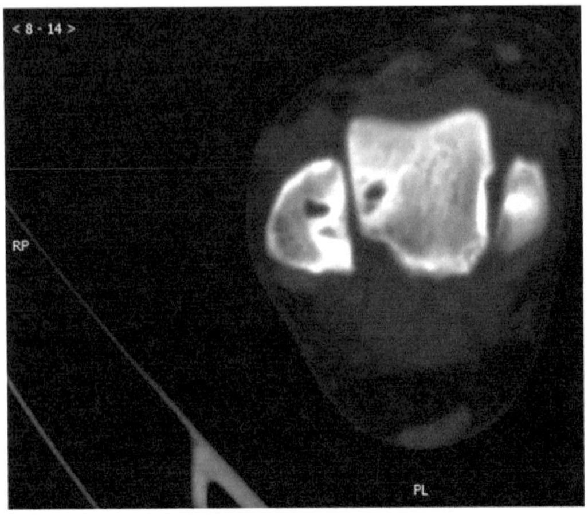

Fig. 49.3 Axial CT image of the right ankle in bone window

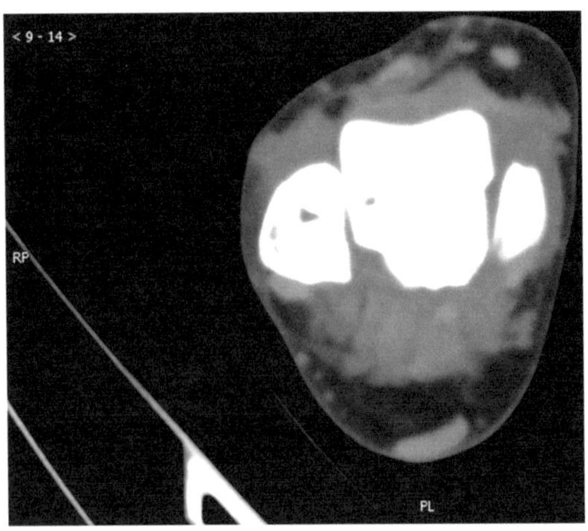

Fig. 49.4 Axial CT image of the right ankle in soft tissue window

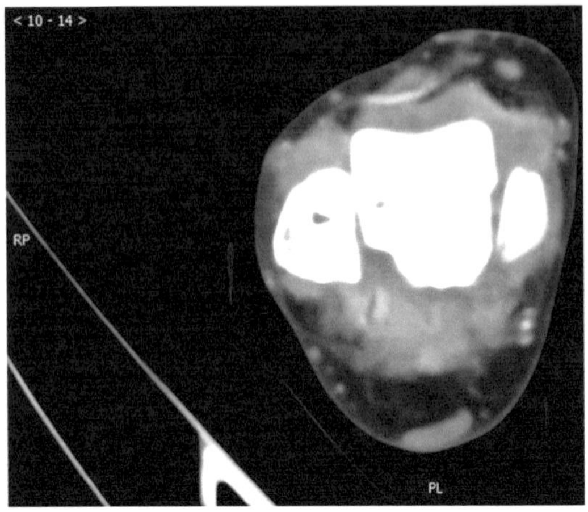

Fig. 49.5 Axial post-contrast CT image of the right ankle in soft tissue window

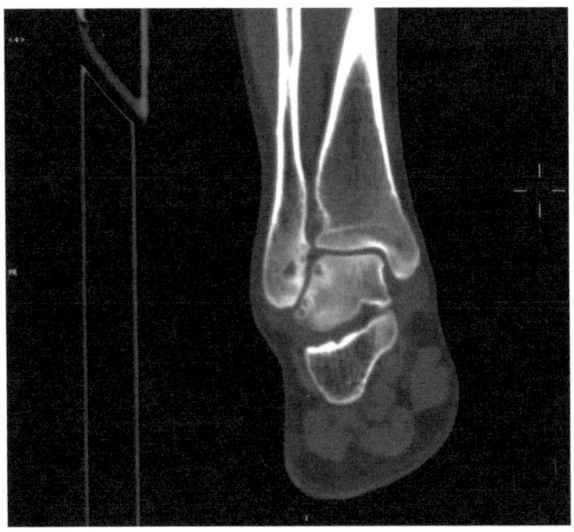

Fig. 49.6 Coronal CT image of the right ankle in bone window

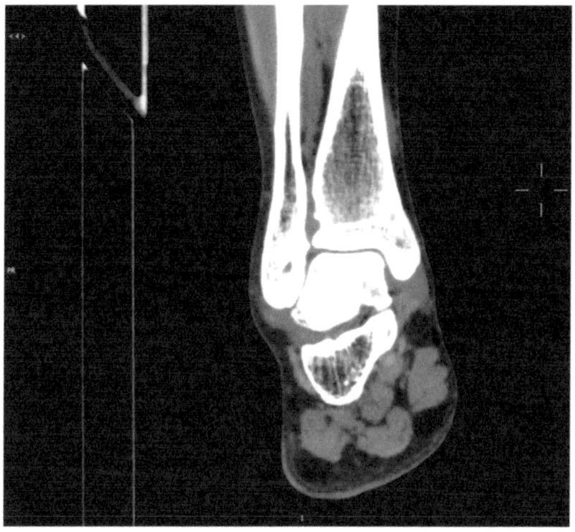

Fig. 49.7 Coronal CT image of the right ankle in soft tissue window

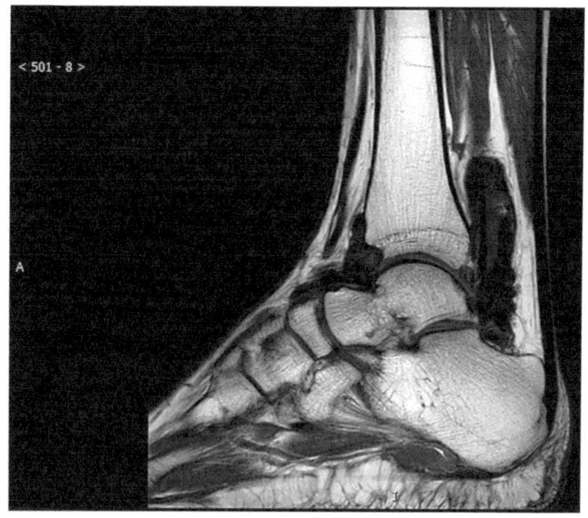

Fig. 49.9 Sagittal T1-weighted MR images of the right ankle

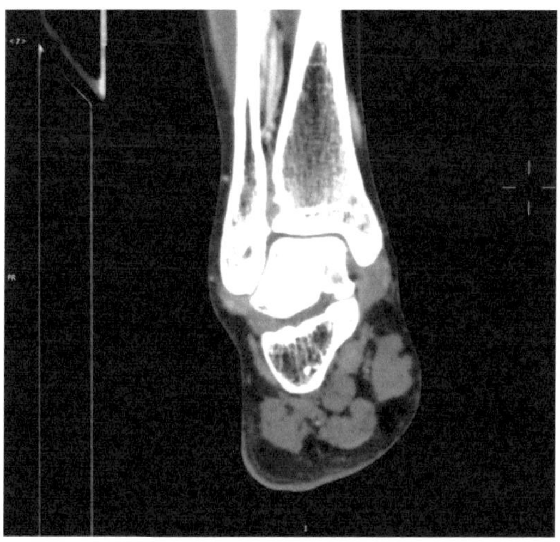

Fig. 49.8 Coronal post-contrast CT image of the right ankle in soft tissue window

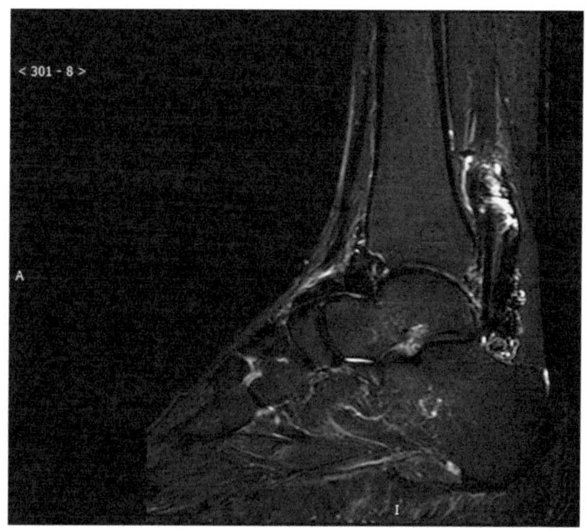

Fig. 49.10 Sagittal fat-suppressed T2-weighted MR images of the right ankle

49.3.3 MR Imaging

MR images of the right ankle demonstrated diffuse synovial thickening with multiple hemosiderin depositions and also involved flexor hallucis longus tendon sheath with erosions to the distal tibia, fibula, and talus. Heterogeneous enhancement was noted (Figs. 49.9, 49.10, 49.11, and 49.12).

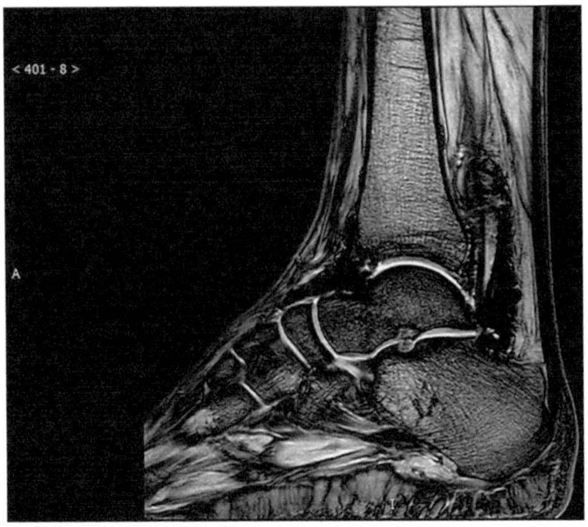

Fig. 49.11 Sagittal gradient echo sequence MR images of the left ankle

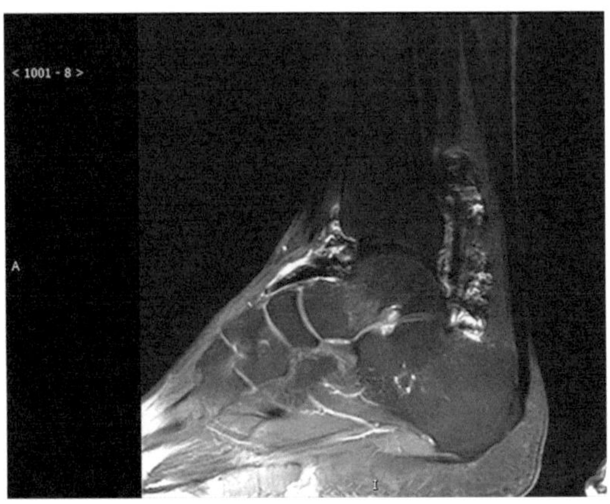

Fig. 49.12 Sagittal post-contrast fat-suppressed T1-weighted MR images of the right ankle

49.4 Description and Discussion from Residents

Radiographs demonstrated distal tibia and fibular bone destruction around the right ankle region with compressive changes. CT images demonstrated bone destruction around the articular surface about the distal tibia, fibula and talus with peripheral sclerosis, consistent with compressive erosions from synovial proliferation. There was heterogeneous signal on MR images with avid enhancement of the synovium. No enhancement was noted of the low signal region, indicating hemosiderin deposition. Given the above findings, our consideration is pigmented villonodular synovitis (PVNS), currently known as tenosynovial giant cell tumor.

49.5 Analysis and Comments from Professor Cheng Xiao-Guang

Patient is a young male. He had repeated right ankle sprain for 8 years. Peri-articular soft tissue mass around the right ankle was noted on the radiographs with osseous destruction about the distal tibio-fibular joint without osteoporosis or joint space narrowing. CT soft tissue window of the right ankle demonstrated heterogeneous densities of the peri-articular soft tissues with peri-articular erosions of the distal tibio-fibular and distal tibio-talar joints with peripheral sclerosis and preserved joint space. Soft tissue mass showed avid enhancement. Given the above growth and distribution characteristics, my consideration is PVNS. MR images showed the characteristics and extent of the lesion more clearly with multiple areas of synovial proliferation within the joint and hemosiderin deposition on T2-weighted images, all consistent with PVNS. The characteristics of PVNS lesions are as follows: (1) accompanied by multiple bone erosions; (2) imaging findings appear more severe than clinical symptoms; (3) no osteoporosis; (4) no joint space narrowing. Typical differential diagnosis includes tuberculous arthritis and rheumatoid arthritis. Osteoporosis is commonly seen with these two entities, and with rheumatoid arthritis, the involvements are usually symmetrical, not consistent with the current case.

49.6 Diagnosis

Tenosynovial giant cell tumor.

Suggested Reading

Cheng XG, You YH, Liu W, et al. MRI features of pigmented villonodular synovitis (PVNS). Clin Rheumatol. 2004;23(1):31–4.

Fraser EJ, Sullivan M, Maclean F, et al. Tenosynovial giant-cell tumors of the foot and ankle: a critical analysis review. JBJS Rev. 2017;5(1):01874474-201701000-00001.

Spindle Cell Lipoma: Case 25

50

50.1 Medical History

Patient is a 29-year-old female. She incidentally noticed right big toe swelling about 6 years ago without pain and seek no medical attention. The swelling has increased in the last 2 months, without pain.

50.2 Physical Examination

A 4 cm × 3 cm palpable soft tissue mass around first phalanx and first metatarsophalangeal joint of the foot with clear margin, soft, rubbery, and mobile, without pint tenderness or vascular murmur.

50.3 Imaging Findings

50.3.1 Radiograph

Radiographs demonstrated soft tissue swelling about the first proximal phalanx and first metatarsophalangeal joint (Figs. 50.1 and 50.2).

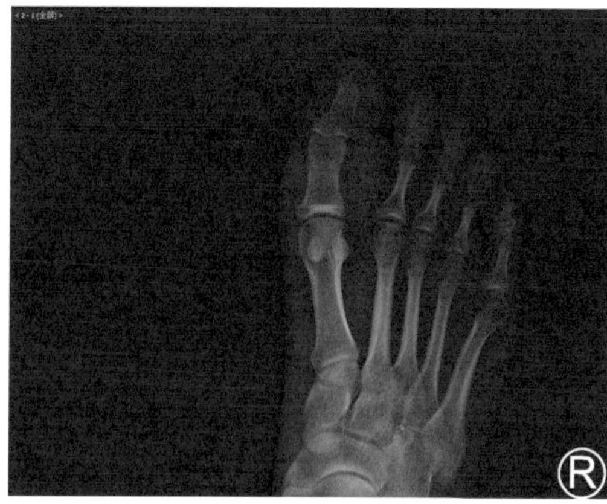

Fig. 50.1 Frontal view of the right foot

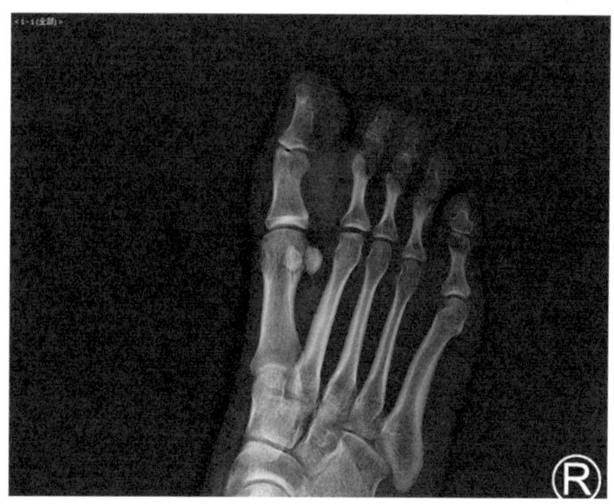

Fig. 50.2 Oblique view of the right foot

X. Cheng et al., *Imaging of Bone Tumors in Wrist, Hand, Ankle and Foot*,
https://doi.org/10.1007/978-981-99-6407-9_50

50.3.2 CT Imaging

CT images of the right foot demonstrated soft tissue mass about the first phalanx, involving the subcutaneous soft tissue with internal heterogeneous densities, containing fat densities. No enhancement was noted. The adjacent osseous structures and joint spaces are preserved (Figs. 50.3, 50.4, and 50.5).

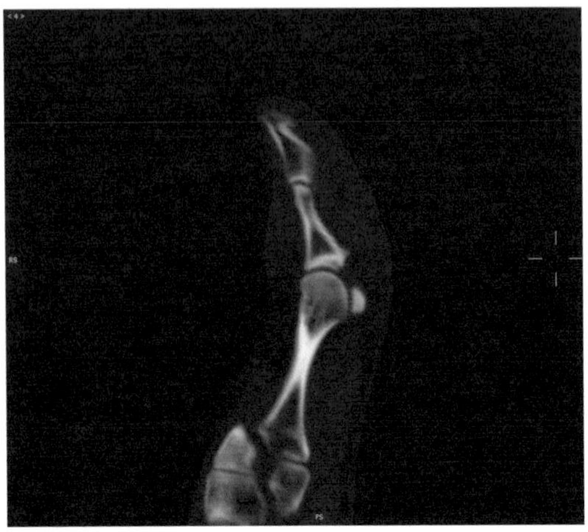

Fig. 50.3 Sagittal CT image of the right foot in bone window

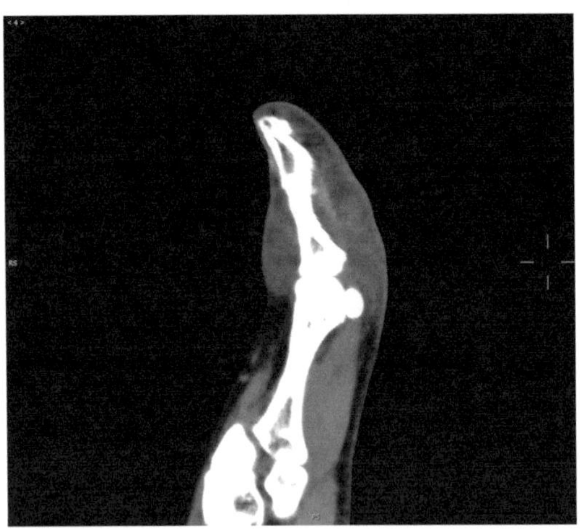

Fig. 50.4 Sagittal CT image of the right foot in soft tissue window

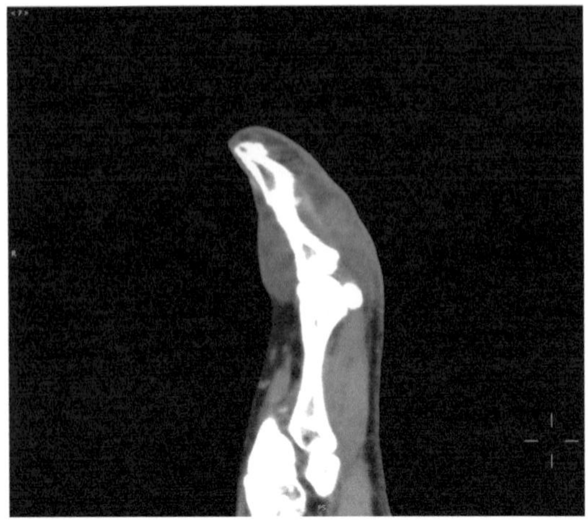

Fig. 50.5 Sagittal post-contrast CT image of the right foot in soft tissue window

50.4 Description and Discussion from Residents

Radiographs demonstrated soft tissue mass about the first phalanx of the right first toe, with homogenous density and no involvement of the first phalanx. CT images show heterogeneous densities of the soft tissue mass with likely fat densities within and no calcification or osseous content and no enhancement. Given the location of the lesion and mild symptoms, our consideration is giant cell tumor of the tendon sheath. However, the enhancement pattern is not consistent with this diagnosis. Lipomatosis of nerve is in the differential diagnosis, but not consistent with the growth pattern of current lesion as surrounding the first phalanx, which usually only extends along one side of the bone.

50.5 Analysis and Comments from Professor Cheng Xiao-Guang

Patient is a young female with a long history. Soft tissue mass along the first phalanx was demonstrated on radiographs without involvement of the first phalanx. CT images showed this soft tissue mass surrounding the first phalanx with internal low densities and no enhancement. My first consideration is megalodactyly. Megalodactyly is a clinical diagnosis, with homogenous thickening of the toe. However, with the current case, there is more focal involvement, not consistent. Angiolipoma is in the differential diagnosis; and if the patient is older, liposarcoma is also in the differential diagnosis. MRI images would be helpful at narrowing down the differential diagnosis.

50.6 Diagnosis

Spindle cell lipoma.

Suggested Reading

Hochman MG, Wu JS. MR imaging of common soft tissue masses in the foot and ankle. Magn Reson Imaging Clin N Am. 2017;25(1):159–181.

Younan Y, Martinez A, Reimer N, et al. Combined classical spindle cell/pleomorphic lipoma spectrum imaging and clinical data. Skeletal Radiol. 2018;47(1):51–59.

Jelinek JS, Wu A, Wallace M, et al. Imaging of spindle cell lipoma. Clin Radiol. 2020;75(5):396.e15–396.e21.

MIX
Papier aus verantwortungsvollen Quellen
Paper from responsible sources
FSC® C105338

If you have any concerns about our products,
you can contact us on
ProductSafety@springernature.com

In case Publisher is established outside the EU,
the EU authorized representative is:
Springer Nature Customer Service Center GmbH
Europaplatz 3, 69115 Heidelberg, Germany

Printed by Libri Plureos GmbH
in Hamburg, Germany